$1.00

DISCARDED
MEDICAL LIBRARY
UNIVERSITY OF CALGARY

JUN 7 1989

RECENT ADVANCES
IN
ORTHOPAEDICS

Recent Advances in
Orthopaedics

EDITED BY

A. GRAHAM APLEY

M.B., B.S.(Lond), F.R.C.S.(Eng)

Consultant Orthopaedic Surgeon, Rowley Bristow Orthopaedic Hospital, Pyrford, Surrey; Surgeon in Charge, Emergency and Accident Centre, St. Peter's Hospital, Chertsey

With 290 Illustrations

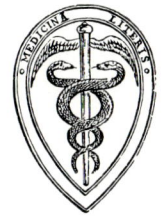

J. & A. CHURCHILL LTD.
104 Gloucester Place, London

1969

First Published......1969
Standard Book Number: 7000 1416 0

© J. & A. Churchill Ltd, 1969. All rights reserved. No part of this publication may be reproduced, stored in a retrieval system, or transmitted, in any form or by any means, electronic, mechanical, photocopying, recording or otherwise, without the prior permission of the copyright owner.

PRINTED IN GREAT BRITAIN

PREFACE

At first glance the title of this book is self-explanatory; but on reflection the meaning of 'recent' varies with the age of the reader, and the 'advances' of yesterday have become the commonplaces of today (or have been discarded already). Since precise definitions were impossible I decided, in selecting the topics, to adopt Humpty Dumpty's famous etymological policy: "when I use a word it means what I choose it to mean—neither more nor less". With this liberal, if somewhat autocratic, editorial attitude 'recent advances' came to mean for me "new enough to be exciting and fresh enough not to be hackneyed, yet not so advanced as to be untested".

The giants of the not-too-distant past (and what giants they were) devoted much energy to dealing with bone infections, deficiency diseases, poliomyelitis and, a laggard fourth, congenital deformities. The first three have been so effectively mastered, in the developed countries at least, that their total absence from this book will surprise no-one. The giants of today (and what giants they are) have different but broader interests. While still retaining their craftsmanship and their humane approach to the individual patient, they are concerned with wider problems: of inheritance, of growth, and of decay.

In a single generation the emphasis has changed from correction and salvage procedures to prevention and replacement. The orthopaedic surgeon is no longer content to be a meticulous carpenter: he has become a precision engineer. His evolution has meant harnessing and exploiting the rapid advances in biochemistry, genetics, physiology, immunology, and, equally, those of metallurgy and the physical chemistry of plastics (the list is far from comprehensive). The 'backroom boys' have been brought into the operating theatre.

The immense scope and potential of the new orthopaedics offer a stimulatingly wide choice of subjects for this present collection. The reader is invited to play the game of picking his own 'top twelve'. My friends and colleagues were subjected to this harassment. They chose an encouraging number of topics in common with each other and with my private list; but, of course, no two lists were alike. How could they be? Surgeons are individualists, not to say guerrilla fighters. Some are interested in fundamental problems of genetics, metabolism or tissue rejection; others are attracted by major advances in technique or delicate refinements of diagnosis. Nearly all seek an authoritative, balanced assessment of the relative merits of differing methods.

Something to suit each of these varying tastes has been included. Clearly an international cuisine was imperative and, though every reader is bound to debate the choice, he will find it harder to criticize the ingredients. Each chapter comes from a master of his subject, combining authority with originality.

It was clearly important to cross the barriers of geography and language. The contributors have been brought together (the list is alphabetical) from Canada, China, France, Great Britain, Hong Kong, Soviet Russia, Switzerland and the United States of America. Some chapters were originally written in languages other than English. In editing and working with translators, I have sought not to impose a cold uniformity of style but, within the limits required for clarity, to retain and enjoy the individual or national flavour.

I welcome this opportunity to offer my sincere thanks to all the contributors; their original work and ungrudging co-operation have brought me many new ideas and a few new friends.

A. G. A.

ACKNOWLEDGEMENTS

It is a pleasure to acknowledge my gratitude to: Margaret Collie, M. A. for her translation from the Russian; Mary Love, B. A. for other translations and help in proof-reading; Mr. G. E. T. Raine, F.R.C.S. and Mr. G. Sadow, F.R.C.S. for their help in checking the text and in proof-reading; and to the publishers whose constant courtesy and kindness made an arduous task into a pleasant one.

CONTRIBUTORS

BURWELL, R. Geoffrey, B.Sc., M.D., F.R.C.S.
  Professor of Orthopaedics, University of London; Honorary Consultant Orthopaedic Surgeon, Royal National Orthopaedic Hospital, London.

CURREY, H. L. F., M.Med. (Cape Town), M.R.C.P.
  Senior Lecturer in Rheumatology, The London Hospital Medical College.

D'AUBIGNÉ, R. Merle, M.D., F.R.C.S.Eng.(Hon), F.A.C.S.(Hon)
  Member Academie des Sciences; Professor of Orthopaedic Surgery, Hôpital Cochin, Paris.

HELAL, B., M.Ch.(Orth), F.R.C.S.
  Consultant Orthopaedic Surgeon, Highlands Hospital, Winchmore Hill and Chase Farm Hospital, Enfield, Middx.

HELFET, A. J., M.D.
  Professor of Orthopaedic Surgery, Albert Einstein College of Medicine, Yefshiva University, Bronx, New York.

HODGSON, A. R., O.B.E., F.R.C.S.(Ed), F.A.C.S.
  Professor of Orthopaedic Surgery, University of Hong Kong.

HORN, J. S., F.R.C.S.
  Formerly Professor of Orthopaedics and Traumatology, Peking, China.*

IMAMALIEV, A. S.
  Head of the Department for the Preparation and Preservation of Organs and Tissues, Central Inst. of Traumatology and Orthopaedics, Moscow.

JAMES, J. I. P., M.S., F.R.C.S.
  Professor of Orthopaedic Surgery, University of Edinburgh.

MASON, Michael, D.M., F.R.C.P.
  Physician, Departments of Physical Medicine and Rheumatology, The London Hospital.

MÜLLER, Maurice E., M.D.
  Professor of Orthopaedic Surgery and Head of the Clinic for Orthopaedic Surgery, University of Bern.

SALTER, Robert Bruce, M.D., M.S.(Tor), F.R.C.S.(C), F.A.C.S.
  Professor of Surgery, University of Toronto; Surgeon-in-Chief and Senior Orthopaedic Surgeon, The Hospital for Sick Children, Toronto.

SHARRARD, W. J. W., M.D., Ch.M.(Sheffield), F.R.C.S.
  Consultant Orthopaedic Surgeon, United Sheffield Hospitals and University of Sheffield.

WYNNE-DAVIES, Ruth, M.B., F.R.C.S.
  Senior Lecturer, Orthopaedic Genetic Research, University of Edinburgh.

YAU, Arthur C. M. C., F.R.C.S.(Ed)
  Senior Lecturer in Orthopaedic Surgery, University of Hong Kong.

* Present address: c/o The British Orthopaedic Association, 82 Portland Place, London.

CONTENTS

1. Genetic Factors in Orthopaedics . . *J. I. P. James and Ruth Wynne-Davies*   1

2. Gout and Chondrocalcinosis ('Pseudogout') . . . *H. L. F. Currey and R. M. Mason*   37

3. The Reattachment of Severed Extremities . . *J. S. Horn*   49

4. Compression as an Aid in Orthopaedic Surgery . . . *Maurice E. Müller*   79

5. Silicones in Orthopaedic Surgery . . . *B. Helal*   91

6. The Fate of Bone Grafts . . *R. Geoffrey Burwell*   115

7. The Preparation, Preservation and Transplantation of Articular Bone Ends . . . . *A. S. Imamaliev*   209

8. The Orthopaedic Surgery of Cerebral Palsy and Spina Bifida . . . . . *W. J. W. Sharrard*   265

9. Anterior Surgical Approaches to the Spinal Column *A. R. Hodgson and A. C. M. C. Yau*   289

10. An Operative Treatment for Congenital Dislocation and Subluxation of the Hip in the Older Child *Robert B. Salter*   325

11. The Concept of Arrest of Osteoarthritis in the Hip and Knee *Arthur J. Helfet*   361

12. Arthroplasty in the Treatment of Degenerative Osteoarthritis of the Hip . . . *R. Merle d'Aubigné*   377

Chapter 1

GENETIC FACTORS IN ORTHOPAEDICS

J. I. P. JAMES and RUTH WYNNE-DAVIES

GENERAL INTRODUCTION TO GENETICS

The Physical Basis of Heredity

During cell division the chromosomes can be visualized, and in man these total 46, 23 from each parent. It is known that they are composed of deoxyribonucleic acid (D.N.A.) molecules strung on a protein framework. The chromosome is in the form of a long chain of D.N.A., divided into segments, each forming a gene. These are the units of heredity. There are thousands of genes to each chromosome and, in man, perhaps 100,000 genes in each cell. Any one gene has a characteristic position, or locus, on its chromosome but its biochemical composition may vary. That is, there are alternative forms of gene at any one locus and these are known as alleles. The genes direct the synthesis of polypeptides which in turn form proteins, each of remarkable specificity. Genetic information is coded by bases which form part of the D.N.A. molecule. The order of the amino acids of a polypeptide chain is specified by a 3-base sequence, and this series of 3-bases forms one segment of a chromosome and constitutes one gene. The protein formed from the polypeptides may be either an enzyme or a structural protein such as collagen.

In man the 23 pairs of chromosomes comprise 22 autosomes and one pair of sex chromosomes, one X derived from the mother and either one X or Y derived from the father. Individuals with XX sex chromosomes are female and XY are male. Chromosomes are classified by their microscopic appearance (Fig. 1).

Patterns of Inheritance

Inheritance in man is immensely complex because very large numbers of interacting genes are concerned. There are, however, four well-defined types which can be described:

(1) Major genes
(2) Alternative genes } Single gene-pairs
(3) Chromosomes
(4) Polygenes } Groups of genes

MAJOR GENES

Each major gene is one of a pair, one derived from each parent. The characteristic of the major gene-pair is that the trait or abnormality

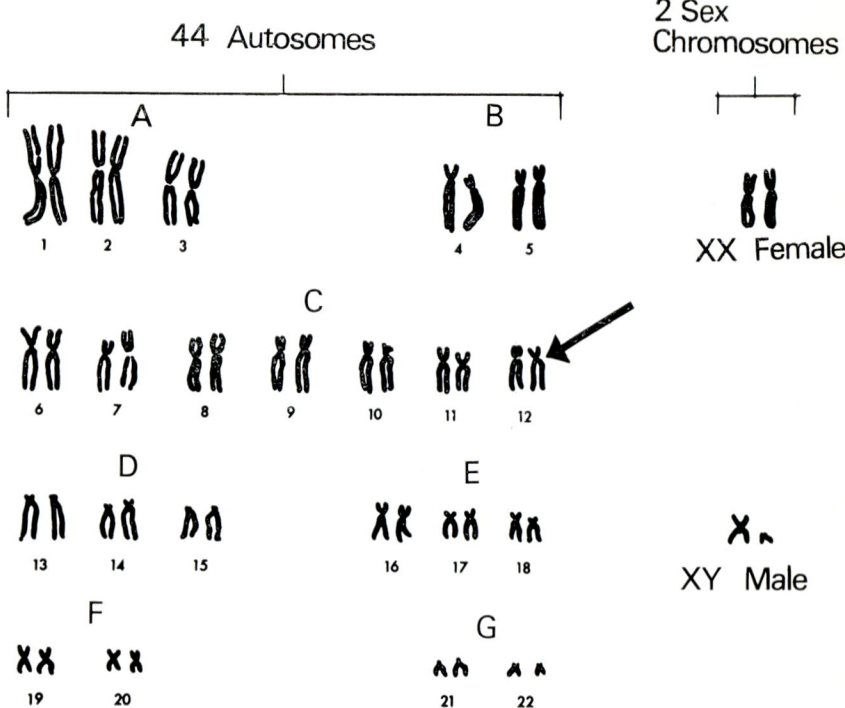

FIG. 1. Human chromosomes are classified on the basis of size and position of the centromere (shown by arrow), which may be central, off centre, or near one end of the chromosome. It is not yet possible to identify with certainty each separate chromosome and thus they are placed in seven groups, A–G. Sex chromosome X belongs with Group C (6–12) and Y, the smallest chromosome of all, to Group G.

associated with it is nearly always manifest in the individual. That is, one gene-pair = one character, which is either present, or is not, and is clinically detectable. The major genes illustrate the simplest patterns of inheritance and follow the ratios described by Mendel for dominant, recessive and sex-linked traits.

If both members of the major gene-pair are identical the individual is homozygous for that particular gene. If the members of the pair are dissimilar then the individual is heterozygous for that gene. If the trait or abnormality is manifest in the heterozygote this is referred to as dominant inheritance (Fig. 2). If the trait is apparent only in the homozygote (two identical genes) then this is recessive inheritance (Fig. 3). It is, however, possible in some cases of recessive inheritance to detect the heterozygote or carrier of only one abnormal gene by chemical tests, identifying a metabolic disorder even though this is not clinically apparent in that individual.

Sex-linked inheritance is better referred to as X-linked, meaning that the gene concerned is on the X chromosome (Fig. 4). An X-linked

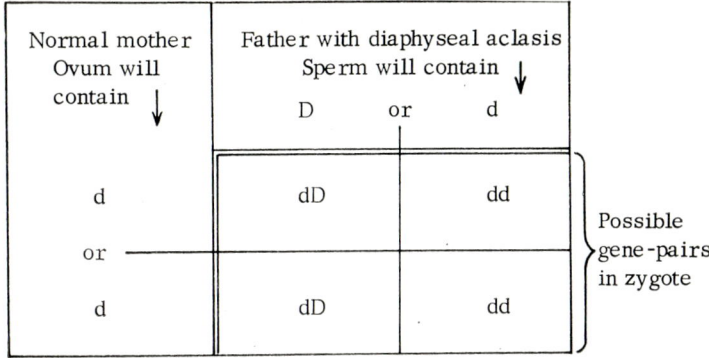

Fig. 2. Dominant inheritance. D = the abnormal gene responsible for diaphyseal aclasis, and d = the normal gene occupying the same locus on the chromosome (i.e. its allele). At reduction division in the testis, when the chromosomes separate there is an equal chance of a sperm containing D or d. Since the mother is normal, all ova will contain d. The children of these parents have an equal chance of carrying dD or dd. Diaphyseal aclasis is apparent in the heterozygote (dD), this being the characteristic of dominant inheritance. Thus, on average, half the children will be affected with the disorder, the other half normal clinically and not carrying any abnormal genes.

gene may be dominant or recessive in character. In the male the X chromosome is partnered by the very much smaller Y chromosome, thus many genes are present without an allele or second member of the pair. The pattern of inheritance is characteristically different from autosomal inheritance because the male gives his X chromosome only to his daughters and the Y only to his sons.

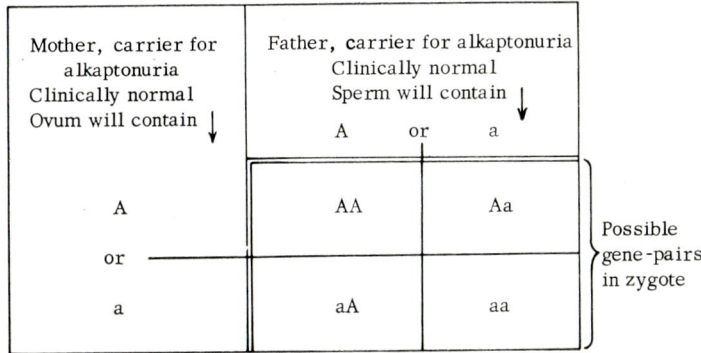

Fig. 3. Recessive inheritance. a = the gene responsible for alkaptonuria, A = the normal gene at the same locus. At reduction division in ovary and testis half the ova and half the sperms will carry A, and half a. The children of these parents have the chance of carrying AA, Aa or aa. Alkaptonuria is clinically apparent only in the homozygote (aa), this being the characteristic of recessive inheritance. Thus, on average, one quarter of the children are completely normal (AA); one half are carriers of the gene (heterozygotes Aa) and one quarter exhibit the disease—i.e. are homozygous for the disordered gene (aa).

In man these major dominant, recessive and X-linked genes are mostly harmful and lead to disease or deformity. Most of the *normal* variation between one man and another (e.g. height, weight, intelligence) is not explicable on the major gene basis. This is discussed in the following sections, but it may be noted here that even when a major harmful gene or gene-pair is acting to produce a disorder the clinical features in different individuals may be far from uniform. This is because the harmful gene is acting on a background of many thousands of normal genes which may tend themselves either to exaggerate or to limit the adverse effect in any one individual.

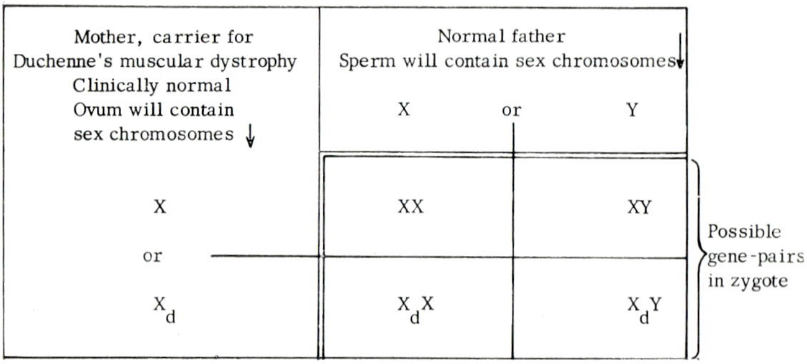

Mother, carrier for Duchenne's muscular dystrophy Clinically normal Ovum will contain sex chromosomes ↓	Normal father Sperm will contain sex chromosomes ↓	
	X or Y	
X	XX	XY
or		
X_d	$X_d X$	$X_d Y$

Possible gene-pairs in zygote

FIG. 4. X-linked inheritance. X and Y are the normal sex chromosomes, and at reduction division in the testis there is an equal chance of sperm containing X or Y. The mother is an asymptomatic heterozygote (carrier), her ova will on average contain half the normal X and half X_d, the gene responsible for Duchenne's muscular dystrophy. This is a recessive condition, all daughters of these parents will appear normal, but half will be carriers ($X_d X$). Half the sons will be normal, and half exhibit the disease ($X_d Y$). The Y chromosome is very small, there is no normal allele to partner the abnormal gene and the disease becomes clinically manifest. In this instance the $X_d X$ daughters can be detected by biochemical tests.

ALTERNATIVE GENES

In the previous section one pair of genes was considered at a single locus, both being normal, one abnormal, or both abnormal. This, however, is not the only possibility in genetic variation. In man there are many examples of multiple alleles, or several alternative possible genes at one locus. Dissimilar genes exist for carrying out the same function in different individuals. This was first demonstrated in the ABO blood groups where one individual may be group A and another group B, but the genes concerned, although dissimilar, are at the same locus on the chromosome (polymorphic inheritance). These alternative genes have themselves a simple (dominant, recessive or X-linked) pattern of inheritance and there are now many examples associated with the red blood cells and with nucleated tissue cells throughout the body. It is, of course, the occurrence of this type of genetic variation which gives the cellular differences between individuals which causes the problems of blood transfusion and, in a degree yet to be determined, of organ transplantation.

IMMUNOGENETICS

The formation of both antigens and antibodies is under genetic control. The antigen–antibody reaction is the method by which the body rejects any foreign cells, proteins or other substances. The basic characteristic of an antigen is its ability to stimulate antibody formation. Antigens are found on the red blood cells and on nucleated cells throughout the body. The antigens of the red blood cells (the blood groups) are mucopolysaccharides and differ in character, as well as being produced by different genes, from the tissue antigens and those of the white blood cells. All antigens are formed during embryonic life, whereas the ability to produce antibody develops only shortly before birth. Thus, at birth the individual is tolerant of its own cells, but henceforth rejects all foreign cells.

Transplantation of tissues between individuals depends on overcoming this immune response, either by using a genetically identical donor (monozygotic twin); by using tissues which do not provoke an immune response (for example, the avascular tissues, cornea or cartilage) or by suppressing the immune reaction. Clearly, a close relative of the recipient must have some antigens in common with him, and so the choice of a donor is important. Tissue antigens are now being intensively studied in relation to organ transplantation.

Autoimmune disease results when the individual starts to form antibody to his own antigens. This may result from mutation in an antigen or, alternatively, the disorder may arise on the antibody side with mutation of a gene controlling antibody formation.

The Inheritance of Groups of Genes

The previous section discussed the simple inheritance of a pair of genes at one locus. However, the inheritance of multiple genes, either in one block or separated, presents different and sometimes more difficult problems in interpretation.

CHROMOSOMES

The normal situation in the germ cells in the ovary or testis at division is for the 46 chromosomes to pair and then to separate at a reduction division giving 23 in each ovum or spermatozoa. This reduction division is unique to gonadal cells. The cell is brought up to its full number again at fertilization (zygote formation). Abnormalities of cell division can occur giving rise to chromosomal aberrations which are visible under the microscope. In each case a large block of genes is concerned and the damage to the body is widespread. The following is the mechanism of the common errors in man:

Trisomy: two members of a chromosome pair fail to separate at reduction division in the gonad and thus give rise after fertilization to a zygote with either three or only one representative of a chromosome pair (Fig. 5). The commonest example is mongolism or Down's syndrome. In these individuals the chromosome count is increased to 47 because there are three chromosomes No. 21 instead of the usual pair. The best name for this disease therefore is 'trisomy 21'.

Deletion indicates the loss of a chromosome, the cell having only one representative of a pair. This is far more damaging to the developing organism than an extra chromosome and deletion of a whole autosome is not compatible with life. Deletion of a sex chromosome (XO) does occur in Turner's syndrome. Partial deletion of an autosome may occur, for example the loss of one arm of a chromosome, but even this has a serious effect on the body.

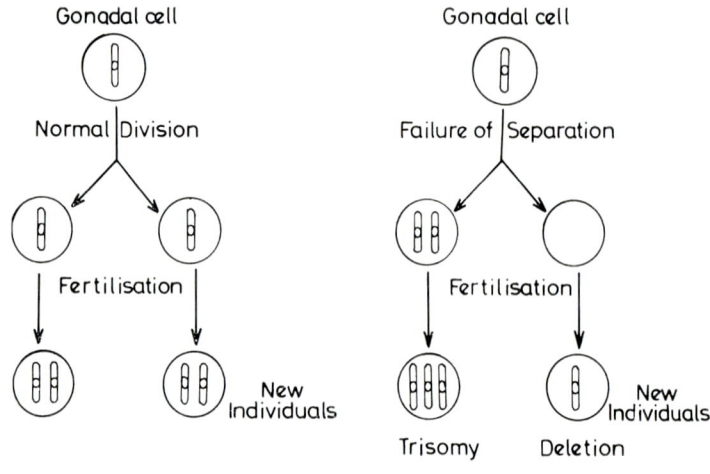

FIG. 5. Trisomy and deletion. At reduction division in ovary or testis there may be an unequal distribution of one pair of chromosomes, leading to new ova or sperms containing both members of a pair, or neither. Thus at fertilization the zygote may contain three representatives of a chromosome instead of a pair (trisomy), or only one (deletion).

Translocation indicates fragmentation of a chromosome with transference of a part to another chromosome. If there is no loss of chromosome material then there is no clinical abnormality, but the individual is a translocation carrier. In a subsequent generation, if this fragment is either additional to the full complement after fertilization or is deficient, then clinical disorder will result.

Chromosomal Mosaics. When the error of cell division or the translocation occurs at reduction division in the ovary or testis of a parent the new individual formed at fertilization will have this error transmitted in every cell in the body. This can be seen under the microscope whichever cell is examined. However, there are individuals in whom the error of chromosome division arises perhaps in the second or third cell division of the fertilized ovum. There are then two lines of cell, normal and abnormal, and these individuals are known as 'mosaics'. There are then difficulties in diagnosis as cells must be taken from several sites for microscopic examination.

Although the mechanism of these chromosomal aberrations is known, in a general way, the reason for their occurrence is not clear. One factor in trisomy 21 (Down's syndrome) is that it occurs in the elderly mother, but this does not seem to be so significant in other trisomies. It is theoretically possible that radiation could be a cause of these chromosomal anomalies, but clear evidence is not available in man. There are probably some genes which influence cell division in man, these have been described in other animals. Families have been reported in which several examples of chromosomal aberration occur, not all of the same kind, which suggests an underlying genetic tendency to this error in some cases.

POLYGENES

In the previous types of single gene inheritance described there is a distinct and clearcut difference between individuals. An individual either has blood group A or has not, and there is no question of gradation.

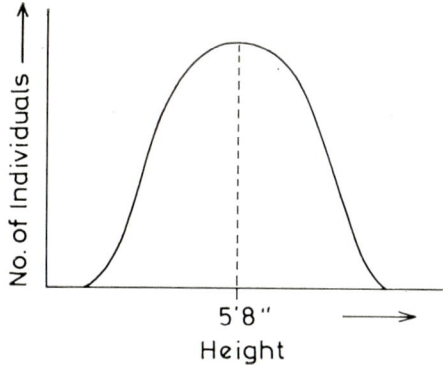

FIG. 6. "Normal" distribution of height. This illustrates the continuous variation characteristic of multiple gene (polygenic) inheritance. Most people are "average". There are a few individuals at each end of the distribution whose height is greatly in excess of the mean, or very much less.

This is known as discontinuous variation. However, the majority of normal human characteristics show continuous variation, changing imperceptibly over a wide range, for example height, intelligence, or birthweight. This cannot be explained on the basis of single genes. Continuous variation must depend on the combined action of many genes and this type of inheritance is called polygenic. Unlike the major genes, the action of any one pair is unimportant, but the combined effect of a large number gives the individual his characteristic make-up or genetic constitution. For example, if the height of an individual is considered (Fig. 6) one knows that most people are 'average', that is, their height will have a mean of between 5 ft. 5 in. and 5 ft. 10 in. There are a few individuals at each end of this distribution whose height is greatly in excess of this, or very much less. There may perhaps be a threshold level beyond which the individual is considered abnormal. This 'normal' distribution of continuous variation in a population arises where multiple factors are involved, each having a small effect some acting one way and some another. It is apparent that half these polygenes must have been derived from one parent and half from the other, thus on average a child will be half like each parent. This is to be distinguished from the inheritance of the single major dominant gene where, in respect of the one trait under consideration, half the children will be exactly like the parent carrying it.

Mutations

Mutation is a change in genetic structure. This may arise spontaneously, or under certain conditions it can be artificially induced. If the mutation occurs in the gonadal cells then the variation will be apparent only in the next generation. A somatic mutation is one occurring in non-gonadal tissues, affecting only the daughter cells of the mutant cell. The individual, therefore, will be a mosaic, with more than one cell line. However, since the gonadal cells are normal the next generation is not affected. The naturally occurring mutation rate varies for different genes but tends to be around 1 in 100,000 per gene locus, though methods of measuring this in man are somewhat inaccurate. A mutant gene in man is usually harmful. Man being a successful animal, the useful mutations have long since been selected and incorporated into his make-up.

Mutation is, of course, a mechanism of evolution. If the genotype were stable without possibility of change then natural selection and evolution could not occur. Mutations can be induced in animals by a number of agents the most powerful being ionizing radiation, but evidence for the occurrence of this in man is not conclusive.

POPULATION GENETICS

Gene frequencies in populations can be disturbed not only by mutation, but by other factors such as non-random mating. The Amish of Pennsylvania provide a classic example of a small religious sect who by intermarrying have caused a striking rise in incidence of an exceedingly rare (autosomal recessive) disorder—chondro-ectodermal dysplasia or the Ellis-Van Creveld syndrome. (Short limbed dwarfism with polydactyly, congenital heart disease and normal intelligence). The incidence elsewhere in the world is considerably less than 1 per million, but among this group of Amish it rises to 50 in 8000 (1 in 160) (McKusick 1966).

Another factor which disturbs the gene frequency of a population is the immigration of individuals carrying a distinct genotype to the population they join. This is well shown by the gradual change in blood group frequencies of the American negroes, which shows that they now have about 30 per cent of Caucasian ancestry.

Age of Onset of the Clinical Disorder

In genetic disorders the abnormal gene must be present at conception (with the rare exception of somatic mutations). However, the associated disease or deformity is not necessarily apparent at birth, but may appear at any time throughout the whole of life. There is very often a characteristic age of onset for various disorders (Fig. 7). The 'congenital' disorders are those which are due to an anomaly of development and are apparent at birth. They may be genetic, or resulting from an adverse intrauterine environment such as rubella or Thalidomide. Thus congenital disorders may or may not be genetic, and genetic disorders may or may not be congenital. This variable age of onset of genetic conditions illustrates the importance of the interaction of the gene and its environment, either physiological or external, at all stages of life.

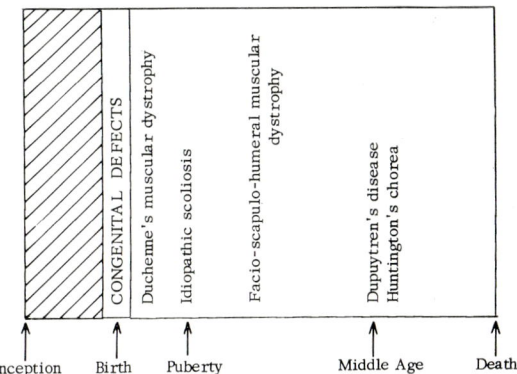

FIG. 7. Age of onset of clinical disorder. If a disorder is genetic in origin then the abnormal genes must be present at conception. However, the disease or deformity may not be clinically apparent until much later in life. "Congenital" defects are those which are present at birth and they may be genetic in origin or due to adverse factors in the intra-uterine environment.

Distinction Between Genetic and Environmental Factors

The major gene disorders are nearly all extremely rare. Many cause early death or such an abnormal individual that marriage and reproduction are unlikely. Congenital abnormalities produced by toxic agents in utero are also extremely rare. The common developmental anomalies are nearly all produced by a multiplicity of factors, both genetic and adverse factors in the uterine environment. Clinical genetic research is largely concerned with elucidating and distinguishing between these genetic and environmental factors.

EVIDENCE FOR GENETIC FACTORS

(1) If there is an increased incidence within a family of a particular deformity, when compared with the general population incidence (as in clubfoot, congenital dislocation of the hip or idiopathic scoliosis) then a genetic factor is suspected, although this evidence alone is insufficient

as a similar environment could be argued as the cause. However, the inheritance within the families may follow a dominant, recessive, X-linked or polygenic pattern which would be clear evidence for a genetic factor.

(2) A high incidence of the disorder in both of identical (monozygotic) twins points to a genetic factor (see page 11).

(3) In the case of a rare disorder, if the parents are related to each other, for example first cousins, then recessive inheritance is probable. The disease alkaptonuria is transmitted as an autosomal recessive condition and it has been shown that between 30 and 40 per cent of the parents are first cousins. The reason for this is that with rare recessive conditions the likelihood of two heterozygote individuals for the abnormal gene mating with each other are greater within a single family where both individuals have derived the abnormal gene from a common ancestor.

(4) Increased age of the parents may indicate a genetic factor, because mutations will occur with increasing age. However, an increased maternal age could be interpreted as evidence for an environmental factor, as the ageing uterus might be of significance.

EVIDENCE FOR ENVIRONMENTAL FACTORS

(1) The incidence of congenital malformations increases with maternal age and theoretically this could perhaps be due to placental insufficiency. Evidence from animal experiments supports this, but it remains conjectural in humans.

(2) The birth history may be suggestive of a pre-natal environmental disturbance, for example the high proportion of breech presentations in babies with congenital dislocation of the hip. Hydramnios and oligamnios cannot be measured with certainty but gross degrees are undoubtedly associated with malformation and pressure signs in the foetus.

(3) A characteristic position in the order of children in the family (the parity) of the deformed individual is indicative of an environmental disturbance. For example, a condition such as talipes calcaneo-valgus which is commoner in first-born than in subsequent children must be associated with an environmental factor. With a disordered gene there is an equal chance of any child in the family being affected.

(4) Seasonal variation in incidence of a deformity has been noted. For example, some reports indicate a rise in incidence of congenital dislocation of the hip among children born in the winter months.

(5) A regional variation in incidence may also indicate some environmental factor. For example, idiopathic scoliosis in the infant is uncommon in North America although the genetic constitution of the population there must be very similar to the European.

(6) The socio-economic status of the family indicates that environmental factors are operating where a disorder proves to be commoner in one particular social class. For example, anencephaly is commoner in families of the lower income groups.

(7) Teratogenic agents are rare in man but such factors as viral infection, ionizing radiation and drugs acting in early pregnancy should be considered.

(8) Finally, there are certain developmental disorders in which characteristically there are no other cases within the family and they are probably caused therefore by some adverse intrauterine environmental factor rather than by a genetic anomaly (arthrogryposis, Ollier's disease, transverse congenital amputations).

Twins

The value of twin investigations is in distinguishing between genetic and environmental factors. The incidence of the defect arising in both members of identical (monozygotic) twin pairs, non-identical (dizygotic) twin pairs and non-twin siblings is compared.

(1) If both of identical twin pairs are always affected then the condition must be solely a genetic disorder (e.g. trisomy 21).

(2) If the incidence of both twins being affected is higher amongst monozygotic than dizygotic twin pairs there must be some genetic factor present but some environmental factor acting as well, as in talipes equino-varus and congenital dislocation of the hip.

(3) If the incidence of both twins being affected is the same in monozygotic and dizygotic twin pairs then environmental factors are probably acting, a situation seen in spina bifida and meningocele.

(4) If the incidence is higher amongst twin pairs than amongst non-twin siblings then clearly this being a twin pregnancy would be relevant because of its additional ante-natal complexities.

Family Surveys

In this method of research a group of patients with a suspected heritable anomaly is selected and the number of cases within their families established. This requires a visit to them to obtain accurate medical information rather than accepting hearsay evidence which is frequently unreliable. The family incidence is then compared with the frequency of the disorder in the general population. If the family incidence is much in excess of the population figure then one may obtain some idea of the nature of any genetic factor involved:

(1) Mendelian ratios for a dominant, recessive or X-linked gene may be immediately apparent, thereby indicating that genetic factors are present.

(2) The family incidence may be in excess of the expected population incidence, but showing no genetic pattern of inheritance. This would indicate that environmental factors are acting.

(3) The family incidence may be in excess of the general population figures and follow a typical pattern of inheritance, though not to the full level of Mendelian ratios. A large survey has to be done to obtain enough cases to see if a pattern becomes apparent.

Multiple gene inheritance clearly may give a complex pattern.

The method of recording a family tree is shown in Fig. 8. The comparison of incidence of the deformity in first, second and third degree relatives is important. For example, polydactyly often has dominant inheritance, in which case, one would expect 50 per cent of the first degree relatives of the selected (index) patients to be affected, 25 per cent of second degree and 12·5 per cent of third degree. This illustrates the typical Mendelian ratios. However, if a condition shows an increased family incidence compared with the general population this pattern may still be apparent although not with the same percentages. For example, in adolescent idiopathic scoliosis it was found that 6·9 per cent of the first degree relatives of the girls were affected, 3·7 per cent of the second degree and 1·6 per cent of the third degree. This illustrates the halving each time characteristic of dominant inheritance though clearly other factors must be operating here as well. The reason for these ratios is that, on average, an individual has half his genes in common with his first degree relatives, one-quarter in common with the second degree and one-eighth in common with the third degree relatives.

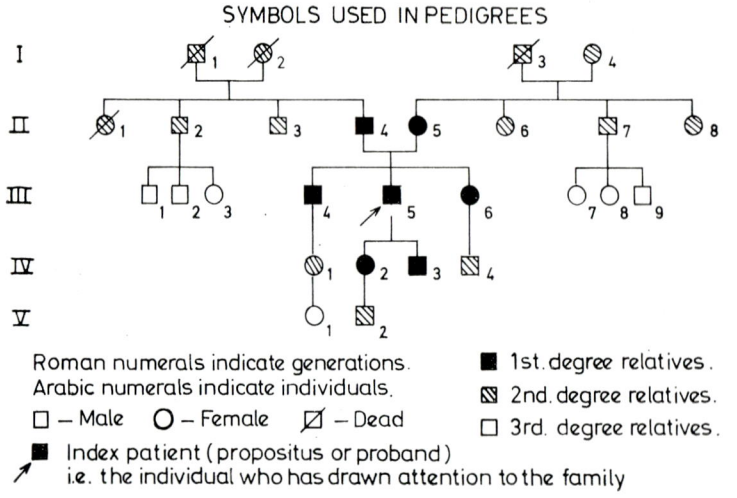

FIG. 8. Symbols used in pedigrees showing 1st, 2nd and 3rd degree relatives.

In addition to establishing the incidence amongst relatives the family survey attempts to uncover some of the environmental factors that may be operating and without which the gene may never manifest itself. Thus, a full history is taken relating to the pregnancy, birth, parity, parental age, date and place of birth, social class and so on, as well as an enquiry relating to possible teratogenic agents which may have acted during pregnancy.

SUGGESTED FURTHER READING:

An Introduction to Medical Genetics—J. A. Fraser Roberts. 4th Edition, Oxford University Press (London), 1967.
Genetics in Medicine—J. S. Thompson and M. W. Thompson. W. B. Saunders and Co. (Philadelphia/London), 1966.
The Thread of Life—John Kendrew. G. Bell and Sons Ltd. (London), 1966. (Based on the series of television lectures).
Human Heredity—C. O. Carter. Pelican Books, 1962 (1967 reprint).

GENETIC PROBLEMS IN ORTHOPAEDIC DISEASE

Clinical Forms of Chromosome Disorders

These may be broadly grouped into anomalies of the autosomes and of the sex chromosomes. It is probable that anomalies of cell division are a great deal more common than would be suspected from the clinical types presenting. Many cases abort in early pregnancy, are stillborn or die within a short time of birth. One survey of abortion material has shown that chromosome anomalies account for some 20 per cent of abortions in early pregnancy (Carr 1963). The mechanism of the error of cell division has been described in the previous section.

Autosomal Aberrations

Trisomy 21 (*Down's syndrome, Mongolism*). This involves chromosome No. 21 and occurs if there are three instead of the usual pair. It is the smallest chromosome but even so the effect on the body is extensive. It is the commonest of the trisomies to occur as a clinical entity. The features are well known and include mental retardation, some degree of dwarfing, a slanting appearance of the eyes, short broad hands with a single palmar crease and incurved little finger, there is a wide gap between the first and second toes. About one-third of cases have a congenital heart defect and expectation of life is dependent on this.

Trisomy 18. This involves a slightly larger chromosome and thus the effects on the body are more serious than in trisomy 21. There are multiple congenital abnormalities including mental retardation, micrognathia, contracture of the proximal interphalangeal joints, 'rockerbottom' feet, occasionally myelomeningocele and also cerebellar, cardiac and renal malformations. About 90 per cent die in the first year of life.

Trisomy of one of the 13–15 group of chromosomes. This is also a syndrome of multiple anomalies with perinatal death. Features include cleft lip and palate, polydactyly, contracture of the interphalangeal joints, absent olfactory bulbs and tracts, absent corpus callosum and again cardiac and renal malformations.

Sex-Chromosome Aberrations

Clinical disorders due to both trisomy and to deletion of the X and Y chromosomes are very much commoner than autosomal aberrations, and although sometimes producing widespread effects in the body may be compatible with a long life. However, the individuals are infertile and often they present for the first time at an infertility clinic.

Additional sex chromosomes. The triple X situation (XXX) is sometimes found on microscopic examination, but does not present with any clinical abnormality. These individuals are normal females. It is thought that only one 'X' is working even in a normal cell and the presence of two extra ones in a female is thus not of clinical significance.

The XXY, XXXY, XXXXY situations exist and individuals with two or more Xs as well as a Y present with Klinefelter's syndrome. They are male but the testes are small, there is no spermatogenesis and hence they are infertile. Gynaecomastia is common, the patients are usually tall and sometimes mentally retarded. Radio-ulnar synostosis is an occasional feature.

Individuals also exist with more than one Y chromosome (XYY, XXYY, XXXYY). These individuals are male and are exceptionally tall. There is evidence of psychotic abnormalities and criminal delinquency (Casey *et al.* 1966). The presence of two or more Xs in addition to two Ys will produce the Klinefelter syndrome as described above.

Deletion of sex chromosomes. As with the autosomes this is a more serious event than the presence of an additional chromosome. The YO situation (i.e. deletion of a whole X chromosome in the male) is not compatible with life.

The XO situation (deletion of one X in a female) gives Turner's syndrome and illustrates the much greater effect on the body of a deletion as opposed to an addition. The clinical features include shortness of stature, webbing of the neck, low set ears and cubitus valgus. Other defects, such as coarctation of the aorta, mental defect and angiomata of the small intestine, are frequent. Secondary sex characters are ill-developed and the ovary is only a streak of connective tissue. The individuals usually have primary amenorrhea and are infertile.

There are two points to be noted in connection with these chromosomal aberrations. One is that the Y chromosome is strongly sex determining and that an individual possessing a Y is invariably male although he may be infertile. Secondly it should be remembered that some individuals with sex chromosome anomalies will be mosaics and that many cells in the body will in that case be normal. The clinical features in mosaicism are transitional between those of the full syndrome and normality.

Major Gene Disorders

(*An alphabetical list of conditions of orthopaedic interest is given in Appendix I together with a note of the clinical features and the type of inheritance concerned.*)

In some instances precise structural details of the abnormal gene are known. A gene is a protein, proteins are made up of amino acids and in the haemoglobinopathies the actual abnormal amino acid is known. In sickle cell anaemia, for example, there is alteration of A_1 haemoglobin (beta chain). This produces various effects on bone such as generalized osteoporosis, aseptic necrosis and multiple infarcts. The inheritance is autosomal recessive.

Proteins derived from the genes form enzymes and in the inborn errors of metabolism there is a specific underlying defect leading to a metabolic block. In a large number of instances a precise enzyme has been defined. For example, in alkaptonuria there is an absence of homogentisic oxidase blocking the breakdown of phenylalanine and tyrosine to aceto-acetic acid. Clinically there is pigmentation of cartilage and ligaments with premature arthritis.

It is of interest that all the enzyme disorders so far elucidated have been recessive conditions and it is possible that enzyme defects are only clinically apparent in the homozygous state. However, the heterozygous carrier although showing no clinical disorder, may sometimes be identified by chemical means. Genes also control the structural proteins such as collagen, but there is as yet no detailed biochemical information regarding these defects.

The type of inheritance is deduced from family surveys, but ultimately one hopes that the precise nature of the protein disturbance will be identified for each disorder and perhaps even become correctable.

The following are short notes on disorders only recently described:

Homocystinuria (autosomal recessive). The presence of homocystine in the urine was noted in 1962 by Carson and Neill in a Northern Ireland survey of mentally backward individuals. The clinical features of the condition are similar to the Marfan syndrome in that there is very often the same overgrowth of long bones, ectopia lentis, pectus excavatum or carinatum, scoliosis and vascular disorders. However, joint laxity is not such a common feature as in Marfan's and there are more often joint contractures of the fingers. Osteoporosis and fractures occur and the patients are frequently mentally retarded. The most characteristic lesion is of the medium-sized arteries and veins which are dilated and subject to thromboses, whereas in the Marfan syndrome it is more usually the aorta which is affected by aneurysmal dilatation. The inheritance of Marfan's syndrome in contrast is dominant.

Pycnodysostosis (autosomal recessive). This was described by Maroteaux and Lamy in 1962. It is similar to cranio-cleido-dysostosis (dominant inheritance). The bones in pycnodysostosis are increased in density and pathological fracture is common. As in cranio-cleido-dysostosis there are Wormian bones in the skull and the terminal phalanges of the fingers are short.

Diastrophic dwarfism (autosomal recessive). This was also described by Maroteaux and Lamy in 1961. It is characterized by severe dwarfism, deformities of the feet and hands, scoliosis and ossification of the cartilages of the ear.

Mucopolysaccharidoses. Under this heading are a number of syndromes including Hurler's and Morquio's, which have in common a disorder of mucopolysaccharides, but are distinguished by various clinical features, their mode of inheritance and by pathological and biochemical findings (McKusick 1966).

Hurler's syndrome (gargoylism) is characterized by dwarfism, progressive mental defect, hepato-splenomegaly and clouding of the cornea. The skeletal manifestations include an enlarged 'shoe-shaped' sella turcica, premature closing of the sagittal suture with hyperostosis in this region, a kyphus at the 12th thoracic—1st lumbar vertebral area, anterior hooklike projections of the vertebrae and broad hands with stubby fingers and incurved little fingers. Stiffness of joints is another feature; there is diastasis recti and umbilical hernia almost invariably and sometimes other herniae. In the urine are found chondroitin sulphate B and heparitin sulphate.

Hunter's syndrome is similar to Hurler's but manifestations are not so severe. The disease runs a longer course and there is no clouding of the cornea. Chondroitin sulphate B and heparitin sulphate are again found in the urine, but the method of inheritance is different, being an X-linked recessive condition.

A third mucopolysaccharidosis is known as the Sanfilippo syndrome in which the patients have severe mental retardation, although the systemic and skeletal changes are not so marked. Heparitin sulphate only is found in the urine. The condition is an autosomal recessive. Morquio's syndrome is characterized by severe dwarfing but the children are usually of normal intelligence. There are obvious skeletal changes and in childhood the lumbar spine may show anterior beaking as in Hurler's syndrome, but later the vertebrae are characteristically flattened with a central tongue. The femoral heads are distorted, and the angle the manubrium makes with the sternum is about 90°. The joints are not usually stiff and there may in fact be joint laxity leading to disorders such as severe genu valgum. Keratosulphate is found in the urine. The inheritance is autosomal recessive.

Two other mucopolysaccharide syndromes have so far been described, each an autosomal recessive and each excreting chondroitin sulphate B only in the urine, but differing in their clinical manifestations. Both are extremely rare.

Over the next decade or two it must be anticipated that a large number of these abnormal metabolic, genetically determined diseases will be described. When the complexity of human metabolism is considered the theoretical number of possible inherited diseases is almost infinite.

Common Developmental Disorders

TALIPES EQUINO-VARUS

In a survey from Exeter (Wynne-Davies 1964) the incidence of talipes equino-varus in the population was found to be 1·2 per 1000 (1·6 males and 0·8 females). One hundred and forty-four patients with the deformity were studied and the incidence of the same deformity amongst their relatives was found to be as follows:

Parents: 4 affected of 288 (1·4 per cent or approximately 10 times the population incidence).
Siblings: 8 affected of 272 (2·9 per cent or approximately 20 times the population incidence).

When the figures were further broken down into those for the male and female relatives of the male and female patients, it was found that the rarer sex to be affected, females, unexpectedly had more relatives with the deformity (Figs. 9a and b).

The incidence of the same deformity in all second degree relatives was 0·6 per cent and in third degree 0·2 per cent.

A survey of twins with talipes equino-varus was carried out by Idelberger (1939). He found that the incidence of both dizygotic twins having the deformity was only 2·9 per cent, the same figure as for siblings in the Exeter survey. However, the incidence of both identical twins having the deformity was 32·5 per cent.

The Exeter survey showed the deformity to be unrelated to the age of either parent or to the patient's position in the family. Associated anomalies of the patients showed an unexpectedly high (17 per cent) proportion of minor connective tissue defects such as hernia (7 per cent of the boys) and generalized joint laxity.

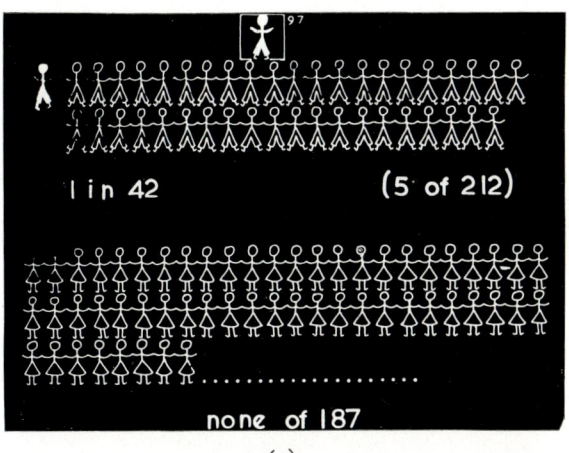

(a)

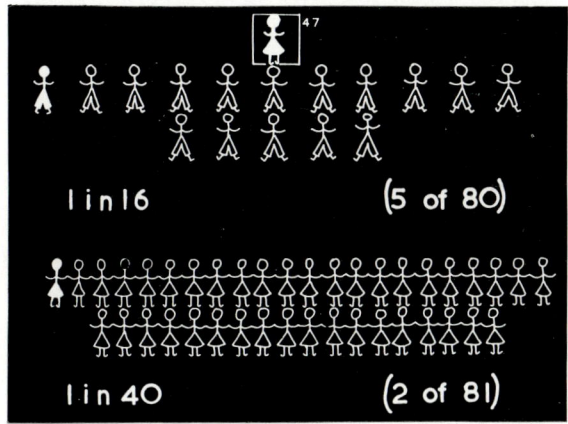

(b)

FIGS. 9a and b. This illustrates the higher incidence of T.E.V. amongst the relatives of the girl patients (Fig. 9b) compared with the boys (Fig. 9a).

Interpretation. There is a (× 20) increase in the family figures over the general population (siblings 2·9 per cent compared with a population incidence of 1·2 per thousand). Theoretically this could be due to a similar family environment or to genetic factors or both. However, the twin figures clearly indicate that some genetic factor is operating because both identical twins are affected in 32·5 per cent of cases compared with only 2·9 per cent of non-identical twins. Because both identical twins did not invariably have the deformity there must clearly be some environmental factor acting as well as the genetic.

The next point is to consider the nature of the genetic factor. The characteristic pattern of sex-linked inheritance is not apparent and can be ruled out. Incomplete expression of a recessive gene is considered, but the evidence is against it. If a recessive gene were acting one would expect a high incidence amongst siblings and low among parents, but the figures here are very similar (1·4 and 2·9 per cent). Also, with recessive inheritance one might expect some instances of related parents, and some instances of the deformity on both maternal and paternal sides of the family. Neither of these was found.

The remaining possibilities are dominant and polygenic inheritance, and in both cases one would expect a similar incidence in parents and

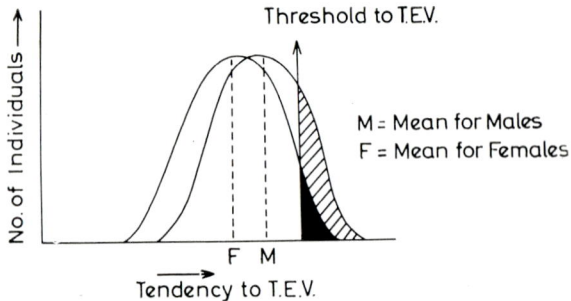

FIG. 10. Polygenic inheritance (after Carter 1964). If a hypothesis of polygenic inheritance in talipes equino-varus is considered, then the underlying tendency to the deformity must be twice as great in males as in females (because they have the deformity twice as often), i.e. the female population is shifted to the left compared with the males. It is seen from the diagram that the affected females are drawn from the extreme of their population range and this is mirrored in the increased number of their relatives affected with the same deformity.

siblings, as is found here. However, the increased incidence amongst the relatives of the females (i.e. the rarer sex to be affected with the deformity) cannot be explained on the basis of inheritance of a single dominant gene, but it is just what would be expected from the concept of polygenic inheritance (Carter 1964, Fraser Roberts 1964) (Fig. 10).

Another point in favour of polygenic inheritance in talipes equino-varus are the figures for the second and third degree relatives. With single dominant gene inheritance one would expect a 'halving' of incidence from first to second and second to third degree relatives, whereas the figures for this survey fall rapidly to the population incidence (first degree relatives 2·9 per cent, second degree 0·6 per cent and third degree 0·2 per cent, which is very little above the population incidence of 0·1 per cent). This is to be expected from polygenic inheritance.

Thus the evidence points to the inheritance of this condition being polygenic with an added environmental factor.

TALIPES CALCANEO-VALGUS

This is a minor, transient deformity and ascertainment of the population incidence and affected relatives must be incomplete as many cases will pass undiagnosed. However, the figures obtained from the Exeter survey showed in some respects a similar pattern to those for talipes equino-varus. The points of difference were the sex ratio, in that the condition was commoner in girls than boys, an association (5 per cent of cases) with congenital dislocation of the hip, and a definite increase in the number of cases amongst first born children compared with the normal population (Table I).

TABLE I

Birth Order in Calcaneo-Valgus and Normal Population

	1st born	2nd	Birth Order 3rd	4th	Total
Calcaneo-valgus	39	8	5	11	63
Normal population	25	19	10	9	63

This evidence indicates an intrauterine environmental factor operating, as genetic factors would have an equal chance of acting in any child and the deformity would not be related to the position in the family. This is with the exception of children born to elderly parents, where there is an increased chance of genetic mutation.

CONGENITAL DISLOCATION OF THE HIP

A number of factors relating to the aetiology of congenital dislocation of the hip (C.D.H.) are known and a large-scale survey is in progress at Edinburgh and Glasgow in an attempt to answer some of the problems.

Population incidence. Until recently the reported incidence of C.D.H. was about 1 per 1000. However, examination of the newborn infant for a dislocating hip is now being increasingly practised. If this examination is carried out in the first half of the first week of life, the incidence rises to 11 per 1000, though approximately half of these stabilize by the end of the first week giving a population incidence of 5 per 1000 (Thieme *et al.* 1968). Barlow (1962) gives an incidence of 15 per 1000 under $3\frac{1}{2}$ days old, but only half this number at the end of the first week of life. It is possible that 'lax hip' in the newborn is not genuinely related to congenital dislocation of the hip, but it could of course be a minor manifestation of a severe deformity (cf. resolving scoliosis).

Breech presentation. The normal population incidence of breech births is between 2 and 3 per cent. It was noted by Muller and Seddon (1953) that 16 per cent of C.D.H. children were born by breech births. Carter and Wilkinson (1964a) also found 16 per cent of C.D.H. children were breech born. They noted that a further 9 per cent had undergone therapeutic version and pointed out that it is the frank breech (with knees extended) which is important in dislocation of the hip rather than breech presentation. This present study confirms the high incidence of breech births or versions, and it is found that this is present in boys more often than girls, although girls have C.D.H. six or seven times more often than boys.

Oestrogen excretion in newborn infants with C.D.H. In 1961 Andren and Borglin reported abnormal oestrogen metabolism in the perinatal period of children with congenital dislocation of the hip. It was suggested that an inborn error of oestrogen metabolism contributed to hip joint laxity and congenital dislocation. The problem was re-examined by Thieme and co-workers (1968) using a more sensitive method of oestrogen assay. The results showed that oestrogen excretion in C.D.H. infants was slightly higher than in a control group of subjects but the difference failed to reach a significant level. They concluded therefore there was no real evidence of abnormal urinary oestrogen excretion in congenital dislocation of the hip.

TABLE II

Siblings with C.D.H.

		Brothers	Sisters
Girl index patients			
Hospital for Sick Children*	143	1 of 115	5 of 109
Edinburgh/Glasgow survey	235	2 of 235	10 of 245
Total	378	3 of 350 (0·9%)	15 of 354 (4·2%)
Boy index patients			
Hospital for Sick Children*	21	4 of 17	1 of 18
Edinburgh/Glasgow survey	36	0 of 40	2 of 35
Total	57	4 of 57 (7%)	3 of 53 (5·7%)

* Carter (1965)

Family studies. There are no figures yet available for neonatal congenital dislocation of the hip but previous surveys of children who had C.D.H. diagnosed later indicate an incidence amongst first degree relatives of about 30 times the population incidence, with similar figures for both siblings and children. The incidence of congenital dislocation of the hip amongst the parents of patients is rather low but this probably indicates a low marriage rate amongst the previous generation of individuals with C.D.H. As with talipes equino-varus there is some evidence that the rarer sex to be affected, boys, have more affected relatives than the girls (Table II).

The figures shown are those for the Hospital for Sick Children, Great Ormond Street (Carter 1965) and preliminary figures from the Edinburgh/Glasgow survey. Carter also reports a rapid drop in incidence amongst the second and third degree relatives.

Twins. Idelberger (1951) studied twins with congenital dislocation of the hip and found that in 10 of 29 monozygotic pairs both had C.D.H. (41 per cent) but only 3 of 109 dizygotic twin pairs (2·8 per cent). This latter figure was obtained for non-twin siblings in other surveys.

Acetabular dysplasia. It is possible that acetabular dysplasia is one of the inherited factors in congenital dislocation of the hip, as suggested by Faber (1937) and Wilkinson and Carter (1960). This requires further investigation.

Joint laxity. It has been suggested (Carter and Wilkinson 1964b) that a familial generalized joint laxity is another inherited factor in congenital dislocation of the hip. The examination of undue joint mobility is somewhat imprecise but examination of C.D.H. patients in the present survey, together with a large group of normal controls, has been carried out. It is apparent that this is indeed a significant factor in many cases, and the heritable nature of the disorder is confirmed by finding a high incidence of joint laxity amongst the first degree relatives of the patients.

Interpretation. It is apparent from twin studies that both genetic and environmental factors must be acting here (41 per cent of monozygotic twins both affected compared with 2·8 per cent of dizygotic twins). Like talipes equino-varus, it is probable that the pattern of inheritance is polygenic as evidenced by a similar incidence among siblings and children; the rapid fall in incidence among second and third degree relatives, and also the probable higher incidence amongst the relatives of the boy patients.

The genetic factors are probably related to joint laxity and to acetabular dysplasia, while the environmental factor which 'triggers off' the dislocation in many cases is probably related to the breech malposition.

IDIOPATHIC SCOLIOSIS

A survey of the families of children attending the Edinburgh Scoliosis Clinic has been completed (Wynne-Davies 1968). This consisted of a detailed examination of 114 index patients and the personal examination of some 2000 first, second and third degree relatives.

In the patients the side of the curve and the age at which it becomes apparent was found to be similar to that described by James (1954) (Fig. 11). In the infant patient the curve was usually to the left (88 per cent), was commoner in boys and the deformity resolved in half the cases presenting at the clinic under one year of age. In the adolescent patient the curve was nearly always to the right (90 per cent), was very much commoner in girls and the curve did not spontaneously disappear.

Thus there are two peaks of incidence, one in infancy and the other in adolescence with less new cases developing during the middle juvenile years. For the purpose of the survey the children were divided into 'early onset' scoliosis (under eight years) and 'late onset' (eight years or over).

It was found during the examination of the relatives of these children that a mild degree (up to 50°) of scoliosis was quite common, particularly after the age of 50 years. Many individuals had a curve without being aware of it, and, conversely, many were aware of having scoliosis but the aetiology was found to be unrelated to idiopathic scoliosis. The commonest misdiagnoses were related to osteoporosis, Scheuermann's disease in which the adolescent kyphosis is quite frequently accompanied by scoliosis, and postural scoliosis resulting from a variety of causes such as a short leg. It was thus necessary to do a population survey in order to establish the true figures of idiopathic scoliosis in the general population so that a comparison could be made between this and the affected relatives of the patients with idiopathic scoliosis. It was carried out in

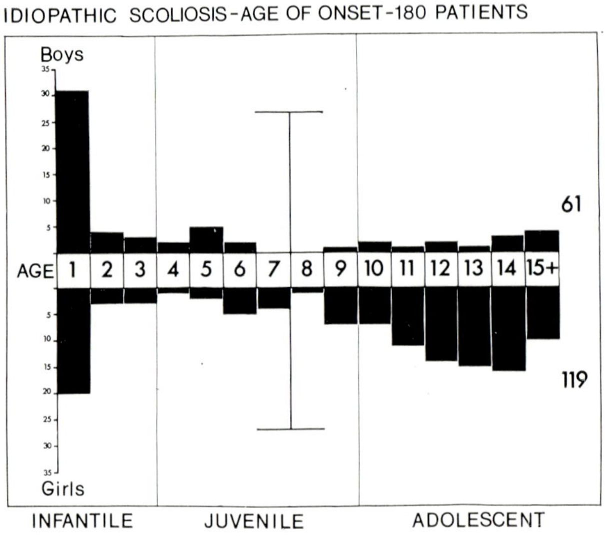

FIG. 11. Age of onset and sex distribution of idiopathic scoliosis.

Edinburgh's schools, nursery schools and infant clinics, and included children from two weeks to 18 years of age. A physical examination was necessary and radiography was carried out when indicated by the clinical appearance of a curve. Amongst 11,000 children examined about 60 were brought to hospital for further examination and X-ray, of whom only 20 were found to have true idiopathic scoliosis (Table III).

It was found that there was a concentration of idiopathic scoliosis within the families of patients, and it is probable that the infantile and adolescent types share the same basic aetiology since families contained instances of each. The highest incidence was among the first degree relatives of the adolescent girl patients, where 6·9 per cent were affected. The second degree relatives of this group had 3·7 per cent affected and the third degree 1·6 per cent. Even in these more distant relatives the incidence was still considerably above the normal population figures (×10 in the third degree) (Fig. 12). The family incidence was also

GENETIC FACTORS IN ORTHOPAEDICS

TABLE III
Idiopathic Scoliosis Population Survey

	11,087 Edinburgh Children		
	Population incidence per 1000		
	Male	Female	Total
Early onset Scoliosis	1·2	1·3	1·3
Late onset Scoliosis	0·3	3·9	1·8

raised in the infantile scoliosis group but not to the same extent and not showing the 'halving' each time characteristic of the relatives of the adolescent girl patients.

The question of 'resolving' scoliosis was considered separately as it was not clear if these children belonged aetiologically to the same

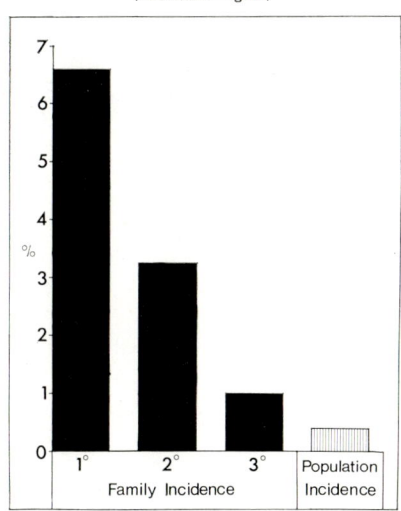

Fig. 12. This shows the number of relatives with idiopathic scoliosis of the adolescent girl patients, and illustrates the "halving" from first to second and second to third degree relatives.

group. The curve was nearly always left-sided, rather more common in boys than girls. Their relatives were affected with scoliosis in the same proportions as in the main infantile group, and much in excess of the population incidence. This suggested that the resolving type of scoliosis is the mildest manifestation of what may be a very severe disorder.

An interesting point in connection with the children with adolescent scoliosis, both boys and girls, was that the maternal age was significantly in excess of the normal by comparison with a control series obtained from the Registrar General's figures on parental age. The paternal age and the position in family of the deformed child showed no significant difference from normal.

The congenital anomalies associated with scoliosis were of some interest. The most striking disorder was plagiocephaly, or moulding of the head, present in all infants with idiopathic scoliosis who were seen under the age of one year (Fig. 13). The deformity was transient and by the age of three years only half showed it and by five years there was only the occasional child with persistent plagiocephaly.

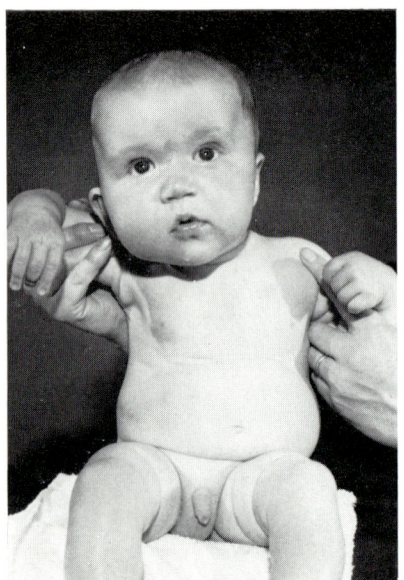

FIG. 13. Left-sided plagiocephaly.

In all cases the plagiocephaly agreed with the side of the curve, i.e. 88 per cent of infants had left-sided curves and the left side of the head appeared pushed back. A control group of infants under one year of age in the city clinics was examined and only 11 per cent were found to have plagiocephaly, equally left- and right-sided.

The only other common anomaly to be associated with scoliosis was mental retardation with and without epilepsy. Other cases presented with congenital dislocation of the hip, clubfoot, various congenital heart disorders and upper limb defects.

Interpretation. Both the infantile and adolescent groups showed an increased incidence amongst the families of the patients as compared with the general population. The figures for the adolescent girls suggest a dominant type of inheritance with the expected halving of incidence from first to second and then to third degree relatives, though other factors must be operating in addition. This pattern was not apparent amongst the relatives of the infant patients and it is probable that here there is a strong environmental factor acting, and this is also suggested by the constant association of infantile scoliosis and plagiocephaly.

NEURAL TUBE DEFECTS

The neural tube defects include anencephaly and spina bifida/meningocele (with or without hydrocephalus). There has been a number of surveys and it is clear that hydrocephalus occurring alone is unrelated to anencephaly and spina bifida. One type of hydrocephalus due to stenosis of the aqueduct of Sylvius is a rare major gene (X-linked recessive) condition. Anencephalus and spina bifida/meningocele are related aetiologically as they often occur together and cases of each appear in the same families and they are therefore considered together here.

There is a high preponderance of females with anencephaly and this is also present though less marked in spina bifida. The population incidence of anencephaly and spina bifida shows some regional variation (Table IV).

TABLE IV

Population Incidence of Anencephaly and Spina Bifida (Family Survey Evidence)

	Incidence per 1000 births	
	Anencephalus	Spina bifida
Belfast (Stevenson and Warnock 1959)	4·6	2·2
Birmingham (McKeown and Record 1960)	2·0	3·0
Northamptonshire (Pleydell 1960)	1·1	2·0
Southampton (Williamson 1965)	1·95	3·22
South Wales (Laurence, David and Carter 1968)	3·54	4·13

The reason for the regional variation may perhaps be associated with the social class of the patient's family. It has been repeatedly shown that anencephaly and spina bifida are commoner amongst the lower social classes. For example, using the Registrar General's classification of social class, based on the father's occupation and graded from I to V Williamson (1965) found for the Southampton area that only 7 per cent of the anencephaly and spina bifida children belonged to the upper social classes (I and II) whereas the expected figure for the general population in that area was 18 per cent.

The incidence of the same deformity amongst the siblings of patients is considerably higher (about 5 per cent) than the general population figures which vary from about one to five per thousand. If two siblings are already affected, then the chances of a third having the same deformity are higher still, being 1 in 10 (10 per cent) (Carter and Fraser Roberts 1967).

Another interesting point is that there appears to be a concentration of cases on the maternal side of the family among the children of the mother's sisters. It is possible that this could be due to the mother giving a more accurate family history than the father, but this is not a feature apparent in other surveys and it is suggested that there may perhaps be some genetic factor which affects the uterine development and so predisposes to these deformities. The incidence in second and third degree relatives falls rapidly towards the population incidence. There are no large scale twin surveys available, but such evidence as there is points to the incidence in identical and non-identical twins being similar.

Interpretation. There is certainly an increased incidence amongst the families when compared with the normal population but there are several factors here which point to environmental influences being of more importance than genetic, namely, the increased incidence amongst patients of a low socio-economic status, the increased number of first-born children affected and the fact that only one of identical twins is characteristically affected. Evidence that there is some rise in incidence on the maternal side of the family suggests a genetic factor which itself is affecting the uterine environment. It is possible that environmental factors 'trigger off' the deformity in individuals with a polygenic predisposition to it.

DUPUYTREN'S CONTRACTURE

A family survey was carried out by Ling (1963) taking 50 patients with Dupuytren's contracture from the Edinburgh Hand Clinic and examining as many relatives as possible of these individuals. It was in this survey that personal examination of the relatives was found to be of great importance. On primary questioning only 8 of the 50 patients gave a positive family history, but when the survey was completed it was found that in fact 34 (68 per cent) actually had relatives affected with Dupuytren's disease. This is a disease which is most common after middle age (Fig. 14) and thus correction had to be made to the figures first obtained to allow for the fact that some of the younger relatives examined might yet develop Dupuytren's disease in later life. Another factor which had to be allowed for was that the population incidence of this disorder is very high, estimated by Ling from various surveys to occur in 25 per cent of all males over the age of 75 years, though rather less often in females. Thus in a survey one would expect that certain relatives of the original patients would be bound to have the disease anyway. When allowance was made for these factors it was found that the inheritance of Dupuytren's disease followed the pattern of a single dominant gene (Fig. 15).

DUPUYTREN'S DISEASE AND EPILEPSY

There has been a number of reports associating Dupuytren's disease with various other conditions, namely epilepsy, tuberculosis, alcoholism, diabetes mellitus and rheumatoid arthritis. This problem has recently been studied by Thieme (1967) who also looked into the question of Dupuytren's disease and epilepsy being connected with barbiturate usage rather than epilepsy itself as suggested by Skoog (1948). He took a group of 131 patients with Dupuytren's contracture from the Edinburgh

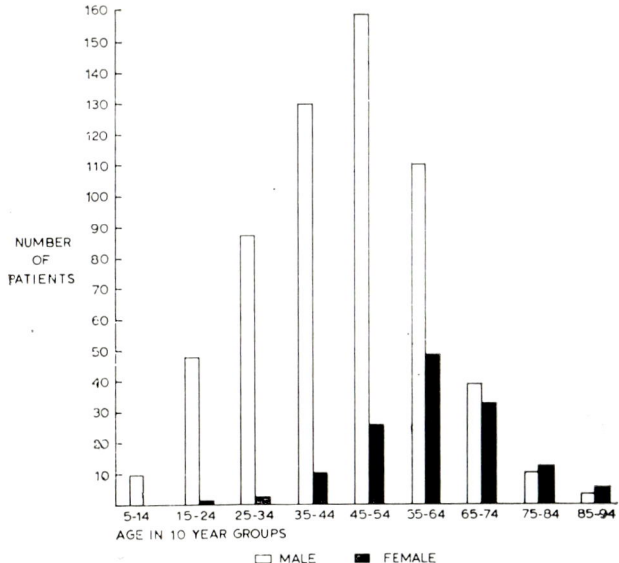

Fig. 14. Age distribution of the onset of Dupuytren's disease.

Hand Clinic and 88 proven idiopathic epilepsy patients from a neurological out-patient clinic. All first degree relatives (parents, siblings and children) were sought and examined personally, and all the suspected associated disorders were looked for in each of the two groups. In all

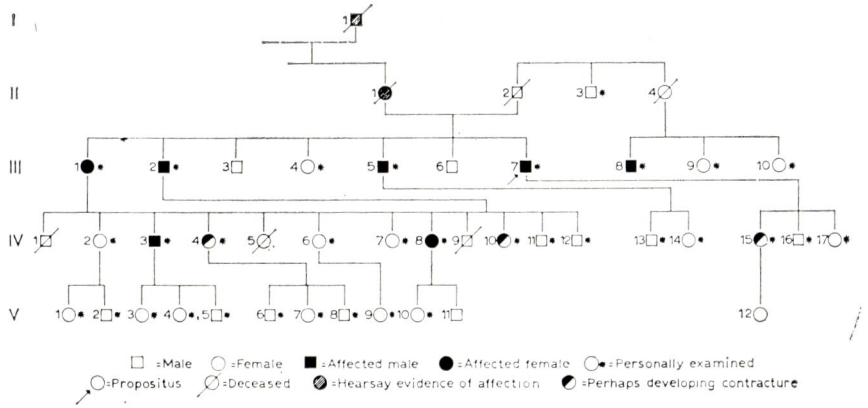

Fig. 15. Pedigree of a family with Dupuytren's disease.

instances there was good medical evidence of the disorders. In the case of epilepsy, children under two years with an occasional fit were excluded.

So far as the inheritance of Dupuytren's disease was concerned he arrived at similar figures to Ling and thus confirmed the probability of single major gene dominant inheritance. He was unable to confirm anything other than chance association with any disease except idiopathic epilepsy. The question of the association with many diseases has clearly arisen because Dupuytren's is so common with advancing age that it will on occasion occur with many long-standing disorders. However, there seemed to be a real association with idiopathic epilepsy. Skoog had earlier noted that 42 per cent of epileptics in a special home had Dupuytren's disease. The epileptic patients in this present survey were taken only from an out-patient clinic and were not therefore so severely affected as his specially selected group. Also, of course, many were young individuals and again correction had to be made for age to allow for the fact that the incidence of Dupuytren's disease in any case increases with age (Tables V*a* and *b*).

TABLE V*a*

Incidence of Idiopathic Epilepsy in Dupuytren's Disease

No. of patients with Dupuytren's disease	No. with confirmed epilepsy in addition to Dupuytren's	Expected incidence of epilepsy for normal population	Increase
131	11 (8·4%)	0·7 (5 per 1000 or 0·5%)	× 15·7

TABLE V*b*

Incidence of Dupuytren's Disease in Idiopathic Epilepsy

No. of patients with idiopathic epilepsy (Corrected to age 75 years)	No. with Dupuytren's disease in addition to epilepsy	Maximum expected incidence of Dupuytren's for normal population at 75 years of age	Increase
88 (Corrected for age 52·5)	19 (36·9%)	13 (25%)	× 1·5

TABLE VI

Dupuytren's/Epilepsy Study. Barbiturate Use in all Patients and Relatives

	With Dupuytren's	%	Without Dupuytren's	%
Total No. of individuals	351		408	
Occasional use of Barbiturates	79	22·5	92	22·5
Barbiturates for more than one year	47	13·4	59	14·4
Barbiturates for more than five years	32	9·1	38	9·3

A history of barbiturate usage was obtained from all individuals in the survey both with and without Dupuytren's disease, grouping into occasional use of the drug, barbiturates taken continuously for more than one year, and taken continuously for more than five years.

The results are shown in Table VI.

The percentages for each group are almost exactly similar, thus quite clearly demonstrating that this drug is in no way concerned with the aetiology of Dupuytren's disease.

Genetic Counselling

Genetic counselling is concerned with giving advice in connection with congenital and developmental defects, either to the affected individual or to his relatives. There will obviously be concern in a family as to the likelihood of further cases occurring and the importance of giving well-informed advice to a deformed individual, his parents or to other relatives can hardly be overemphasized. The problem may not be simple in that there are several genetic conditions which while presenting the same clinical picture have on occasion different modes of inheritance. There are sporadic cases from new mutations and clinical conditions which mimic genetic disorders without being heritable. There is the possibility of identifying heterozygotes carrying harmful recessive genes by biochemical tests.

Patients can obtain as accurate information as is available from the various Genetic Counselling Centres in the country and a list of these is given in Appendix II.

APPENDIX I: MAJOR GENE DISORDERS

(The Authors have Drawn Heavily on 'Mendelian Inheritance in Man' (McKusick 1966). This is a Computer Compiled Encyclopaedia of Genetic Disorders to which the Reader is Referred for Further Information Including Key References)

Disease	Inheritance	Notes
Achondroplasia	Dominant	Short-limbed dwarfism, with short proximal segment of limbs. Bulging frontal region of skull, flattened bridge of nose, small foramen magnum. Sometimes internal hydrocephalus.
Acrocephalosyndactyly (Apert's syndrome)	Dominant	Deformity of skull with syndactyly of fingers and toes.
Acrocephalosyndactyly with polydactyly	Dominant	As above with polydactyly and progressive synostosis in the feet, hands, carpus, tarsus, cervical vertebrae and skull.
Alkaptonuria	Autosomal recessive	Urine turns dark on standing and alkalinization, pigmentation of cartilage, disc calcification and premature arthritis.

Disease	Inheritance	Notes
Brachydactyly	Dominant	Various types with shortening of one or more phalanges.
Calcaneo-navicular fusion	Dominant, some cases only	
Diaphyseal aclasis (multiple exostoses)	Dominant	Exostoses typically at the growing ends of long bones, also in the hand. Occasional malignant change particularly in central tumours.
Diastrophic dwarfism	Autosomal recessive	Calcification of pinnae, scoliosis, foot and hand deformities, some cases cleft palate.
Dupuytren's contracture	Dominant	Typically in the hand, may affect plantar fascia, also associated with knuckle pads. Onset usually in middle age. Association with epilepsy.
Ectrodactyly	Dominant	'Lobster claw' deformity of hand.
Ehlers-Danlos syndrome	Dominant	Marked joint laxity, lax skin, bruise easily, poor scar tissue.
Ellis-Van Creveld syndrome (Chondroectodermal dysplasia)	Autosomal recessive	Dwarfism, polydactyly, congenital heart defect, normal intelligence.
Engelmann's disease	Dominant sometimes	Gross thickening of the cortex of long bones.
Fanconi's anaemia	Autosomal recessive	All marrow elements affected, pigmentation in the skin; heart and kidney malformations, radial club hand and thumb deformities.
Fanconi's syndrome (see 'rickets')		
Flexion contracture of fingers	Dominant sometimes	Usually affecting the little finger.
Gout	Dominant	
Haemophilia (classical)	X-linked recessive	Recurrent haemarthroses lead to joint destruction in young adults.
Heart/hand syndrome (Tabatzik syndrome)	Dominant	Cardiac arrhythmia and malformation of upper extremities, particularly 'stub thumb'.
Homocystinuria	Autosomal recessive	Simulates Marfan's but more commonly associated with mental retardation and epilepsy, which appear late in childhood, absence of joint laxity.
Hydrocephalus (due to congenital stenosis of aqueduct of Sylvius)	X-linked recessive (some cases)	Occurs alone without spina bifida or meningocele. Males only.

Disease	Inheritance	Notes
Joint laxity, familial	Dominant, some cases only	
Madelung's deformity	Dominant	Also occurs in Turner's syndrome.
Marfan's syndrome	Dominant	Ectopia lentis, aortic aneurysm, excessive length of extremities—particularly distally, joint laxity, sometimes finger contractures.
Metaphyseal dysostosis	Dominant, also recessive sometimes	Irregularity of the metaphyseal ends of long bones
Mucopolysaccharidoses		
(1) Hurler's syndrome (gargoylism)	Autosomal recessive	Progressive mental retardation, dwarfism, hepato-splenomegaly, and clouding of cornea. Chondroitin sulphate B and heparitin sulphate in the urine.
(2) Hunter's syndrome	X-linked recessive	As above but without corneal clouding and a slower course. Chondroitin sulphate B and heparitin sulphate in the urine.
(3) Sanfilippo syndrome	Autosomal recessive	Severe mental defect, few skeletal changes. Heparitin sulphate only in the urine.
(4) Morquio's syndrome	Autosomal recessive	Dwarfism, not usually mental retardation, flattening of vertebral bodies, deformed femoral heads, kerato-sulphate in the urine.
(5) Scheie's syndrome	Autosomal recessive	Stiff joints, clouding of cornea, no mental retardation, chondroitin sulphate B in the urine.
(6) Maroteaux-Lamy syndrome	Autosomal recessive	Osseous and corneal changes without mental retardation, chondroitin sulphate B in the urine.
Multiple epiphyseal dysplasia	Dominant	Maldevelopment of many epiphyses leading to premature osteoarthritis.
Muscular dystrophy		
(1) Duchenne's	X-linked recessive	Onset in early childhood. Formerly called pseudo-hypertrophic type. Males only.
(2) Resembling Duchenne's	Autosomal recessive	Both sexes affected.
(3) Limb girdle	Autosomal recessive	Onset in adult life.
(4) Facio-scapulo-humeral	Dominant	Adult onset, slow course.
Myositis ossificans progressiva (Fibro-dysplasia ossificans progressiva)	Dominant	Progressive extra-skeletal ossification usually starting in head, neck and trunk, with short great toes and thumbs.

Disease	Inheritance	Notes
Nail-patella syndrome	Dominant	Dysplasia of nails, absent or small patellae which lead to recurrent dislocations, iliac horns, sometimes dislocation of head of radius. Linked to ABO blood groups.
Neurofibromatosis (von Recklinghausen's disease)	Dominant	Cafe-au-lait spots, multiple neurofibromata, scoliosis, pseudarthrosis of the tibia, fibrous replacement of other bones sometimes.
Osteogenesis imperfecta (Fragilitas ossium)	Dominant	Fragile bones, blue sclerotics, otosclerosis developing in the second or third decades, joint laxity in 45% of cases.
Osteopetrosis	Dominant and recessive types	Increased density and fragility of bones with encroachment on marrow cavities leading to severe anaemia.
Osteopoikilosis	Dominant	'Spotted bones' near the ends. Of no clinical significance.
Polydactyly, postaxial	Dominant	Frequent in negroes.
Polydactyly, preaxial	No clear genetic basis	
Pseudo-hypoparathyroidism (Albright's hereditary osteodystrophy)	Dominant, perhaps X-linked dominant	Symptoms of hypoparathyroidism without response to parathormone. Short usually third and fourth metacarpal and metatarsal bones, epilepsy, mental retardation.
Pycnodysostosis	Autosomal recessive	Bone sclerosis with fragility, wide cranial fontanelles, micrognathism, hypoplasia of clavicles and osteolysis of terminal phalanges.
Radio-ulnar synostosis	Dominant sometimes.	Also occurs in Klinefelter's syndrome.
'Rickets'		
(1) Hypophosphatasia	Autosomal recessive.	Absent alkaline phosphatase.
(2) Organic aciduria	X-linked recessive	Aminoaciduria, alkaline urine, proteinuria, renal tubular acidosis.
(3) Renal tubular acidosis	?Dominant	Inability to acidify urine.
(4) Hypophosphataemia (Vit. D resistant)	?X-linked dominant	Disordered renal phosphate transport with decreased intestinal calcium ion absorption.
(5) Fanconi's syndrome	Autosomal recessive	Glucosuria, amino-aciduria, and hyperphosphaturia.
Sickle cell anaemia	Autosomal recessive	One of the haemoglobinopathies with generalized osteoporosis, aseptic necrosis, and multiple infarcts.
Spondyloepiphyseal dysplasia	Dominant and X-linked	Delayed dwarfism, head and face not involved.
Symphalangism	Dominant	Fusion of distal or proximal interphalangeal joints.
Syndactyly	Dominant	Probably several different genes.
Thalassemia	Autosomal recessive	Osteoporosis, thickened trabeculae.

APPENDIX II: GENETIC COUNSELLING CENTRES

An International Directory of Genetic Services has been compiled by Henry T. Lynch, M.D. (editors: Daniel Bergsma, M.D., Henry T. Lynch, M.D.). This directory, published in May 1968 by the National Foundation—March of Dimes, contains the addresses of centres in all parts of the world. A new edition is due in 1969 and further information can be obtained from:

Daniel Bergsma, M.D., The National Foundation—March of Dimes, 800 Second Avenue, New York, New York 10017.

The addresses of the Counselling Centres in Great Britain are:

ABERDEEN	Human Genetics Laboratory, Room 208, Aberdeen Royal Infirmary, Foresterhill, Aberdeen.
BIRMINGHAM	The Institute of Child Health, Francis Road, Birmingham, 16. Department of Medicine, The Children's Hospital, Ladywood Road, Birmingham, 16.
BRISTOL	Department of Child Health, Bristol Royal Hospital for Sick Children, St. Michael's Hill, Bristol.
DUNDEE	Department of Pathology, University of Dundee, Dundee.
EDINBURGH	Department of Human Genetics, University of Edinburgh, Western General Hospital, Crewe Road, Edinburgh, 4.
GLASGOW	Department of Medical Genetics, Royal Hospital for Sick Children and Queen Mother's Hospital, Glasgow, C.3.
INVERNESS	Paediatric Unit, Raigmore Hospital, Inverness.
LEEDS	Department of Paediatrics and Child Health, 27 Blundell Street, Leeds, 1.
LIVERPOOL	The Heredity Clinic, David Lewis Northern Hospital, Great Howard Street, Liverpool, 12.
LONDON	Institute of Child Health, 30 Guildford Street, London, W.C.1. Paediatric Research Unit, Guy's Hospital, London, S.E.1. Genetic Clinic, University College Hospital, Gower Street, London, W.C.1.
MANCHESTER	Department of Medicine, Manchester Royal Infirmary, Oxford Road, Manchester, 13. Royal Manchester Children's Hospital, Pendlebury, near Manchester.
NEWCASTLE	Laboratory of Human Genetics, University Department of Child Health, 19 Claremont Place, Newcastle-upon-Tyne.
OXFORD	Population Genetics Research Unit, Old Road, Headington, Oxford.
SHEFFIELD	Department of Genetics, University of Sheffield, Langhill, Manchester Road, Sheffield, 10.
SOUTHAMPTON	Genetic Counselling Centre, Children's Hospital, 154 Winchester Road, Shirley, Southampton.

References

ANDREN, L. and BORGLIN, N. E. (1961). Disturbed urinary excretion pattern of oestrogens in newborns with congenital dislocation of the hip. I. The excretion of oestrogen during the first few days of life. *Acta endocr.*, **37**, 423.

BARLOW, T. G. (1962). Early diagnosis and treatment of congenital dislocation of the hip. *J. Bone Jt. Surg.*, **44B**, 292.

CARR, D. H. (1963). Chromosome studies in abortuses and stillborn infants. *Lancet*, **ii**, 603.

CARSON, N. A. J. and NEILL, D. W. (1962). Metabolic abnormalities detected in a survey of mentally backward individuals in Northern Ireland. *Archs. Dis. Childh.*, **37**, 505.

CARTER, C. O. (1964). The genetics of common malformations. In "Congenital Malformations". Papers and discussions presented at the Second International Conference on Congenital Malformations. Ed. M. Fishbein. International Medical Congress, New York. Page 311.

CARTER, C. O. (1965). The inheritance of common congenital malformations. In "Progress in Medical Genetics". Vol. 4. p. 59. Ed. A. G. Steinberg and A. G. Bearn, New York: Grune and Stratton.

CARTER, C. O. and WILKINSON, J. A. (1964a). Genetic and environmental factors in the aetiology of congenital dislocation of the hip. *Clin. Orthop.*, **33**, 119.

CARTER, C. O. and WILKINSON, J. A. (1964b). Persistent joint laxity and congenital dislocation of the hip. *J. Bone Jt. Surg.*, **46B**, 40.

CARTER, C. O., DAVID, P. A. and LAURENCE, K. M. (1968). The genetics of the major central nervous system malformations, based on the South Wales socio-genetic investigation. *J. med. Genet.* **5**, 81.

CARTER, C. O. and FRASER ROBERTS, J. A. (1967). The risk of recurrence after two children with central nervous system malformations. *Lancet*, **i**, 306.

CASEY, M. D., SEGALL, L. J., STREET, D. R. K. and BLANK, C. E. (1966). Sex chromosome abnormalities in two state hospitals for patients requiring special security. *Nature*, **209**, 641.

FABER, A. (1937). Erbbiologische untersuchungen uber die anlage zur hangeborenen huftverrenkung. *Z. Orthop.*, **66**, 140–166.

FRASER ROBERTS, J. A. (1964). Multifactorial inheritance and human disease. In "Progress in Medical Genetics". Vol. 3. p. 178. Ed. A. G. Steinberg and A. G. Bearn, New York. Grune and Stratton.

IDELBERGER, K. (1939). Die ergebnisse der zwillingsforschung beim angeborenen klumpfuss. *Verh. dt. orthop. Ges.*, **33**, 272.

IDELBERGER, K. (1951). Der erbpathologie der sogenannten angeborenen heift vervenkung. Urban and Schwarzenberg. Munchen and Berlin.

JAMES, J. I. P. (1954). Idiopathic scoliosis. *J. Bone Jt. Surg.*, **36B**, 36.

LAMY, M. and MAROTEAUX, P. (1961). Le nanisme diastrophique. *Presse med.*, **68**, 1977.

LAURENCE, K. M., DAVID, P. A. and CARTER, C. O. (1968). The major central nervous system malformations in South Wales. I. Incidence with local variations and geographical factors. *Brit. J. prev. soc. med.* **22**, 146.

LING, R. S. M. (1963). The genetic factor in Dupuytren's disease. *J. Bone Jt. Surg.*, **45B**, 709.

MAROTEAUX, P. and LAMY, M. (1962). La pycnodysostose. *Presse med.* **70**, 999.

McKEOWN, T. and RECORD, R. G. (1960). Malformations in a population observed for five years after birth. Ciba Foundation Symposium on Congenital Malformations. Ed. G. E. Wolstenholme and C. M. Connor. London: J. and A. Churchill Ltd.

McKUSICK, V. A. (1966). Mendelian inheritance in man. London: William Heinemann Medical Books Ltd.

McKUSICK, V. A. (1966). Heritable disorders of connective tissue. 3rd Edition. St. Louis: The C. V. Mosby Company.

MULLER, G. M. and SEDDON, H. J. (1953). Late results of treatment of congenital dislocation of the hip. *J. Bone Jt. Surg.*, **35B**, 342.

PLEYDELL, M. J. (1960). Anencephaly and other congenital abnormalities: An epidemiological study in Northamptonshire. *Br. med. J.* **1,** 309.

SKOOG, I. (1948). Dupuytren's contracture, with special reference to aetiology and improved surgical treatment. Its occurrence in epileptics. Note on knuckle pads. *Acta chir. scand.* Suppl, No. 139, p. 96.

STEVENSON, A. C. and WARNOCK, H. A. (1959). Observations on the results of pregnancies in women resident in Belfast. I. Data relating to all pregnancies ending in 1957. *Ann. hum. Genet.* **23,** 382.

THIEME, W. T. (1967). Personal communication.

THIEME, W. T., WYNNE-DAVIES, R., BLAIR, H. A. F., BELL, E. T. and LORAINE, J. A. (1968). Clinical examination and urinary oestrogen assays in newborn children with congenital dislocation of the hip. *J. Bone Jt. Surg.* **50B,** 546.

WILLIAMSON, E. M. (1965). Incidence and family aggregation of major congenital malformations of the central nervous system. *J. med. Genet.*, **2,** 161.

WILKINSON, J. and CARTER, C. O. (1960). Congenital dislocation of the hip. The results of conservative treatment. *J. Bone Jt. Surg.*, **42B,** 669.

WYNNE-DAVIES, R. (1964). Family studies and the cause of congenital club-foot. *J. Bone Jt Surg.*, **46B,** 445.

WYNNE-DAVIES, R. (1968). Familial (idiopathic) scoliosis. *J. Bone Jt Surg.*, **50B,** 24.

Chapter 2

GOUT AND CHONDROCALCINOSIS ('PSEUDOGOUT')

H. L. F. CURREY and R. M. MASON

Introduction

The past ten years have seen important advances in the understanding and treatment of gout. It is now established that it is the urate crystal itself which provokes the synovial inflammation in acute gouty arthritis. Following upon this has come the recognition that urate crystals are not the only cause of 'crystal synovitis'. Thus, acute 'pseudogout' attacks may occur during the course of a newly described syndrome in which a calcium salt is deposited in joint cartilage, which also gives a very characteristic radiological appearance—'chondrocalcinosis articularis'. At the same time there have been significant improvements in the treatment of gout resulting both from the introduction of new drugs and from a better understanding of the place of established remedies. Together these now provide much more adequate control of the disorder.

For the orthopaedic surgeon these advances offer firstly, two valuable aids in the diagnosis of arthritis—polarized light microscopy of synovial fluids for the detection and identification of crystals, and radiological screening for joint cartilage calcification. Secondly, awareness that pseudogout may mimic suppurative arthritis, makes it possible to avoid a very real pitfall in the diagnosis of acute joint disease. Finally, the more sophisticated drug control now obtainable in gout has enhanced the importance of surgery in this condition.

The Mechanism of Acute Gouty Arthritis

Over a hundred years ago the observations of Garrod (1848) showed that the underlying metabolic defect in gout is an elevation in the level of serum uric acid. The natural assumption which followed was that urate, precipitated in the joint space, acted as an irritant, producing acute inflammation. However, for over a century, experiments (with one exception which was ignored) attempting to prove this were unsuccessful. Urate solutions injected into the joints and other tissues of experimental animals produced no inflammation. The only successful experiments were those of Freudweiler (1899, 1901) who was able to produce an acute arthritis indistinguishable from gout by the injection of uric acid crystals in suspension into a joint. These experiments were ignored, perhaps because of the 'almost unbelievable verbosity and repetition' which characterized these reports (Brill and McCarty 1964). The problem was resolved however when Hollander (1960) showed that the synovial fluid from acutely inflamed gouty joints did actually contain microscopic urate crystals and following this Faires and McCarty (1962), by injecting sodium urate crystals into their own knee joints, reproduced a gouty attack in a dramatically acute and quite convincing form!

The Concept of Crystal Synovitis

Analysis of the factors concerned in experimental urate synovitis (Seegmiller, Howell and Malawista 1962) showed that urate provokes inflammation only when it is in microcrystalline form. In solution, on the other hand, or as amorphous urate, it is relatively non-irritant. This suggested that urate crystals act by virtue of their physical rather than their chemical properties; and it is now known that other compounds may be equally irritant provided they are injected as crystals of the same order of size. Hence 'crystal synovitis' is used to describe this type of inflammation. Acute gout is one example, 'pseudogout' another, and the reaction which occasionally follows intra-articular injection of crystalline corticosteroids, is yet a third type (McCarty and Hogan 1964). There may well be others.

The final common pathway whereby crystals produce inflammation is not finally settled. The balance of evidence favours a sequence in which crystals are phagocytosed by polymorphonuclear leucocytes, which then die and disintegrate, releasing enzymes contained in their lysosomes to act as chemical mediators of inflammation. In this scheme, colchicine (specifically suppressive in acute gout, yet without effect on urate metabolism) may act by modifying the phagocytic activity of leucocytes (Seegmiller, Howell and Malawista 1962a). Much remains to be explained; for example, the electron microscope appearance suggesting that urate crystals may be precipitated in leucocytes rather than being engulfed by them (Riddle, Bluhm and Barnhart 1967). The kinins also have a claim as the chemical mediators of inflammation in gout, for urate crystals can activate Hageman factor (Kellermeyer and Breckenridge 1965). There is however strong experimental evidence against this factor being of major importance (Phelps, Prockop and McCarty 1966).

Pseudogout and Chondrocalcinosis

The screening of synovial fluids for urate crystals led to the discovery by McCarty and Hollander in 1961 that some fluids from acutely inflamed joints contained crystals of an entirely different substance, now known to be calcium pyrophosphate dihydrate (CPPD). Patients showing this phenomenon were observed to have another feature in common— radiological calcification of joint cartilage (McCarty, Kohn and Faires 1962). The radio-opaque material laid down in cartilage proved to have the same chemical composition as the synovial crystals (Kohn *et al.* 1962, Lagier, Baud and Bucks 1966) and it is now clear that 'calcium pyrophosphate deposition disease' is a pathological entity and an important cause of joint pathology. The terminology remains unsatisfactory. Currently, 'pseudogout' is used to describe the acute crystal synovitis and 'chondrocalcinosis articularis' the radiological appearance.

Clinically the condition may present as an acute crystal synovitis affecting one or a few joints. The knee is the commonest site, and, in general, large rather than small joints are involved. Podagra, so characteristic of classical gout, is uncommon. Attacks may last a few days and tend to recur at the same site. Typically the acute attack is associated with synovial effusion and may be aborted by a local injection of a corticosteroid preparation or even by simple aspiration of the fluid. Colchicine is of doubtful value. Joints the site of acute attacks may later develop degenerative changes, and in some patients osteoarthrosis, without acute attacks, may be the only manifestation of the disease. Intermediate forms are common. Occasionally, widespread small and large joint involvement may produce a picture mimicking rheumatoid arthritis (Currey *et al.* 1966). Systemic disturbances occur in proportion to the acuteness of the attack and may include pyrexia, leucocytosis, and a raised blood sedimentation rate.

The aetiology is unknown, and the deposition of CPPD may well represent the end result of various different pathological processes. Žitnaň and Sit'aj (1963) from Czechoslovakia reported a number of families in which there was a high incidence of chondrocalcinosis which appeared at a relatively young age—the onset being in the third decade. In their series, no biochemical abnormalities were discovered, but other investigators (McCarty and Gatter, 1964; Serre and Simon 1966; Currey *et al.* 1966) not only found that the condition occurred amongst a generally older age group with less marked family grouping, but many of the subjects demonstrated some biochemical abnormality. Thus there now seems to be a significant association with hyperparathyroidism (*Brit. Med. J.* 1964), haemochromatosis (de Sèze *et al.* 1964); and perhaps with classical gout (Dodds and Steinbach 1966), and diabetes (McCarty and Gatter 1964).

Polarized light microscopy of synovial fluids. The application of modern crystallographic methods to the study of gout and pseudogout has contributed much to the understanding of these conditions. For example, the composition of CPPD crystals was determined using X-ray diffraction methods. But of greater importance to the clinician is the fact that polarized light microscopy of synovial fluids provides a rapid and relatively simple method of diagnosing crystal synovitis, and often of differentiating between urate and CPPD crystals In the simplest terms the polarizing microscope has two 'polars' (which transmit light only in one plane) placed one above and one below the sample. If the polars are adjusted until their planes are at right angles to each other, no light can pass through, and the field appears dark. However, crystals which exhibit the property of birefringence (such as urate and CPPD) will appear as bright objects. This phenomenon is perhaps best illustrated in Figs. 1a and 1b in which material from a gouty tophus is seen using ordinary light (Fig. 1a) and with 'crossed polars' (Fig. 1b). This technique makes possible the rapid screening of fluids for crystals which may be detected even when present in small numbers. The property of birefringence can be further studied by simple optical methods which compare the crystal under examination to a standard quartz plate. Crystals may add to or subtract from the optical properties of superimposed quartz and are

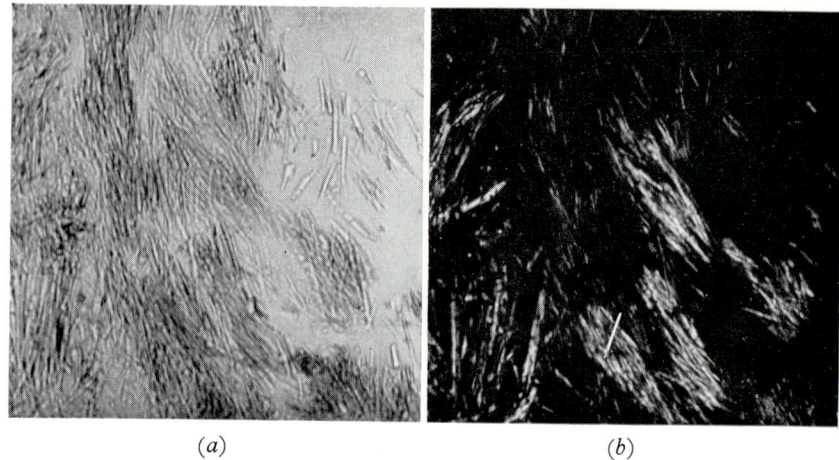

FIGS. 1a and 1b. Urate crystals from a gouty tophus seen (*a*) by ordinary light microscopy, and (*b*) using a polarized light technique with crossed polars.

hence classified as being positively or negatively birefringent. By this test, which provides a rapid method of differentiation, urate crystals are strongly negative, and most forms of CPPD weakly positive. Morphologically, urate crystals are generally needle-like, as shown in Figs. 1a and 1b, while CPPD tends to be shorter and square-ended (Fig. 2b).

Synovial fluid from a joint which is the site of acute crystal synovitis usually contains numerous crystals, many of which are intracellular

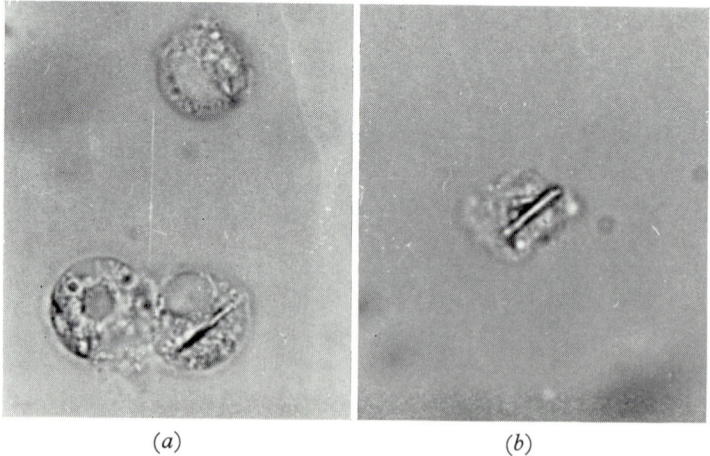

FIGS. 2a and 2b. Typical appearance of CPPD crystals lying within leucocytes. The specimen of synovial fluid came from a knee joint which was the site of acute crystal synovitis (pseudogout). These photomicrographs were taken with partially crossed polars, hence both the birefringent crystals and the non-birefringent leucocytes can be seen.

(Figs. 2a and 2b). Such an appearance provides a positive diagnosis of crystal synovitis and enables gout and pseudogout to be differentiated. Polarized light-microscopy is now indeed an essential procedure in the diagnosis of acute arthritis. Crystals may be observed by non-polarized light microscopy but this is more difficult and less informative (Fig. 3). Examination of joint fluids between attacks generally shows fewer crystals which are mainly extracellular, or often none at all. A few crystals may also be found in joints the site of unrelated arthropathies (Currey et al. 1966). Thus, firm conclusions should never be drawn from a finding of occasional crystals only. Specimens of synovial fluid for polarized light microscopy should not have any anticoagulant added and they are best examined fresh. Nevertheless, it has occasionally been

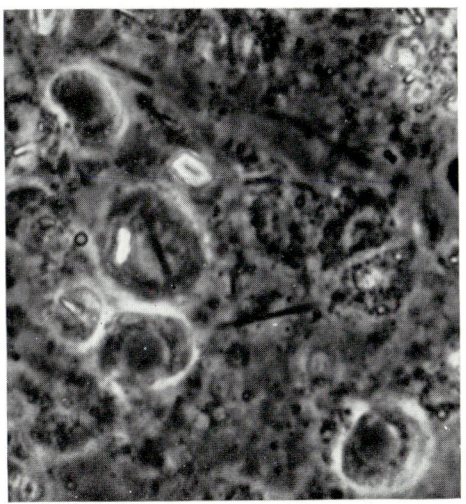

FIG. 3. Synovial fluid from a case of acute crystal synovitis viewed by phase contrast microscopy. Numerous crystals are present, but they are less clearly seen than when their birefringent properties are exploited by using polarized light (cf. Fig. 2b).

found possible to make a positive diagnosis even on specimens sent through the post. Crystals can also be identified in sections of biopsy material (Figs. 4a and 4b). Because of the solubility of these crystals in formalin solution, tissue for crystallographic study must be put into absolute alcohol.

The diagnostic significance of joint cartilage calcification. The appearance of chondrocalcinosis is a relatively gross radiological sign, unlikely to be missed by an observer aware of the condition, although doubtless often ignored in the past. Figures 5 to 10 show the typical appearance in some commonly affected joints. Much the commonest site is the knee meniscus where the fibrocartilage shows irregular opacification (Figs. 5 and 6). A similar pattern may be seen in fibrocartilage of the wrist joint (Fig. 7), the symphysis pubis (Fig. 8) and the intervertebral discs. CPPD laid down in hyaline cartilage appears as a thin punctate line close to, but separate from, the bone cortex. This is most commonly seen in relation to the femoral condyles (Fig. 6) and the heads of the femur (Fig. 8) and humerus (Fig. 9). The high frequency with which the knee joint is involved radiologically suggests that radiographs of both knees provide an adequate screening test for this condition.

The significance of this radiological sign requires consideration. Is it always to be equated with CPPD deposition disease? Or may, for

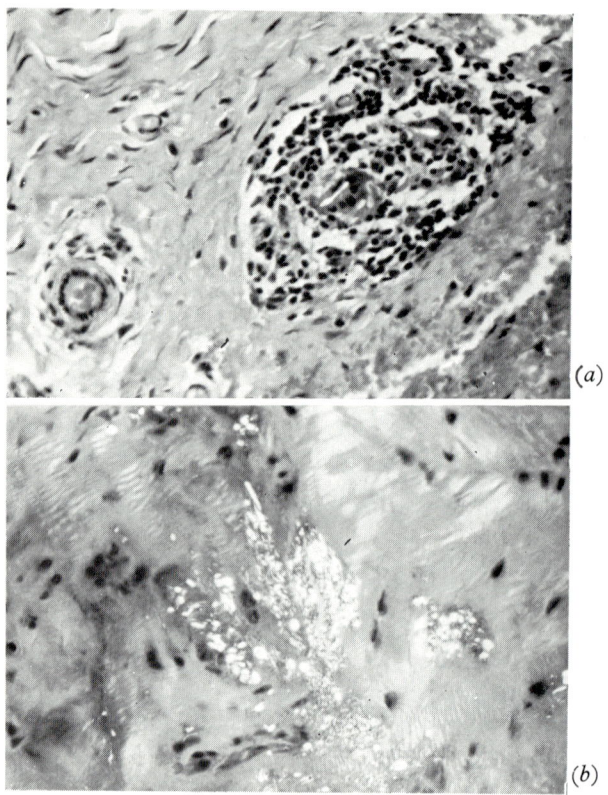

FIGS. 4a and 4b. Crystals in fixed histological sections: (a) Chondrocalcinosis; synovial biopsy from a shoulder joint showing one CPPD crystal within a giant cell. (b) Birefringent crystals in an excised meniscus. Both photomicrographs were taken with partially crossed polars. (Currey, H. L. F. et al., Ann. rheumat. Dis., 1966, 24, 295, reproduced by permission.)

example, isolated calcification of one meniscus be merely secondary to degenerative changes? It has to be said that the frequency with which calcified menisci are found amongst the elderly (Bocher et al. 1965) suggests that, at least in this age group, calcification of menisci alone is not very significant. In this connection McCarty and his co-workers (1966) have studied the knee menisci in 215 cadavera. Seven per cent had calcific deposits which would probably have been visible on clinical

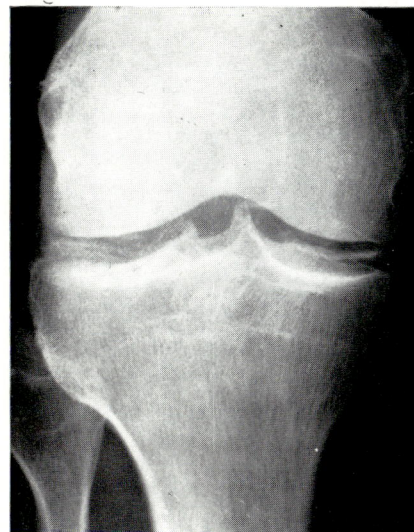

FIG. 5. Chondrocalcinosis in a knee joint. Irregular opacification of both menisci.

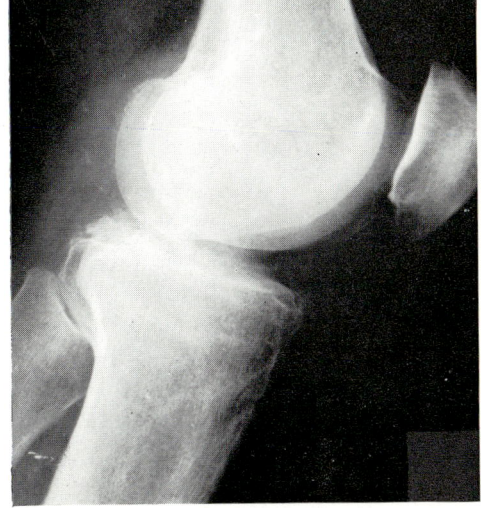

FIG. 6. Lateral view of knee joint showing chondrocalcinosis affecting the menisci and hyaline cartilage overlying the femoral condyles (posteriorly).

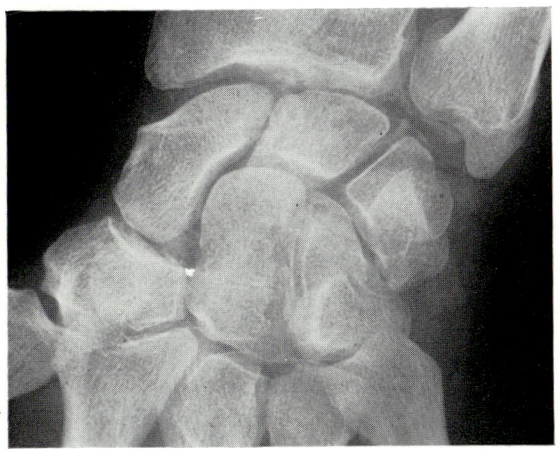

FIG. 7. Chondrocalcinosis of the wrist joint.

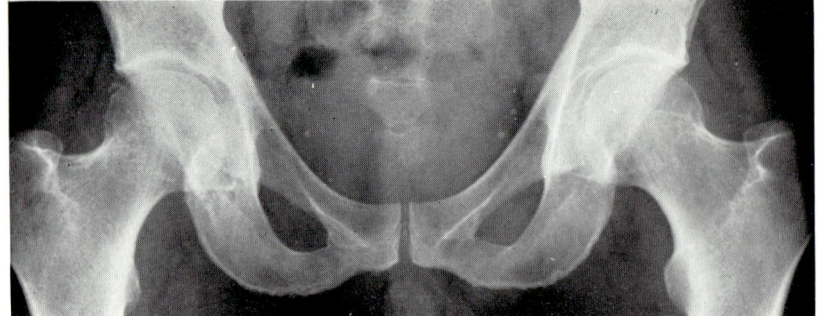

FIG. 8. Pelvis; in addition to the obvious calcification of the symphysis, there is a thin line of calcification over both femoral heads.

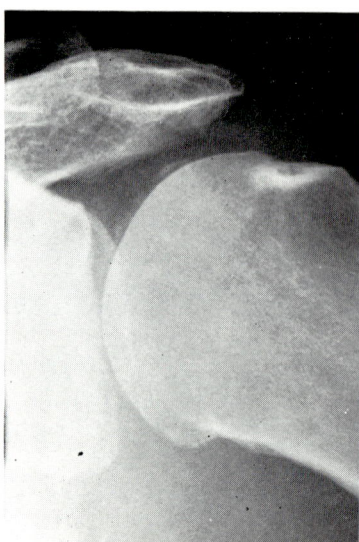

FIG. 9. Chondrocalcinosis round the head of the humerus.

FIG. 10. Chondrocalcinsosis of the elbow joint.

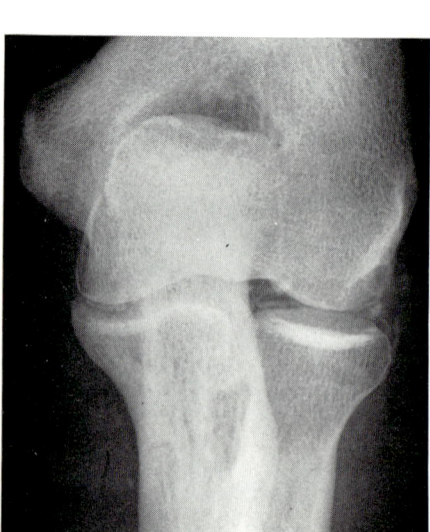

X-rays. Of these, 1·4 per cent had what were clearly secondary deposits—either small isolated plaques, or calcification in the walls of blood vessels. Analysis of these proved them to consist of hydroxyapatite. Deposits of a primary type were found in multiple cartilages in 5·6 per cent of cadavera however. In 3·3 per cent these proved to be CPPD, in 2·3 per cent the calcific material was identified as dicalcium phosphate dihydrate. The significance of the latter type of deposit is not yet established. Like CPPD it has been found in joint cartilage away from the knee. Unlike CPPD, however, its presence has not yet been correlated with pseudogout or other clinical joint disease.

Thus, while slight, particularly isolated, meniscal calcification may not be significant, more pronounced or widespread calcification should be regarded as evidence of a generalized disorder. The incidence of this probably increases with age and in the elderly it is less often associated with significant arthritis.

The finding of chondrocalcinosis is not only an aid in the diagnosis of joint disease, it indicates the need to exclude conditions such as hyperparathyroidism, haemochromatosis, and classical gout.

Pseudogout simulating septic arthritis. Clinically, acute crystal synovitis presents an appearance similar to acute suppurative arthritis. In the case of classical gout, confusion between these two conditions is usually (but by no means invariably) avoided because of the frequency with which the initial gouty attack affects the first metatarso-phalangeal joint. In the case of pseudogout, however, where the knee or other large joints are commonly affected, the observer unaware of this condition is likely to regard the hot and acutely painful joint in a febrile patient, with a leucocytosis and a high sedimentation rate, as septic. Aspiration of a highly cellular fluid may then appear to confirm the need for antibiotic treatment, even in the face of negative bacteriological reports. Hamblen, Currey and Key (1966) have reported such cases. This pitfall in diagnosis is avoided if the investigation of any acute monarticular arthritis always includes microscopy of synovial fluid for crystals and radiographic examination of both knee joints for cartilage calcification.

Drug Therapy in Gout

The considerable advances which the past few years have brought in the treatment of gout by drug therapy, have been reviewed by Barnes and Mason (1967). Only a brief summary of the present position will be given here.

Colchicine, hallowed by tradition as the drug of choice in the treatment of acute attacks, has now given place to phenylbutazone and indomethacin. Used in relatively high doses (phenylbutazone 600 mgms. daily or indomethacin 150 mgms. daily) for a few days, and then reduced in dose as symptoms allow, these drugs have proved highly effective. Colchicine has thus been relegated to use as long-term interval treatment in order to prevent the acute episodes. Given in doses of 1 mgm. daily it considerably reduces the frequency of attacks and should be used in addition to other measures as long-term 'background' prophylaxis. It is particularly useful during periods, such as the stage of introducing uricosuric drugs or allopurinol, when there is an extra liability to acute exacerbations. In these small doses there is little risk of producing the gastro-intestinal symptoms which so limit the usefulness of this drug in the treatment of acute attacks.

For patients experiencing frequent acute attacks, for those with tophi, and for those with plasma uric acid levels averaging over 8 mgm./100 ml., treatment designed to lower the plasma urate level should be instituted. This may be achieved either by the use of uricosuric drugs, which paralyse renal tubular reabsorption of urate, or by allopurinol. This recently introduced drug acts by inhibiting xanthine oxidase, the enzyme leading directly to the formation of uric acid (Rundles et al. 1963; Yü and Gutman 1964):

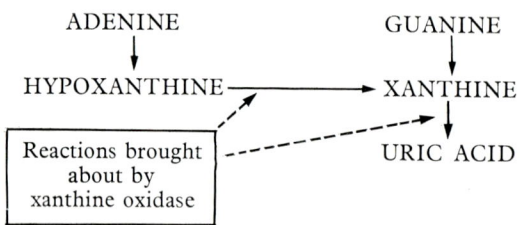

It follows that, while uricosuric drugs increase the load of urate in the urine with a greater hazard of stone formation, allopurinol reduces this load and leads, instead, to an increased elimination of the more soluble oxypurines. Clearly, this is a major factor which may govern the choice of drug. Another factor is the greater effectiveness of allopurinol when renal failure is present.

For these reasons, allopurinol is tending increasingly to replace the uricosuric drugs in the treatment of hyperuricaemia. That it is not yet automatically first choice is due to reservations about long-term toxicity which attend the introduction of any new drug. Our present view is that it seems prudent to use a uricosuric drug for the uncomplicated case, selecting from the following (showing the average daily dose):

> Probenecid (Benemid) 1–2 Gm.
> Ethebenecid (Urelim) 1–2 Gm.
> Sulphinpyrazone (Anturan) 0·4–0·6 Gm.

Allopurinol, however, is indicated in the following circumstances:

> Failure of uricosuric therapy.
> Increased risk of urate urolithiasis.
> The presence of renal failure.

As with the uricosuric drugs, the dose should be titrated against the serum level of uric acid, aiming to reduce this below 6·0 mgm. per cent. This is usually achieved with a dose of approximately 300 mgms. daily. Where metabolic control cannot be achieved with either the uricosuric drugs or with allopurinol used alone, an additive effect may be obtained by using these drugs simultaneously. To date, the toxic effects of allopurinol, except for skin eruptions, appear to be rare.

Surgery in Gout

Prior to the ability of drug therapy to achieve metabolic control of gout operative treatment tended to be a disappointing exercise; the removal of tophi being commonly followed by reaccumulation of the urate deposits and occasionally by a legacy of discharging sinuses. Better drug therapy has altered this. Now that it is possible in the majority of gouty subjects to achieve sufficiently good metabolic control for the process of urate deposition to be reversed, tophi tend to diminish in size. But the process is inevitably slow, and in these circumstances surgery becomes a much more attractive proposition. Once good metabolic control is obtained and urate begins to leave the tophi, it would seem sound practice to resect any large and unsightly deposits or those producing mechanical interference with function, for simple calculations show that even the most vigorous and successful drug therapy would take many years to dissolve away the extensive deposits seen in advanced tophaceous gout.

Acknowledgement

We are indebted to Dr. J. J. Key, Mr. K. V. Swettenham and Mr. R. F. Ruddick for preparing the illustrations.

References

BARNES, C. G. and MASON, R. M. (1967). The treatment of gout. *J. Roy. Coll. Physcns, Lond.*, **1**, 428.
BOCHER, J., MANKIN, H. J., BERK, R. N. and RODNAN, G. P. (1965). Prevalence of calcified meniscal cartilage in elderly persons. *New Eng. J. Med.*, **272**, 1093.
BRILL, J. M. and MCCARTY, D. J., JR. (1964). Studies on the nature of gouty tophi. *Ann. Int. Med.*, **60**, 486.
BRIT. MED. J. (1964). **2**, 889. Editorial. Pseudogout.
CURREY, H. L. F., KEY, J. J., MASON, R. M. and SWETTENHAM, K. V. (1966). Significance of radiological calcification of joint cartilage. *Ann. rheum. Dis.*, **25**, 295.
DODDS, W. J. and STEINBACH, H. L. (1966). Gout associated with calcification of cartilage. *New Eng. J. Med.*, **275**, 745.
FAIRES, J. S. and MCCARTY, D. J., JR. (1962). Acute arthritis in man and dog after intrasynovial injection of sodium urate crystals. *Lancet*, **ii**, 682.
FREUDWEILER, M. (1899). Studies on the nature of gouty tophi. *Deutsch. Arch. f. klin. Med.*, **63**, 266. Translated by Brill, J. M. and McCarty, D. J., Jr. (1964). *Ann. int. Med.*, **60**, 486.
FREUDWEILER, M. (1901). Experimentelle untersuchungen uber die entstehung der gichtknoten. *Deutsch Arch. klin. Med.*, **69**, 155.
GARROD, A. B. (1848). Observations on certain pathological conditions of the blood and urine in gout, rheumatism and Bright's disease. *Med. chir. Trans.*, **31**, 83.
HAMBLEN, D. L., CURREY, H. L. F. and KEY, J. J. (1966). Pseudogout simulating acute suppurative arthritis. *J. Bone Jt. Surg.*, **48B**, 51.
HOLLANDER, J. L. (1960). Arthritis and Allied Conditions. Ed. 6. Philadelphia. p. 77. Lea & Febiger.
KELLERMEYER, R. W. and BRECKENRIDGE, R. T. (1965). The inflammatory process in acute gouty arthritis. I. Activation of Hageman factor by sodium urate crystals. *J. Lab. Clin. Med.*, **65**, 307.
KOHN, N. N., HUGHES, R. E., MCCARTY, D. J., JR. and FAIRES, J. S. (1962). The significance of calcium phosphate crystals in the synovial fluid of arthritic patients: The 'pseudogout syndrome' II. Identification of crystals. *Ann. Intern. Med.*, **56**, 738.

LAGIER, R., BAUD, C. A. and BUCKS, M. (1966). Crystallographic identification of calcium deposits as regards their pathological nature, with special reference to chondrocalcinosis. In 'Third European Symposium on Calcified Tissues'. Ed. Fleisch, H., Blackwood, H. J. J., and Owen, M., Springer-Verlag, Berlin. p. 158.

MCCARTY, D. J., JR. and GATTER, R. A. (1964). Pseudogout syndrome (articular chondrocalcinosis). *Bull. rheum. Dis.*, **14**, 331.

MCCARTY, D. J., JR. and HOGAN, J. M. (1964). Inflammatory reaction after intrasynovial injection of micro-crystalline adrenocorticosteroid esters. *Arthritis rheum.*, **7**, 359.

MCCARTY, D. J., HOGAN, J. M., GATTER, R. A. and GROSSMAN, M. (1966). Studies on pathological calcifications in human cartilage. I. Prevalence and types of crystal deposits in the menisci of two hundred fifteen cadavera. *J. Bone Jt. Surg.*, **48A**, 309.

MCCARTY, D. J., JR. and HOLLANDER, J. L. (1961). Identification of urate crystals in gouty synovial fluid. *Ann. intern. Med.*, **54**, 452.

MCCARTY, D. J., JR., KOHN, N. N. and FAIRES, J. S. (1962). The significance of calcium phosphate crystals in the synovial fluid of arthritic patients: The 'pseudogout syndrome'. I. Clinical aspects. *Ann. Intern. Med.*, **56**, 711.

PHELPS, P., PROCKOP, D. J. and MCCARTY, D. J., JR. (1966). Crystal induced inflammation in canine joints. III. Evidence against bradykinin as a mediator of inflammation. *J. Lab. Clin. Med.*, **68**, 433.

RIDDLE, J. M., BLUHM, G. B. and BARNHART, M. I. (1967). Ultrastructural study of leucocytes and urates in gouty arthritis. *Ann. rheum. Dis.*, **26**, 389.

RUNDLES, R. W., WYNGAARDEN, J. B., HITCHINGS, G. H., ELION, G. B. and SILBERMAN, H. R. (1963). Effects of a xanthine oxidase inhibitor on thiopurine metabolism hyperuricaemia and gout. *Trans. A. Am. Physicians*, **76**, 126.

SEEGMILLER, J. E., HOWELL, R. R. and MALAWISTA, S. E. (1962). The inflammatory reaction to sodium urate. *J. Amer. med. Ass.*, **180**, 469.

SEEGMILLER, J. E., HOWELL, R. R. and MALAWISTA, S. E. (1962a). A mechanism of action of colchicine in acute gouty arthritis. *J. clin. Invest.*, **41**, 1399.

SERRE, H. and SIMON, L. (1966). Chondrocalcinoses articulares diffuses secondaires. *Méd. Hyg. (Genèva)*.

SÈZE, S. DE, HUBAULT, A., WELFLING, J., KAHN, M. F. ET SOLNICA, J. (1964). Les arthropathies des hémochromatoses. Hémochromatose et "chondrocalcinose" articulaire. Leur place dans le cadre des arthropathies métaboliques. *Rev. Rhum.*, **31**, 479.

YU, T. F. and GUTMAN, A. B. (1964). Effect of allopurinol (4-hydroxypyrazolo-(3,4-d) pryrimidine) on serum and urinary uric acid in primary and secondary gout. *Am. J. Med.* **37**, 885.

ŽITNAŇ, D. and SIT'AJ, Š. (1963). Chondrocalcinosis articularis. *Ann. rheum. Dis.*, **22**, 142.

Chapter 3

THE REATTACHMENT OF SEVERED EXTREMITIES

J. S. HORN

Introduction

This report is based on the work of Chinese surgeons who, during the past five years, have gained extensive experience in the reattachment of severed extremities.

The first successful case in January 1963 has been reported elsewhere (Ch'en et al. 1963; Horn 1964). The patient was a 27-year-old factory worker who sustained a traumatic amputation just above the right wrist when his hand was caught in a machine. A workmate found the severed hand, still in its protective glove, lying beneath the machine, himself took it to the hospital to which the patient had been sent and suggested to the surgeon that they should sew it back on. They did so and the result was spectacularly successful.

This event was widely publicized throughout China and surgeons were urged to study it and make plans to deal with similar cases. My own hospital in Peking sent a group of surgeons to Shanghai to see the patient and to discuss details with the surgeons who had been involved. On their return, we organized a surgical team to be available at any time and ensured that the necessary instruments and drugs were always kept ready for use. We carried out a series of animal experiments to familiarize ourselves with the technique of vascular anastomosis. Within a short time we had reattached a number of rabbits' ears and dogs' legs, and had designed some surgical instruments. At our request, a synthetic fibre plant manufactured a small diameter fibre of high tensile strength and an optical instrument factory made us an excellent operating microscope.

Soon we had the opportunity to reattach a completely severed forearm. We made a colour film of the operation, of the post-operative care and of the functional result and in 1965 I showed this film in the Royal Society of Medicine, the British Orthopaedic Association and elsewhere.

Before long it became common knowledge in China that under suitable conditions severed limbs could be reattached with some likelihood of success and surgeons were being flown out to see patients in remote areas and patients, together with their severed limbs, were being flown into the larger centres. In this way, experience was rapidly accumulated.

It is impossible to provide up-to-the-minute statistics for successes and failures in this field or to be dogmatic about the indications or technique. The subject is still developing and there are differences of opinion.

I propose to deal with this subject under the following headings:

(1) The reattachment of amputated limbs: statistics, indications, technique.
(2) The reattachment of amputated fingers: statistics, indications, technique.
(3) The post-operative management of reattached extremities.
(4) Some remaining problems.
(5) Some illustrative cases.
(6) Conclusion.

The statistics given will be those of the Shanghai Sixth Municipal Hospital where the first success was achieved and which has, I believe, reattached more severed extremities than any other hospital in China. I must record my indebtedness to the staff of this hospital for allowing me to present their material and I must make it clear that my own role in this work has been largely that of an admiring spectator while Chinese surgeons have opened up this new and important field of surgery.

The Reattachment of Amputated Limbs

STATISTICS OF THE SHANGHAI SIXTH MUNICIPAL HOSPITAL

Completely severed limbs.

Jan. 1963–Aug. 1966.
10 cases. Male 7. Female 3.
Average age 30·8 years.
Youngest 14. Oldest 48.

Level of amputation:
Avulsion of entire upper limb including the scapula from the chest wall 1
Through upper arm 1
Through forearm 3
Through palm of hand 4
Through middle third of lower leg 1

Average time from injury to restoration of circulation 5·7 hours.
Average unrefrigerated time from injury to restoration of circulation 3·9 hours.

Results. All 10 cases were successful.

Incompletely severed limbs (that is limbs in which the main blood vessels have all been divided and in which the distal part remains attached only by a narrow bridge of viable soft tissue).

Jan. 1963–Jan. 1966.
Number of cases. 18. All males.
Level of amputation: Upper arm 1
Forearm 11
Palm of hand 3
Lower leg 3

Average time from injury to restoration of circulation in 15 cases 6·6 hours (not recorded in 3 cases).

Results. 14 successes.
4 failures.

INDICATIONS FOR REATTACHING AMPUTATED LIMBS

It is considered that all traumatically amputated limbs should be reattached in the following circumstances:

(1) Providing the condition of the patient permits of a long operation which may be associated with significant blood-loss.

(2) Providing the patient is not senile, or suffering from vascular disease of the extremities or from diabetes.

(3) Providing the amputated part is relatively intact. If it has suffered an explosive type of injury or has been severely crushed, reattachment is unlikely to succeed.

(4) Providing the condition of the proximal stump offers the prospect of reasonable restoration of function. If nerves or muscles have been extensively lost, it may not be worthwhile to reattach the limb.

(5) Providing, in the case of the lower limb, that there has not been excessive bone loss. The maximal acceptable shortening has not yet been worked out and knowledge of the late results of reattachment of the lower extremity is too limited to permit firm conclusions.

(6) Providing the time interval between injury and operation has not been too long. It is impossible to define precise time limits because other factors such as the ambient temperature, the condition of the amputated part, the degree of contamination and the level of amputation, also affect viability. Under climatic conditions usually prevailing in South China, 8 hours is considered to be the maximal time interval beyond which reattachment will fail. In cooler climates, this period may be longer while if the amputated part is refrigerated soon after injury, it may be greatly prolonged. The longest delay in a patient to be followed by successful reattachment in China is 18 hours; in this case the severed extremity was kept in a vacuum bottle surrounded by ice-lollies. Owing to inadequate refrigeration in this case, the forearm flexor muscles underwent liquefaction although the limb as a whole survived and gives useful function.

Technique of Limb Reattachment

Anaesthesia. Full anaesthesia is usually unnecessary throughout these prolonged operations. At different stages of the operation, brachial plexus block, infiltration anaesthesia and intravenous anaesthesia may be employed.

Treatment of the Amputated Part

In order to save time, the amputated part is dealt with by a separate surgical team. It is thoroughly cleansed and its vascular bed is irrigated with saline and heparin until the return flow is quite clear. Devitalized or contaminated tissues in the cut end are excised layer by layer until only healthy tissue remains. Lacerations are excised and sutured.

If surgical preparation of the stump takes a long time, the amputated part may be kept in a refrigerator at 2–4°C pending reattachment.

Treatment of the Stump

Tourniquet. No tourniquet is used for limb reattachments. Haemorrhage is controlled by the use of rubber covered vascular clips applied very close to the severed ends of the blood vessels.

Wound excision. Thorough wound excision is essential for success and in general it should aim at removing a complete segment from the cut end of the stump. Retracted muscles are pulled down for inspection and any muscle which is hopelessly denervated or devascularized is excised *in toto*. The excision proceeds with functional restoration in mind and tendons which are likely to be of value in functional rehabilitation are preserved.

If there has been excessive delay between injury and operation, it may be inadvisable to delay vascular anastomosis until thorough wound excision has been completed. In such cases, grossly crushed or contaminated tissue may first be rapidly excised postponing meticulous wound excision until after the circulation has been restored.

Treatment of Bone

Contaminated or splintered bone is removed and the bone is shortened sufficiently to ensure that it can be covered by healthy muscles and that the nerves and blood vessels can be approximated without excessive tension.

Internal fixation is employed to restore rigidity to the limb and to protect the vascular anastomosis from strain. If it is necessary to shorten the limb, a step-cut and cross-screw type of fixation may be the most satisfactory. If only minimal sacrifice of bone length is necessary, plate and screws or intramedullary nail fixation may be preferable. In forearm amputations it is common to fix one bone with a steel plate and screws and the other with an intramedullary Kirschner wire.

If conditions are favourable, bone chips may be placed around the osteosynthesis to expedite union, for non-union is not uncommon.

Whether to deal first with the bones or first with the blood vessels depends on the time interval since injury. If it has been short, it is better to deal with the bones first for the restoration of rigidity to the limb facilitates vascular anastomosis. If, however, the time interval has been long, then the restoration of circulation must take priority.

Treatment of Blood Vessels

Order of Anastomosis. At first there was a tendency to be in a hurry to restore the arterial circulation and so arteries were usually anastomosed before veins. However, this created certain difficulties for following arterial anastomosis, the reattached limb flushed with blood and brisk retrograde haemorrhage occurred from the severed veins. This necessitated the application of vascular clips which were liable to traumatize the thin-walled veins and predispose to subsequent thrombosis. Moreover, while the clips were in place, the reattached extremity became engorged with blood leading to a vicious cycle of congestion and oedema. To avoid these disadvantages it seems preferable to anastomose the veins before the arteries but if there has been long delay, if it has not been possible thoroughly to wash out the vascular bed of the amputated extremity, or if its subcutaneous venous plexus has been extensively damaged, then priority must be given to restoring the arterial inflow.

Number of vessels to be anastomosed. Experience taught the importance of guaranteeing a good venous return. The blood flow per unit crosssection of artery is much greater than that per unit cross-section of vein and therefore, in order to avoid an imbalance between arterial inflow and venous drainage with consequent swelling of the reattached part it is necessary to anastomose two or three veins for every artery anastomosed (Ch'en *et al.* 1965). Post-operative swelling is one of the most important causes of failure and everything possible should be done to avoid it.

In forearm amputations if, after either the ulnar or the radial artery has been anastomosed, the whole hand flushes pink and starts to warm up, then the other artery may be safely ligated.

Blood vessel débridement. Thorough excision of the damaged ends of severed blood vessels is essential for the prevention of thrombosis at the anastomotic site. It is not always easy to identify signs of damage in the wall of a blood vessel, especially when there has been a blunt injury which damages the intima more extensively than the adventitia. Signs of blood vessel wall damage include haematomata in the vessel wall, subintimal petechiae and roughness or kinking of the intima as seen in the cut end. If fissuring of the intima is suspected, the vessel can be distended with saline under pressure to see whether saline leaks out into the subadventitial tissues (Ch'ien *et al.* 1966).

TECHNIQUE OF ANASTOMOSIS

Ts'ui and his colleagues carried out a series of experiments in dogs to compare the results of the following alternatives: anastomosis by suture with anastomosis by coupling; suturing under direct vision with suturing under magnification; interrupted silk with interrupted monofilament nylon; the use or non-use of postoperative anticoagulant therapy; synthetic prostheses with autogenous vein grafts for bridging defects in arteries.

The results were clear-cut.

In arteries with an average diameter of 2·5 mm. or less anastomosis by suture was much superior to anastomosis by coupling. It took slightly less time to accomplish (15·4 minutes as compared with 21·3 minutes) and the patency rate after 118 days observation was 86·4 per cent as compared with 36·4 per cent in the coupling group.

The patency rate in the coupling group fell sharply as the diameter of the blood vessel decreased. This is because eversion of the cut end of a small vessel over a coupling ring inevitably stretches and traumatizes the intima and predisposes to thrombotic occlusion.

The use of magnification had very little effect on the patency rate but since it limited the visual field and restricted manoeuverability, it slowed down the procedure and prolonged the occlusion time.

Monofilament nylon gave slightly better results than 7-0 silk, especially with vessels below 2 mm. in diameter. It is stronger, excites less tissue reaction and passes more smoothly through the vessel wall, with less tendency to drag fragments of adventitia into the lumen. However, it ties less well and there is more chance of leakage from the suture line.

Systemic anticoagulant therapy, which is of little or no value after anastomosis of fairly large vessels, was found to be markedly effective in preventing thrombotic occlusion of vessels with a diameter of less than 1 mm. The patency rate after anastomosis of 17 arteries with an average diameter of 0·77 mm. was only 41 per cent if no anticoagulant was used while it was 73 per cent in a series of 21 anastomoses with an average diameter of 0·67 mm. in which sufficient anticoagulants were given to maintain the prothrombin time at 40–60 per cent of normal for 16 days.

Autogenous vein grafts were markedly superior to synthetic prostheses.

On the basis of these findings and our own clinical experience, we mainly rely on anastomosis by direct suture, reserving the coupling method for the anastomosis of fairly large veins or for vein grafting.

Before anastomosing a vessel by direct suture every trace of adventitia for 1 cm. above and below the anastomosis is removed. This reduces the risk of spasm and ensures that no fragments of adventitia are dragged into the lumen of the vessel where they would be likely to initiate thrombosis.

To facilitate suture and prevent spasm, the ends of the vessels are stretched with mosquito forceps so as to make them funnel-shaped as shown in the accompanying illustration. Two stay sutures are inserted and, for vessels having a diameter greater than 2 mm. a continuous suture

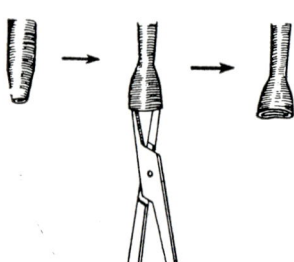

Method of stretching severed end of artery before anastomosis.

entered from the intimal surface and tied to the stay sutures is used. Vessels smaller than 1·5 mm. in diameter are anastomosed with interrupted sutures which enter 0·5 mm. from the cut end, the bites being 0·5 mm. apart. Most Chinese surgeons do not use magnifying loupes but the assistant often uses one to check on the accuracy of the suturing.

The preferred suture material is 9-0 monofilament Capron.

If, after blood vessel débridement, the gap is too big to be closed by direct suture, an autogenous vein graft, usually taken from the other arm, is used. Its direction is reversed to avoid obstruction to blood flow by its valves and it is inserted under slight tension since if it is too long it is liable to kink and thrombose. A segment of vein removed for use as a graft, invariably goes into spasm which can be overcome by distending it with procaine or saline before use.

Delayed vein anastomosis. The importance of anastomosing an adequate cross-section of veins has already been stressed. However, the subcutaneous veins usually go into spasm and may be difficult to find. In such cases, delayed vein suture may be performed on the second post-operative day when spasm has passed off and the veins are easy to handle. This has been done on three occasions with good results.

TREATMENT OF NERVES

In clean amputations, it is usually possible to resect enough of the nerve ends to carry out primary nerve suture and it is advisable to do this because delayed nerve suture is difficult and dangerous on account of the mass of scar tissue which forms around the neuro-vascular bundles. In doing so it is important to ensure complete haemostasis of the cut ends of the nerves and to avoid torsional deformity. If a considerable segment of a nerve is judged to have been irremediably destroyed, an accurate drawing is made of the location and extent of the injury and the nerve ends are anchored with black silk to an easily identified structure. This facilitates subsequent nerve grafting. If both ulnar and median nerves have sustained extensive tissue loss, the first stage of a pedicle nerve graft may be performed by anastomosing their healthy proximal stumps (Strange 1947).

TREATMENT OF MUSCLES AND TENDONS

Muscles and tendons which can play no useful role in recovery of function are removed. Others are sutured. It is sometimes necessary to re-route a muscle so as to fill a dead space or to provide good soft tissue cover for anastomosed blood vessels.

TREATMENT OF DEEP FASCIA

Since post-operative swelling is likely to occur, it is advisable to slit the deep fascia widely so as to prevent tension from developing at a time when it could produce disastrous effects.

SKIN CLOSURE

To minimize the risk of infection, it is essential to effect complete skin closure. If it has been necessary to excise a considerable amount of skin or if the injury itself has caused skin loss, skin closure by direct suture may be impossible. In such cases rotation flaps, abdominal flaps or free skin grafting are employed either singly or in combination. On a number of occasions a free skin graft placed directly over the site of a vein anastomosis or over a vein graft has taken normally without affecting the patency of the underlying veins.

DRESSINGS

A minimum of dressings are applied, no circumferential bandages are used and the fingers are left exposed. Padded plaster splints maintain the position of the limb.

Reattachment of Severed Fingers

After more than 20 failures, surgeons at the Shanghai Sixth Municipal Hospital successfully reattached a completely severed finger on January 8, 1966.

In the following 14 months, they reattached more than 40 completely or almost completely severed fingers. This shows that numerically at least, traumatic finger amputations provide a bigger challenge than limb amputations and I therefore present our experience in this field separately.

STATISTICS FROM THE SHANGHAI SIXTH MUNICIPAL HOSPITAL IN RE-ATTACHMENT OF SEVERED FINGERS FROM JANUARY 1966 TO MARCH 1967.

Completely severed fingers. No. of patients 20. Average age 30 years. Males 15. Females 5. Total number of digits amputated 43.

Analysis of digits amputated:

Thumb 1. Index 17. Middle 11. Ring 8. Little 6.

Of the 43 completely amputated digits, 34 were reattached and 9 were amputated. All the re-attached digits had been amputated through the proximal segment. Of the 34 reattached digits, 24 survived and 10 became necrotic and were subsequently amputated.

Incompletely severed fingers. Number of patients 11, average age 28. Male 8. Female 3. Number of digits 24.

Analysis of digits:

Thumb 4. Index 6. Middle 6. Ring 5. Little 3.

Twenty fingers were reattached and four were primarily amputated. Seven of the reattached fingers became necrotic. One developed skin necrosis over the pulp which necessitated free skin grafting.

The remaining 12 fingers succeeded completely.

Indications. At present, it is considered that all amputated fingers should be reattached providing:

(1) There is no systemic contraindication to a very prolonged operation.

(2) The amputation is relatively clean without excessive bone splintering or soft tissue damage.

(3) Providing the disability likely to result from the injury warrants reattachment. If only either the fourth or fifth finger has been amputated and the other fingers are intact, then unless the patient particularly asks for the finger to be reattached, the operation is not normally advised.

Technique

Anaesthesia. Since finger reattachment operations are usually very prolonged, continuous high epidural anaesthesia supplemented when necessary by intravenous anaesthesia is used. Each finger takes from 3–5 hours and one operation in which four fingers were reattached, took 17 hours.

Tourniquet. In contradistinction to operations for reattachment of severed limbs, a pneumatic tourniquet is usually used for finger reattachment since a bloodless field is essential for anastomosis of digital vessels and to achieve this by the use of vascular clips would increase the risk of thrombosis. The tourniquet must be frequently released and in practice no tourniquet is used for the greater part of the operating time.

Wound excision. Since the fingers contain no muscle tissue, wound excision is a much simpler procedure than in limb amputations. It is enough to remove jagged bone spikes, protruding tendons and a thin layer of tissue from the proximal and distal cut surfaces. The cut ends of the blood vessels are trimmed according to principles described above and the vascular bed in the amputated part is thoroughly irrigated with heparin and saline.

Internal fixation. In nearly every case, bony rigidity is restored by the use of intramedullary Kirschner wires passed either through the proximal interphalangeal joint or through the metacarpophalangeal joint according to the level of amputation. Sometimes it is more convenient to secure internal fixation by Kirschner wires which transfix adjacent metacarpals and occasionally an intramedullary bone peg is used. Kirschner wires are usually left in place for six weeks and they have not resulted in serious infection or joint stiffness.

BLOOD VESSEL ANASTOMOSIS

The aim is to anastomose two dorsal veins and one digital artery in each finger. The veins are sutured first for otherwise, if many fingers are being reattached, blood loss from retrograde bleeding may necessitate blood transfusion. If the cross-section of anastomosed veins is insufficient, serious swelling of the finger is likely to develop.

Anastomosis of dorsal digital veins is usually the most difficult part of the operation. They may be in spasm and one or more of them may have been damaged or destroyed by the injury. In such cases it may be necessary to mobilize and reroute veins from the dorsum of the hand or from an adjacent intact finger, in order to bridge the gap. The only alternative to such methods is a tedious vein grafting operation which carries a high failure rate.

Both veins and arteries are anastomosed by interrupted sutures inserted from inside the blood-vessel within 0·5 mm. of the cut edge. Four sutures can easily be inserted into a digital artery and on one occasion 12 sutures were used. The adventitia is thoroughly removed from both ends of the artery before anastomosis. If spasm is present it is relieved by vigorous distension with saline and heparin and by keeping the blood vessel warm with a jet of warm saline.

If the plane of amputation is oblique, it may be convenient to perform a cross anastomosis, re-routing the vessels from one side of the finger to the other.

DIGITAL NERVES

The traumatized nerve ends are resected in the usual way. It is unnecessary to suture the nerves for, as the author has previously pointed out (Horn 1959) digital nerves regenerate very satisfactorily providing their ends are nearly in apposition and providing they are lying in a well defined tissue plane. If, after resection, the nerve ends cannot be brought into contact, it may be possible to bridge the gap by swinging a nerve from one side of the finger to the other. If necessary, the digital nerve from one side may be used as a free graft to restore continuity in the other and when this is done, the importance of restoring sensation to the radial sides of the index, middle and ring fingers and to the ulnar sides of the thumb and little finger should be borne in mind.

TENDONS

The extensor tendon and the flexor retinaculum are sutured in order to ensure soft tissue coverage at the level of osteosynthesis. Flexor tendons are drawn into the wound, trimmed and anchored to the flexor sheath. Primary suture of flexor tendons has not yet been attempted, but later, with increasing experience, it probably will be.

WOUND CLOSURE

The wound is closed without drainage by careful suture of the skin and subcutaneous tissue.

For reasons which are made plain below, a stab wound is made in the pulp of the finger at the conclusion of the operation and the colour and rate of flow of blood from it is noted.

No dressings are used.

Postoperative Management of Reattached Extremities

BLOOD TRANSFUSION

Blood vessels in reattached extremities are very prone to go into spasm and a fall in blood pressure may precipitate this. It is advisable to maintain the systolic blood pressure at 100 mm. or higher throughout the operation and the best way to do this is by blood transfusion. More blood is lost in multiple finger reattachments than in limb reattachments and it is found that finger reattachments often need 500 c.c. of blood transfusion per finger. Before the tourniquet is released it is advisable to have a transfusion running in order to be able to forestall a fall in blood pressure. Hypotension in the post-operative period may also necessitate blood transfusion.

ANTICOAGULANTS

Anticoagulants are not used after reattaching amputated limbs, but in finger reattachments, anticoagulants are started during the operation and continued for 10 days post-operatively. Heparin, in sufficient amounts to prolong the clotting time to 20 minutes, is given for the first four days, the usual dose being 300 mgm. or 30,000 units of heparin daily. Dicoumarol, in sufficient doses to reduce the pro-thrombin time to 20–30 per cent of normal, is started on the first post-operative day and by the fourth day replaces heparin.

During anti-coagulant therapy, if bleeding from the suture line and from the stab wound in the pulp of the finger is troublesome, it is treated by local applications and by blood transfusion.

Position. The reattached extremity is usually kept at the level of the heart. If there is a tendency to swell, it is raised slightly and if the arterial supply is precarious it may be lowered.

Swelling. Until it was realized that it was necessary to anastomose a larger cross-section of veins than of arteries, post-operative swelling was common. It was usually dealt with by making multiple incisions into the reattached part so that blood and oedema fluid could drain away but the incisions sometimes became infected and adversely affected the functional result.

Swelling is now much less common and can usually be controlled by adjusting the position of the limb. If necessary, intravenous hypertonic low molecular Dextran or 20 per cent human albumen may be given.

EARLY DETECTION OF THREATENED CIRCULATORY FAILURE

Regular skin temperature recordings from the reattached part provide a valuable guide to the condition of the circulation. The normal and the operated limbs are kept, as far as possible, under identical environmental conditions and the temperature of selected parts is measured with an electric skin thermometer every two hours. Usually the temperature in the reattached part is higher than on the normal side for the first two weeks; then it becomes cooler and finally, over a period of several months, it reaches the same temperature.

A fall in the temperature of the reattached part in the early post-operative period is a warning sign while a fall of 6°C is a danger signal demanding immediate attention.

Apart from skin temperature, the colour, the presence or absence of mottling, the briskness of the capillary return after local pressure and the response to pricking, all provide information about the state of the circulation. Pallor and mottling on elevation suggest an arterial deficiency. Cyanosis with or without mottling when the limb is at heart level suggests inadequacy of the venous return. The capillary reflux after local pressure is usually exaggeratedly brisk if there is moderate venous obstruction but it becomes sluggish if there is arterial obstruction or capillary thrombosis. If the venous return is obstructed, a prick causes a flow of thick, cyanosed blood which clots rapidly unless anticoagulants are being used. If the arterial supply is threatened, a prick either draws more blood or a very small quantity of blood of normal colour.

THE MANAGEMENT OF THREATENED CIRCULATORY FAILURE

There are four main causes of circulatory embarrassment in a reattached extremity and, for correct treatment, it is essential to diagnose which of them is playing the main role.

They are:

(1) Excessive tension proximal to the reattachment.
(2) Venous thrombosis.
(3) Arterial thrombosis.
(4) Arterial spasm.

Excessive tension proximal to the reattachment may be due to external pressure from splints or encircling bandages, to traumatic swelling within the fascial envelope or to a deep haematoma in the proximal part of the limb. The first is treated by removing all splints and dressings, the second by fasciotomy and the third by exploration, evacuation of the haematoma and haemostasis.

Venous thrombosis may occur at the site of anastomosis or in the venous plexus in the reattached part. It manifests itself by a falling skin temperature, swelling and cyanosis. Treatment depends on whether blockage is complete or partial and on whether small vessels in the distal venous plexus are thrombosed. If the circulation does not improve after a short period of elevation, exploration is indicated. If the vein is found to be thrombosed, it is incised and the clot is removed. The intima is inspected and if it is abnormal, the affected segment is resected. Then, if direct re-anastomosis is not possible, a vein graft is performed.

Partial thrombosis and thrombosis of veins in the distal venous plexus, is a common cause of failure or threatened failure after finger reattachment. That is why a stab wound is made in the pulp of the finger at the conclusion of the operation and why anticoagulants are used. If a reattached finger presents signs of venous thrombosis, it is gently squeezed and massaged so as to cause bleeding from the stab wound. This temporarily empties the distal venous plexus and may break up or dislodge a thrombus for long enough for a collateral venous return to open up. If after treatment there is temporary improvement, it may be repeated, but if the condition fails to improve, there should be no hesitation in exploring the dorsal veins.

Arterial thrombosis results in a pallid, bloodless, rapidly cooling extremity. As soon as the condition is diagnosed, the artery should be explored. Unless a technical fault is found to be responsible for the thrombosis, it is not enough to remove the thrombus, for there is usually a lesion of the intima which will result in another thrombosis. In such cases the traumatized segment of the artery is radically excised and a vein graft is performed.

Arterial spasm may be difficult or impossible to differentiate from arterial thrombosis. Ultra-sonics have been used in differential diagnosis but its reliability is still unproved. If spasm is suspected anti-spasmodic drugs such as Papaverine, Pethidine or Priscol are given and sympathetic procaine block may be tried although its value is very doubtful. Occasionally changing the position of the limb may result in the sudden relief of spasm. Local warming is of undoubted value for reattached fingers.

If there is no result from such conservative measures, no time should be lost in exploring the vessels. It is wiser to assume that the cause of the circulatory deficiency is thrombosis rather than spasm.

Threatened failure in a reattached extremity demands patience, tenacity and a determination to leave nothing undone which might snatch victory from defeat. Some of the successful limb reattachments in China were re-operated on three or four times with a total operating time exceeding 24 hours.

HYPERBARIC OXYGEN

The first finger to be successfully reattached in Shanghai showed signs of threatened circulatory failure on the ninth day. No cause could be found except for mild infection and it was decided to try the effect of hyperbaric oxygen before exploring the digital artery. The patient was placed in a tank of oxygen at three atmospheres pressure and the colour of the finger immediately improved. He stayed in the tank for 30 minutes and after removal from it, the circulation in the finger remained good. For the next three days the patient spent $\frac{1}{2}$ hour daily in the tank and he made an excellent recovery.

Our experience with hyperbaric oxygen is as yet very limited but it may prove to be a valuable adjunct to treatment.

Some Remaining Problems

Refrigeration. Experimental work in China in the role of refrigeration of amputated extremities was stimulated by the empirical use of partial refrigeration of amputated limbs during transit from remote regions. Although the more sophisticated means of refrigeration are lacking in parts of China, iced lollies and large thermos bottles are readily available in most areas. These have, on a number of occasions, provided a convenient, even if somewhat unreliable means of cooling during transit.

A series of experiments on dogs' legs showed that refrigeration could definitely prolong the permissible interval between amputation and reattachment. Providing the vascular bed is thoroughly washed out with heparin and saline, amputated dogs' limbs can be stored at between 2–4°C for 24 hours with a fair certainty that reattachment will succeed. Refrigeration for 48 hours was followed by successful reattachment in most cases. The longest successful experimental interval in China to date is 102 hours.

There is no doubt that refrigeration is useful in this work but the precise conditions of refrigeration have still to be worked out. In some experimentally refrigerated dog's limbs, the heparin and saline filling the vascular bed froze and it was necessary to apply external heat before the circulation could be restored.

Problems of Muscle Contractility

We have encountered two problems of muscle contractility in limbs which have been successfully reattached. One is the problem of scar replacement of the distal part of those muscle bellies which have been divided by the traumatic amputation. For example, a traumatic amputation through the upper arm, must divide the muscle bellies of biceps, brachialis and triceps and the distal stump of each of these muscles may undergo scar replacement. If the level of section is below the middle of the upper arm, this is not important for there is sufficient contractile muscle in the proximal stump to provide active flexion and extension of the elbow, albeit with reduced power. The proximal stump of the muscle, which is normally innervated and vascularized, pulls through the scarred remnant of the distal stump which acts as a tendon. Naturally it lacks the gliding property of a true tendon and a further operation may be necessary to free adhesions and increase its excursion.

However, if the level of amputation is through the upper third of the arm, the problem is more serious, for the greater part of the muscle bellies involved may lose their contractility and develop widespread and dense adhesions. The triceps usually suffers less severely than the biceps or brachialis because a larger proportion of its muscle belly is likely to be proximal to the level of section and because it is supplied by arteries which enter the muscle at widely separated points.

We have encountered cases in which active elbow flexion has been completely lost as a result of scar replacement of biceps and brachialis and have treated them by pectoralis major transfer after total excision of the scarred muscles.

Most muscles in the upper limbs are supplied with blood either by a single artery or by a leash of arteries which enter close together near the proximal end. For this reason, amputations just below the elbow or the shoulder are most likely to result in scar replacement of muscle bellies. Case 3 (Fig. 3), however, shows that even with high amputations, scar replacement is not inevitable.

The second problem is mummification of muscles in reattached limbs.

Scar replacement of muscles is due to ischaemia severe enough to cause the death of muscle cells but not sufficiently severe or prolonged to cause the death of more resistant types of cells such as fibroblasts. The distal stump of a divided muscle may still get enough blood from vessels penetrating from the deep fascia or running upwards from its point of insertion, to prevent total cellular death so that the surviving fibroblasts can proliferate and gradually replace the dead muscle fibres.

Mummification results from muscle ischaemia severe enough to kill all the cells in the muscle including fibroblasts so that there are no surviving cells to invade the dead muscle and replace it by scar tissue.

In such cases, the tissues surrounding the dead muscle belly gradually encase the dead muscle in a tomb of scar tissue. The dead muscle itself may remain histologically relatively unchanged for many years and that is why the term 'mummification' has been used in this connection (Horn and Sevitt 1951).

The author has seen a few reattached limbs in which while the overall nutritional state of the limb has been good, groups of muscles have become indurated and remained noncontractile. The words *'remained non-contractile'* are used because they were, of course, denervated as a result of the traumatic amputation and it is difficult clinically to differentiate between non-contractility due to denervation and non-contractility due to death of muscle fibres. These were cases of traumatic amputation at a high level and it is possible that their persisting non-contractility was largely due to defective or delayed re-innervation. However, the induration and absence of wasting strongly suggested that mummification was at least partly responsible. Theoretically it should be possible to differentiate between denervation and muscle death by electromyography or by taking muscle biopsies. In practice, both of these methods have the drawback that they give information only about a small part of the muscle and do not necessarily reflect the condition of the muscle as a whole. Since the few limbs which have shown this phenomenon have all been re-attached rather recently, we have not felt justified in performing an exploration in order to establish the precise pathology. Instead a wait and see policy has been adopted, maintaining joint mobility by passive movements, in expectation that patchy mummification would be followed by sufficient muscle regeneration from the periphery of the dead muscle tore store useful function. If this does not eventuate, such surgical methods as muscle transfers and tenodeses to restore function may be used.

A notable feature of this condition which differentiates it from Volkmann's ischaemic contracture, is precisely the absence of contracture. Deformity does not develop and the range of passive movement remains full or nearly so. Moreover, the indurated muscles, unlike the scarred muscles of Volkmann's ischaemic contracture, do not shrink but maintain their full bulk.

A further period of observation will be necessary in order to clarify this unusual and interesting phenomenon.

Restoration of Nerve Function

The only purpose of re-attaching an amputated extremity is to restore function. At present, one of the main obstacles to restoration of useful function is not the viability of the limb as a whole but the functional viability of nerves.

Nerves present little problem if a limb has been amputated by a clean cut, for they can be treated by well established procedures with reliable and predictable results. It has been shown that nerves are less sensitive to the effects of ischaemia than are muscles. The problems arise where a limb has been avulsed rather than cut off and the nerves have been pulled out from either the proximal or the distal part or both. (See cases 2 and 3.) In such cases the main nerve trunks have been extensively traumatized and they may become functionless strands of scar tissue. Three questions arise in these cases. Firstly, how can one ascertain which nerves are capable of recovery and which will become hopelessly scarred? The naked eye appearance provides no answer to this question. Can electrophysiological or histological methods provide an answer? Secondly, what is the best way to deal with nerves which have sustained extensive loss of tissue? Nerve autografting is a valuable procedure but it is subject to great limitations imposed by the non-availability of the necessary quantity of autograft material. We have been trying to tackle this problem by using irradiated homografts (Marmor 1963) but the results so far have been disappointing.

Thirdly, is there any way in which we can prevent scar replacement of traumatized nerves? If, for example, such nerves were to be removed from the limb, irradiated and stored in a refrigerator under suitable conditions, would this eliminate the otherwise inevitable scar response to trauma so that they could later be used as autografts?

At present we are unable to answer any of these questions but we hope to be able to do so in the future.

Toxaemia

I know of two patients who developed severe toxaemic symptoms after successful limb reattachment. One of them, an amputation just below the shoulder, developed a mental disorder which persisted for several weeks. The other, an amputation through the midthigh, also developed mental symptoms and in addition he showed signs of progressive renal failure. When the reattached limb was removed, he made an uneventful recovery.

In neither case was there marked swelling, necrosis or infection of the reattached limb.

The causes, treatment and prevention of systemic toxaemia following limb reattachment are still not clear and warrant further research work. It does not appear, however, that toxaemia after reattachment of amputated extremities is as big a problem as indicated by Shorey et al. (1965). We have seen no toxaemia after reattachment of low amputations and it is possible that the serious toxaemia in his case was due to the fact that part of the reattached hand became necrotic.

Tendon Repair in Reattached Fingers

It is only just over a year since the first success in the reattachment of amputated fingers and a policy in relation to tendon repair has not yet been worked out. If the interosseus-lumbrical mechanism is intact, movements at the metacarpo-phalangeal joints are retained and, in such cases, and especially if it has been injured, it is usual to fuse the proximal interphalangeal joint in a position of function. However, while one is reluctant to fuse joints in fingers showing full or nearly full passive movements one hesitates to carry out tendon grafting in a finger which relies on a single digital artery and on a limited number of venous channels. With careful technique, these misgivings may prove to be unjustified and it is hoped to perform some tendon grafting operations on reattached fingers and also, in favourable cases, to perform primary flexor tendon suture at the time of reattachment.

Homografting

It is often the case that a technical advance opens the way to theoretical advances. A number of Chinese surgeons have now mastered the technique of limb and digit reattachment and inevitably this raises the question of the possibility of transferring a limb or part of a limb from one individual to another. The theoretical implications of homografting impinge on some of the most basic problems of biology and early or easy successes are not to be expected. However, a research approach to this problem is being widely discussed and we hope to make some progress in this sphere of biology.

Arterial Spasm

We still do not understand the mechanism of arterial spasm and are not always able to relieve it. In some cases of reattached fingers, to relieve spasm of the digital arteries, we have exposed the radial artery in order to distend it with saline under pressure. To our surprise we have sometimes found that the radial artery too is in spasm and we have even found the spasm to extend as high as the brachial artery. Relaxant drugs, local applications, sympathetic block and even mechanical distension may all be unavailing. Periarterial sympathectomy may merely transfer the spasm to the upper limit of the zone of removal of adventitia.

This is a troublesome and baffling condition which has been responsible for the loss of a number of reattached extremities.

Some Illustrative Cases
(From the Shanghai Sixth Municipal Hospital and from Chi Shui Tan Hospital, Peking.)

Case 1. The first successful limb reattachment has been fully reported elsewhere (1 and 2). The only reason for referring to this patient again is that I had the opportunity to re-examine him nearly 4 years after the injury and to get an idea of the possible long term results (Fig. 1).

His reattached hand is in extraordinarily good condition. Its colour, temperature and texture are normal and he is doing his original work without difficulty. He states that function in the hand is still improving and except when he is reminded by others of the fact that the hand had once been lying on the factory floor, he is apt to forget his injury.

On examination the following abnormalities could be detected: There is wasting of the hypothenar muscles with slight weakness of abduction and opposition of the little finger.

Subjectively there is hypersensitivity of the skin supplied by the median nerve while objective testing shows moderate impairment of two-point discrimination.

Wrist movements are limited both actively and passively.

There is a contracture of the first volar interosseus muscle resulting in slight limitation of extension of the metacarpophalangeal joint and deviation of the index towards the middle finger. It is planned to correct this by tenotomy or by lengthening the tendon of the first volar interosseus.

He presented me with a prawn made of plastic tubing which he had specially made for me (Fig. 1d). It is a minor masterpiece from both the artistic and technical viewpoints and shows a high degree of recovery of dexterity.

Case 2. The case shown in Fig. 2 is, I believe, the highest traumatic amputation that has been reattached in China. The arm had been caught in a conveyor belt and completely avulsed, together with the scapula, through the acromio-clavicular joint. Though the axillary artery and vein had been torn apart, it was quite possible to anastomose them. As shown in Fig. 2c, nerves had been avulsed from the upper arm for 6 or more inches and it was clear that only very limited return of function would be possible. However, the posterior cord of the brachial plexus had been neatly divided and it was considered worthwhile to reattach the limb even if only to provide an amputation stump that could manipulate a prosthesis.

Accordingly the vessels were anastomosed, the posterior cord and the musculo-cutaneous nerves sutured, the soft tissues repaired and the scapula fixed to the

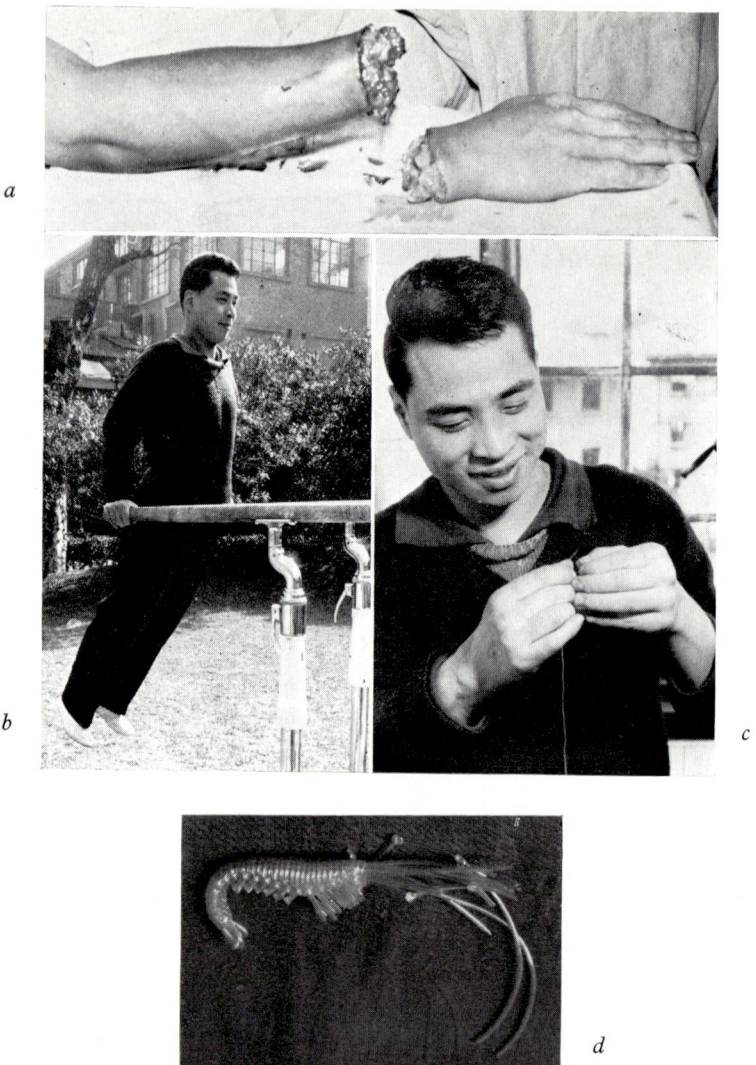

Fig. 1 (Case 1). (*a*) Pre-operative. (*b* and *c*) Condition nearly 4 years after reattachment. (*d*) Model prawn made by patient out of plastic tubing.

clavicle and to the fifth rib by wire sutures. The limb survived and the post-operative course was uneventful. The wire suture between the scapula and the fifth rib has been removed and movements in the scapulo-thoracic plane are being regained. He has regained some power in the triceps and biceps and if necessary, it will be possible to supplement the power of elbow flexion by a pectoralis major transfer. Even if no function returns below the elbow a forearm amputation will enable him to use a working prosthesis, which would otherwise have been impossible. However, he may recover power in the wrist extensors, in which case a flexor tendon tenodesis will restore the grip. Even in such an unfavourable case as this, I think reattachment has been fully justified.

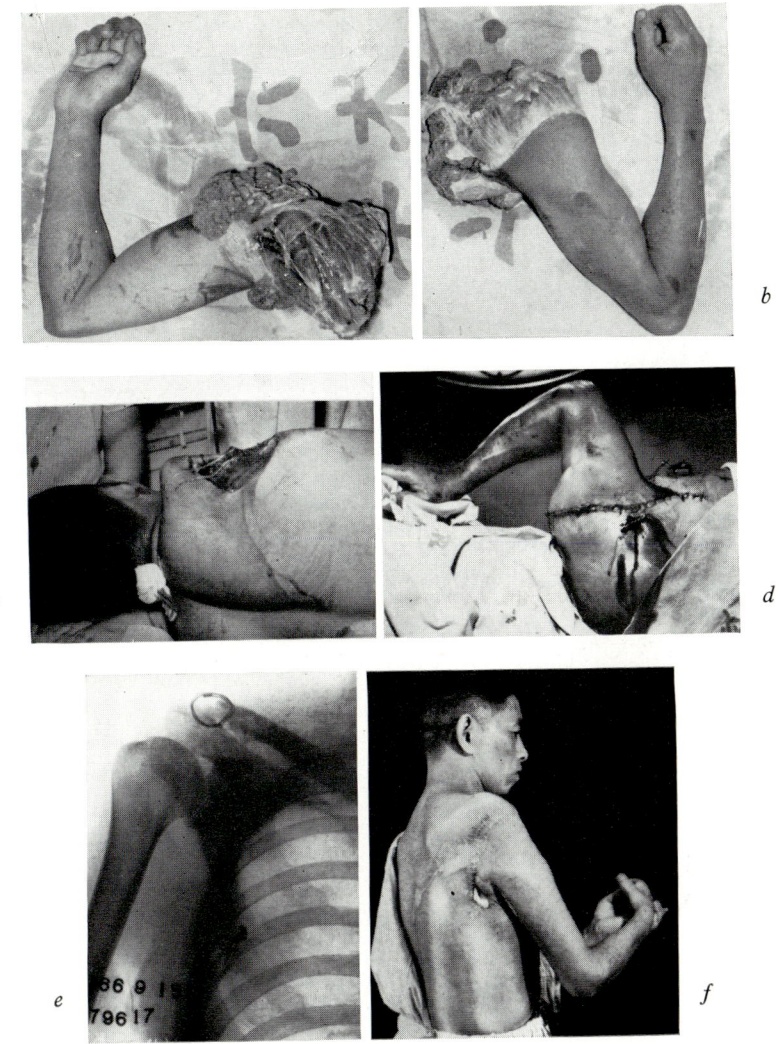

FIG. 2 (Case 2).

(a and b). Pre-operative views of the avulsed limb showing its anterior and posterior aspects. The entire upper limb together with the scapula has been avulsed.
(c) Preoperative view of the traumatic defect on the chest wall. Two nerves have been avulsed from the limb and can be seen lying in the wound and overlying its posterior border.
(d) Immediately after reattachment. The forearm veins are well filled.
(e) Post-operative radiograph showing a wire suture through the acromioclavicular joint and another wire suture fixing the scapula to the 5th rib.
(f) Condition one month after reattachment.

Case 3. The patient illustrated in Fig. 3, caught his right arm in a textile machine as a result of which the limb was avulsed through the neck of the humerus. Fig. 3*a* shows the avulsed limb. Two nerves, the ulnar and the musculo-cutaneous, which had been avulsed from the proximal stump, can be seen protruding from the amputated limb. Fig. 3*b* shows the proximal stump with the musculo-spiral nerve, which had been avulsed from the elbow region, protruding from the wound and lying against the chest wall. The median nerve had been similarly avulsed but it is not clearly seen in the photograph.

The limb was reattached within 3 hours of injury. The upper end of the shaft of the humerus, after shaping, was spiked into the neck of the humerus where it was fixed with two transfixing screws (Fig. 3*c*).

The brachial artery and two veins were anastomosed, the muscle bellies of deltoid, biceps, brachialis and triceps were sutured and the avulsed proximal segments of the median and musculo-spiral nerves were pulled down into the reattached limb through subcutaneous tunnels and anchored at the level of the elbow joint. The avulsed distal segments of the ulnar and musculo-cutaneous nerves were likewise inserted into the proximal stump alongside the neuro-vascular bundle. The wound was closed by primary suture.

No external fixation was used.

The post-operative course was uneventful.

Eight months later the proximal ends of the median and musculo-spiral nerves were exposed, suitably trimmed and sutured to the distal ends. The level of anastomosis in each case was 2 cm. above the point of division into muscular branches. At the same operation an attempt was made to suture the ulnar and musculo-cutaneous nerves but their proximal ends could not be found.

Eight months after this operation and 16 months after the original injury he had regained enough power in the triceps and biceps to flex and extend the elbow against gravity (Fig. 3*d*, *e* and *f*). The wrist flexors had also started to recover. Electromyography confirmed re-innervation of biceps, triceps and the wrist flexors and also showed commencing re-innervation of flexor pollicis longus.

Two years and four months after the original injury the limb was in very good condition. Colour and temperature were normal, the radial and ulnar pulses were strong and shoulder movements were normal. Sweating and sensation had recovered in the median nerve innervated part of the hand. He had recovered powerful flexion and extension of the elbow and powerful flexion of the wrist, fingers and thumb. The thenar muscles were still wasted and weak but they were capable of enough voluntary activity to enable him to abduct and oppose the thumb. The interosseus, hypothenar and extensor muscles of the wrist, fingers and thumb were still paralysed. Fig. 3*g* and *h* show the range of active flexion of the fingers and thumb with the wrist supported.

In view of the extensive avulsion of nerve trunks, recovery in this case has been surprisingly good. Since it had not been possible to suture the musculo-cutaneous nerve recovery in the biceps had not been expected. A possible explanation is that during the reattachment operation, the avulsed distal segment of the nerve had fortunately been placed close to its proximal end and spontaneous regeneration occurred across the gap.

The good recovery of triceps was also surprising since its muscular branches must have been avulsed.

Another noteworthy feature of this case is that the distal stumps of the bellies of biceps and triceps did not undergo scar replacement. It may be that the level of amputation was above that at which the muscular branches to these muscles leave the brachial artery so that anastomosis of the main artery restored a normal blood supply to the divided muscle bellies.

Since no further recovery can be expected in the extensors of the wrist, thumb and fingers, he will need further operative treatment to improve function.

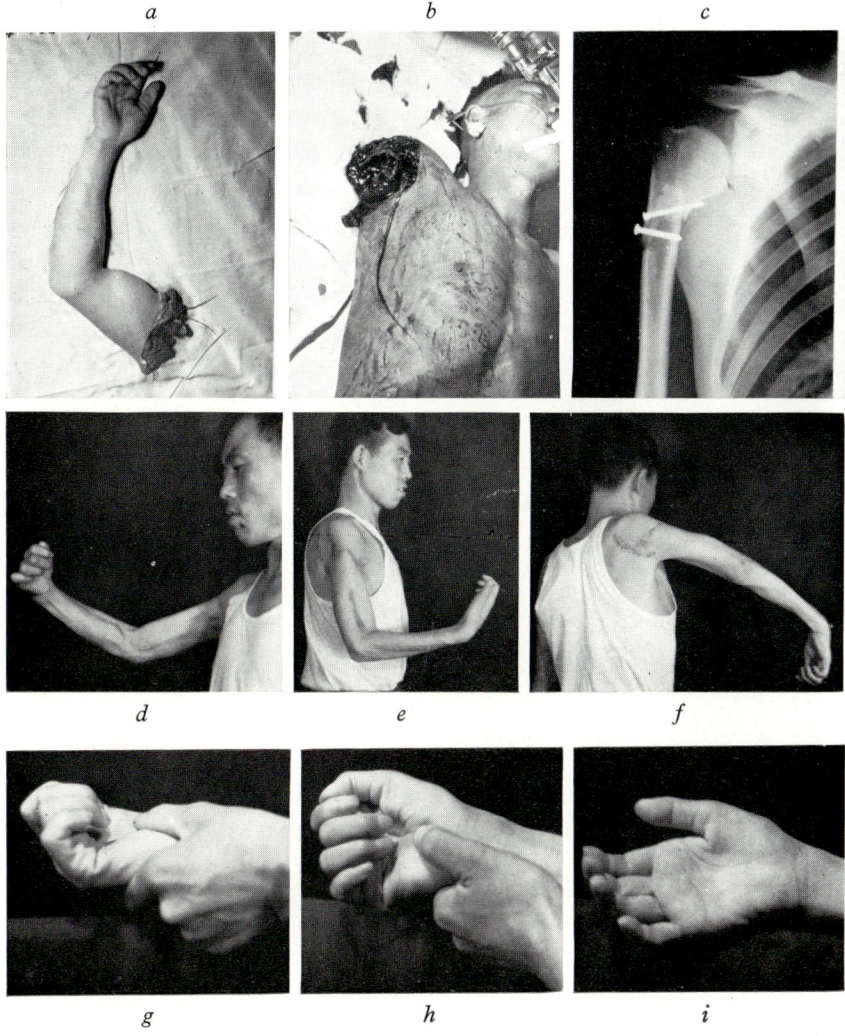

FIG. 3.

(a) The avulsed limb. Two nerves can be seen protruding from the cut surface.
(b) The proximal stump. An avulsed nerve can be seen protruding from the wound and lying against the chest wall.
(c) Post-operative radiograph showing the distal segment of the humerus spiked into the proximal segment and held by two transfixing screws.
(d and e) One year post-operatively showing active flexion of the wrist and elbow against gravity. The operation scar on the lateral aspect of the arm indicates the neurorrhaphy incision.
(f) Showing active extension of the elbow against gravity.
(g and h) Two years and four months post-operatively. With the wrist supported to prevent flexion he has a good range of active flexion of the fingers and thumb.
(i) Showing the hand in the relaxed position.

70 J. S. HORN

Case 4. The case shown in Fig. 4 illustrates the problem of devascularization and denervation of large muscle bellies. As shown in Fig. 4*a*, the flexor muscles of the wrist, fingers and thumb had all been avulsed from the forearm and since there was no possibility of their acquiring a blood or nerve supply, they were excised. Moreover, extensive bone comminution resulted in considerable shortening of the forearm. Function is therefore rather poor but since the intrinsic muscles have recovered, he can flex and extend the metacarpo-phalangeal joints and oppose the

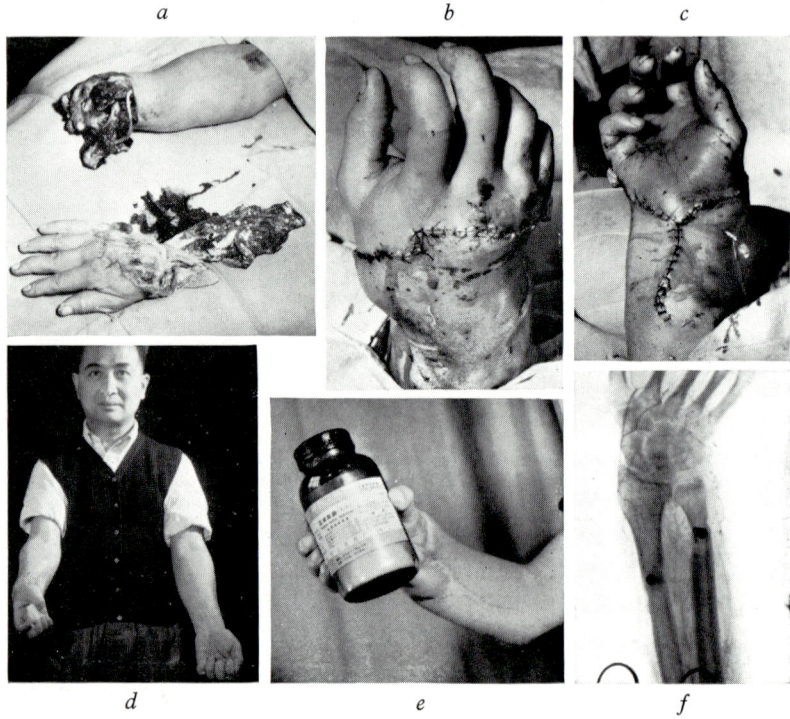

FIG. 4.

(*a*) Pre-operative. The hand has been amputated just proximal to the wrist joint. Most of the flexor muscles have been avulsed from the forearm.

(*b* and *c*) Appearance immediately after reattachment. The skin which had been avulsed from the dorsum of the hand has been sutured back. Later much of it sloughed and was replaced by a free skin graft.

(*d* and *e*) Post-operative. The thumb can be opposed to the fingers and the patient can grasp a jar.

(*f*) Arteriogram showing numerous blood vessels crossing the plane of amputation.

thumb. Sensation has returned throughout the hand and there is no doubt that function is much better than anything which could be provided by a prosthesis. There is still the possibility of further improving function by tendon transfers (See Case 5.)

The arteriogram of this patient is reproduced in Fig. 4*f* because it disproves the assertion that collateral blood vessels do not cross the scar tissue barrier which develops after a circumferential injury (Eiken 1964). Only the radial artery had been anastomosed in this case but numerous arteries can be seen crossing the plane of reattachment.

Case 5. By contrast with the preceding case, this case (Fig. 5), a mid-palm amputation which left the thumb intact, shows that extensive muscle loss is not necessarily incompatible with good recovery. The bellies of flexor digitorum sublimis and profundus and extensor digitorum communis had been completely avulsed from the forearm together with several inches of the ulnar nerve (Fig. 5a). The extensors and flexors of the wrist and the thumb muscles were all intact. The median nerve had not been avulsed.

Since the avulsed muscles could not possibly regain any function, they were excised in toto.

The transverse palmar arch and several dorsal veins were anastomosed and the common digital nerves supplying the index and middle fingers were sutured. Short incisions were then made on the dorsal and volar aspects of the lower third of the forearm and through them, subcutaneous tunnels were made through which the tendons of extensor digitorum communis and flexor digitorum profundus were

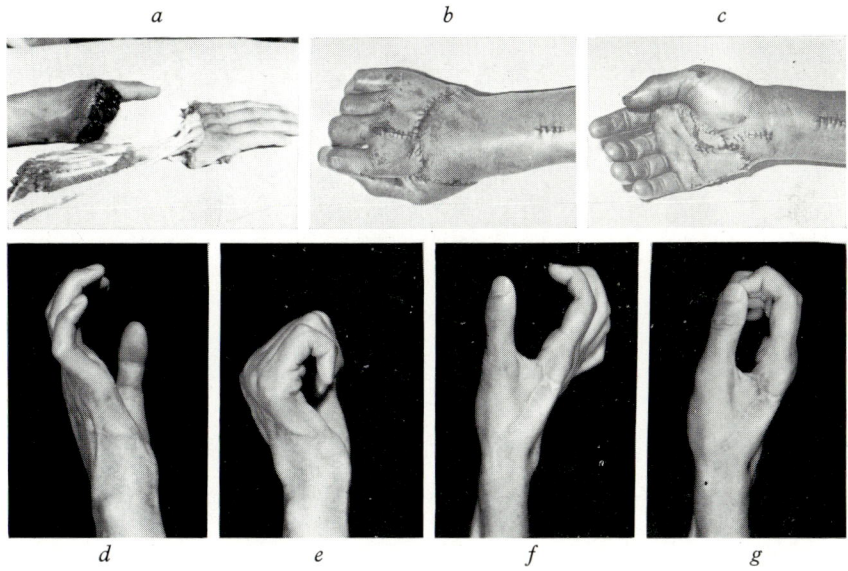

Fig. 5.

(a) Pre-operative. The hand has been amputated through the midpalm level. All the flexor and extensor muscles of the fingers and several inches of the ulnar nerve have been avulsed from the forearm.

(b and c) Immediate post-operative appearance. The incisions on the volar and dorsal aspects of the lower third of the forearm were made for the purpose of returning the avulsed tendons to the forearm for subsequent reattachment to intact muscles.

(d, e, f and g) Showing function one year after injury and after tendon transfers to restore flexion and extension of the fingers. The wasting of the first dorsal interosseus and hypothenar muscles is apparent.

pulled up into the forearm. The stumps of the tendons of flexor digitorum sublimis were excised.

The reattached hand survived and three months later the tendons of flexor digitorum profundus were attached to flexor carpi radialis. Two months after this operation, when active finger flexion had been regained, another operation was performed to attach the tendons of extensor digitorum communis to extensor carpi radialis longus.

A year after injury he had regained powerful flexion and extension of the fingers and sensation in the index and middle fingers was almost normal.

The good result in this case shows that extensive muscle loss is not, in itself, a contraindication to limb reattachment.

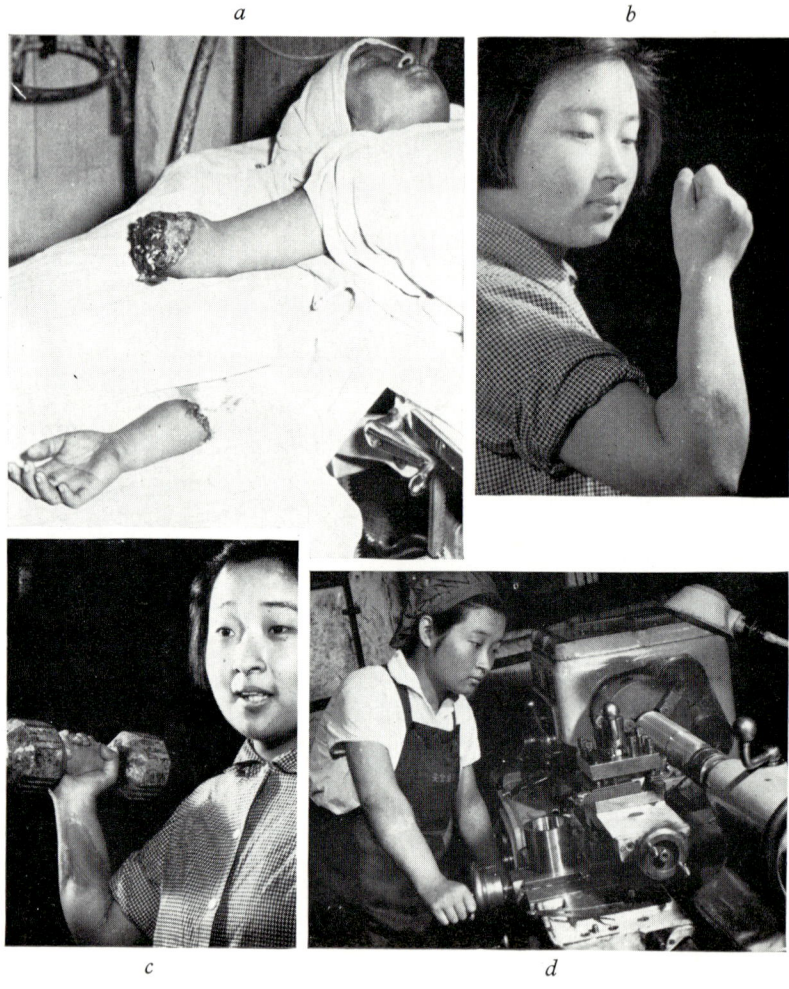

FIG. 6.

(a) Blunt amputation through the middle of the forearm.

(b, c and d) Photographs showing degree of functional recovery. Although a considerable amount of muscle has been destroyed, she can open and close her fist and has resumed her job as a lathe worker.

Case 6. Fig. 6 shows a typical result of reattachment of a blunt amputation through the middle of the forearm. Such an injury destroys a considerable amount of muscle and in this case bone comminution made significant shortening of the forearm inevitable. Although a full range of finger movements is unlikely to be regained, she has recovered sufficient power and sensation to permit resumption of work.

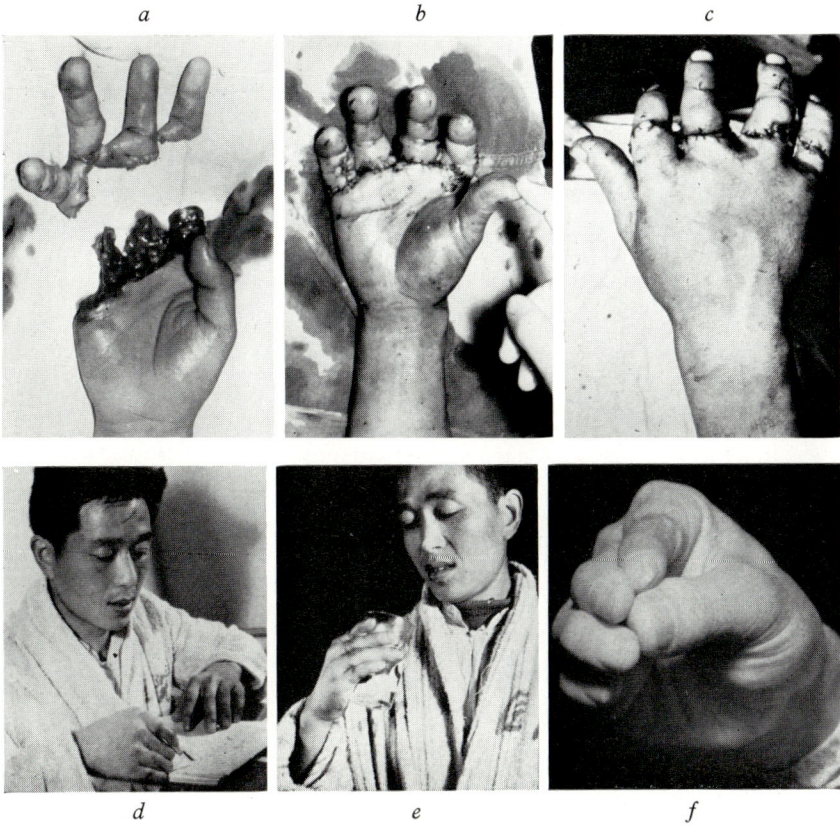

FIG. 7.

(a) Pre-operative. All four fingers have been amputated just distal to the metacarpo-phalangeal joints. The plane of amputation is oblique.
(b and c) Immediate post-operative appearance. In (c) the Kirschner wires in the 3rd and 4th fingers can be seen.
(d, e and f) Ten weeks after reattachment. The patient can write, hold a glass and has a good pinch.

Case 7. The case shown in Fig. 7 shows the result of reattaching an oblique traumatic amputation of all four fingers just distal to the metacarpo-phalangeal joints. Most of the interosseus tendons have been severely traumatized and this impairs function at the metacarpo-phalangeal and inter-phalangeal joints. Nevertheless, the photographs taken within two months of injury, show that the patient had already recovered a good pinch, could write and safely hold a glass.

Case 8. Fig. 8 shows an amputation of all four fingers through the proximal phalanges. All fingers were reattached but the little finger became gangrenous and was later removed. Fig. 8b shows the immediate post-operative condition with the Kirschner wires in place. Fig. 8c and d show the function two months later.

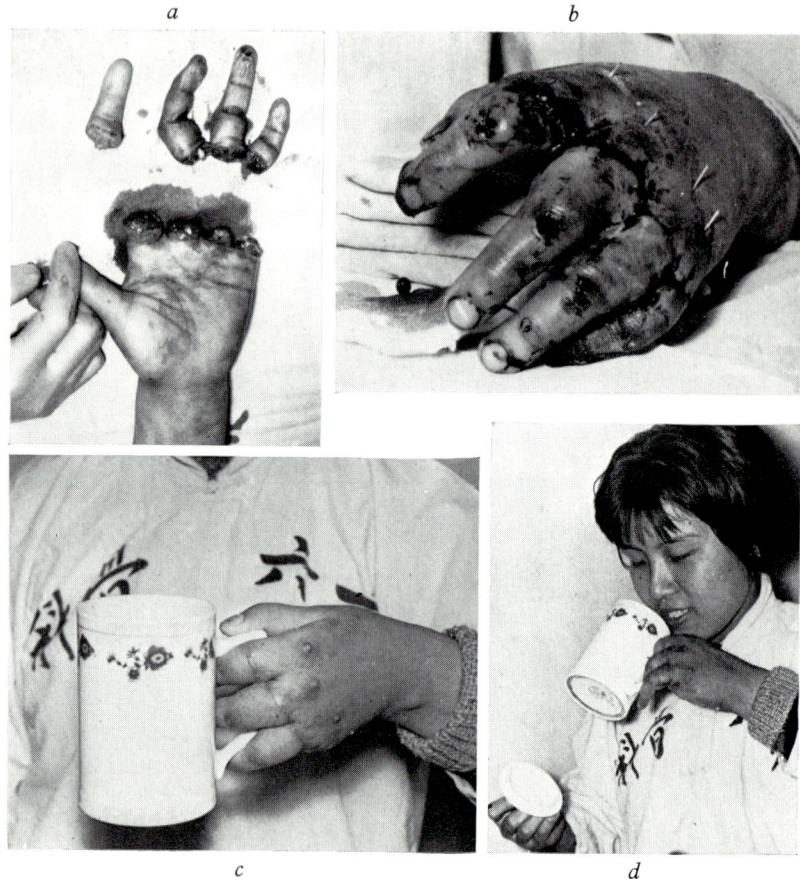

Fig. 8.

(a) Pre-operative. Four fingers have been amputated transversely through the proximal phalanges.
(b) The immediate post-operative appearance. All four fingers have been reattached and the Kirschner wires can be seen emerging on the dorsum of the hand.
(c and d) Two months later. The 5th finger became necrotic and was removed. The other fingers are in good condition and movements at the metacarpophalangeal joints are returning.

Case 9. Fig. 9 shows an amputation through the proximal part of the palm. Two common digital arteries, the arteria princeps pollicis and a number of deep and superficial veins were anastomosed. The thumb and all the fingers survived but a good deal of skin on the dorsum of the hand became necrotic and was replaced by a free skin graft. This tethered the extensor tendons and impaired the function of the hand. The free skin graft was therefore excised and replaced by an abdominal tube pedicle flap. This patient is still undergoing treatment but he has already regained sensation in all digits except the fifth and he can use the hand for writing.

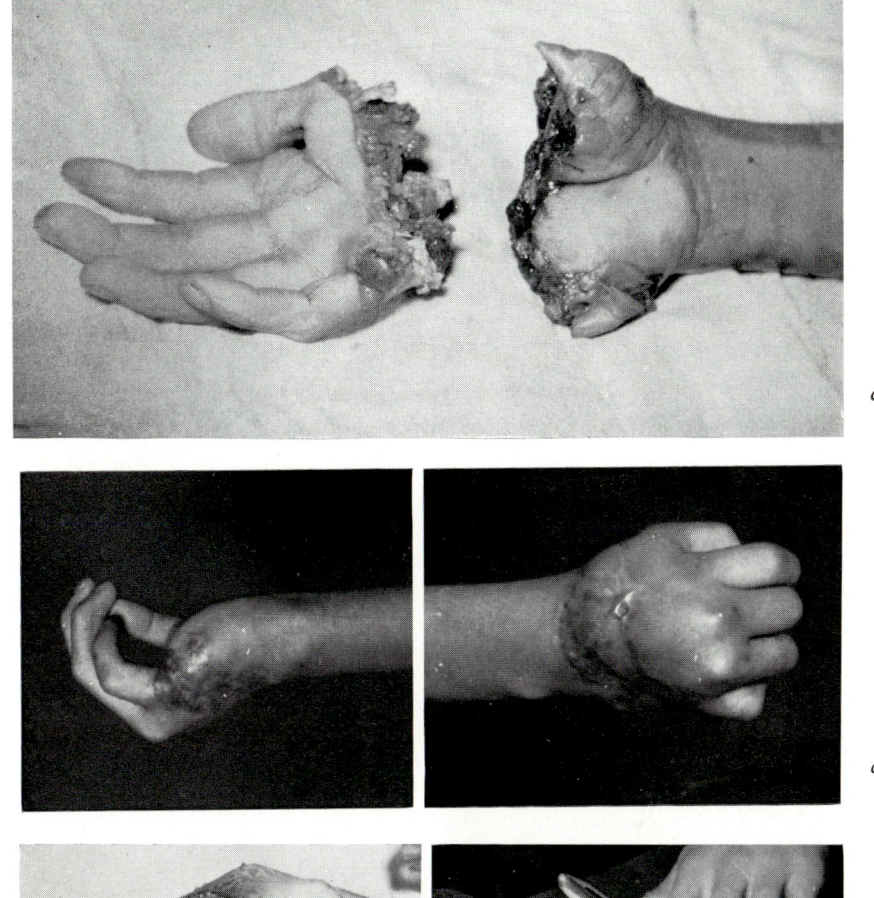

Fig. 9.

(a) Pre-operative. All four fingers and the thumb have been amputated by a blunt injury at the mid-palm level.

(b and c) The reattached fingers and thumb survived but some skin on the dorsum of the hand sloughed and was replaced by a free skin graft which tethered the extensor tendons and prevented flexion at the metacarpophalangeal joints.

(d) The free skin graft has been excised and replaced by an abdominal tube pedicle flap. Photograph shows condition immediately after separation of the flap.

(e) Condition two months later. Movements at the metacarpophalangeal joints have improved and the patient can write.

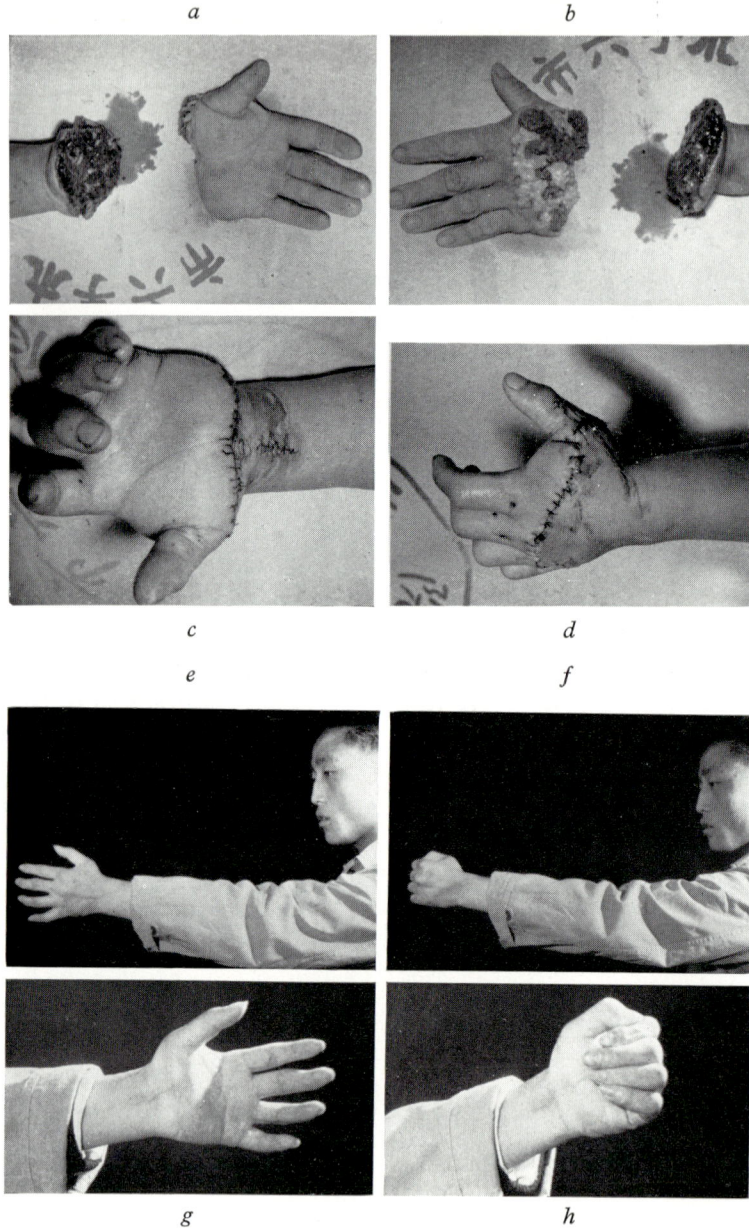

Fig. 10.

(*a* and *b*) Pre-operative. The hand has been amputated through the carpal tunnel.
(*c* and *d*) Immediate post-operative condition. No internal fixation was used. Primary suture of nerves and tendons was performed.
(*e*, *f*, *g* and *h*) Four months later. Function is excellent. The intrinsic muscles have been reinnervated.

Case 10. Fig. 10 shows an amputation through the carpal tunnel just distal to the wrist. The radial and ulnar arteries and four veins were anastomosed. The median and ulnar nerves, the deep flexor tendons, the flexor pollicis longus and the extensor tendons of the fingers and thumb were sutured. The whole hand survived and excellent function was regained.

The success of primary tendon suture in this case suggests that this is the procedure of choice in amputations through the palm of the hand.

Conclusion

I have been asked by non-Chinese colleagues, and I have also asked myself, why have Chinese surgeons been so successful in reattaching severed extremities?

This is a difficult question to answer and an interesting one to ponder over for it involves finding the common denominator which has made possible China's extraordinarily rapid progress in many fields of science and technology since 1949.

In the West, it is usually maintained that politics and medicine are quite separate from each other but in China they are held to be inextricably linked.

Certainly one cannot explain the success of Chinese surgeons in reattaching severed limbs on any theory that they are born with more patience and tenacity than other peoples, or that they have better eyesight or a gentler touch.

I believe that the basic reasons for their success are the political system which removes all obstacles to giving whole-hearted service to the people and the prevailing atmosphere, largely stemming from the teachings of Mao Tse-tung, which impels Chinese people from all walks of life to strive to throw off the stagnation and backwardness of several hundred years, to build their country as quickly as possible into a politically, economically and culturally advanced one and in doing so, unreservedly to place all their energy and all their ability at the disposal of their country and their fellow men.

To put it in a nutshell, they succeed largely because they try very hard and they try very hard because of the nature of the dynamic, forward-moving, purposeful society of which they form an integral part; a self-confident society whose self-confidence is based on a record of solid achievements in many spheres.

There are, of course, other factors but they are of secondary importance. Chinese surgeons enjoy conditions which are conducive to such advances. They work in teams, co-operating with and helping each other. They are given adequate time and facilities for experimental work. They are provided with all necessary equipment. Their work is appreciated and encouraged by the whole people. The practice of flying patients in to the larger cities makes it possible for them to accumulate experience rapidly.

In conclusion, I would like to express my gratitude to my Chinese colleagues for what they have taught me in this field and to express my admiration to them for having opened up a new and worthwhile chapter in the history of surgery.

References

CH'EN, C. W., et al. (1963). Restoration of a completely severed hand; report of a successful case. *Chinese Med. Journ.*, **82,** 632.

CH'EN, C. W., et al. (1965). Further experiences in the restoration of amputated limbs. *Chinese Med. Journ.*, **84,** 225–231.

CH'IEN, Y. C., et al. (1966). Some problems concerning small vessel anastomosis in the reattachment of complete traumatic amputations. *Chinese Med. Journ.* **85,** 79–86.

EIKEN, O., et al. (1964). *Arch. Surg.*, **88,** No. 1., 66.

HORN, J. S. (1959). Modern trends in accident surgery and medicine. p. 308. London: Butterworth.

HORN, J. S. (1964). Successful reattachment of a completely severed forearm. *Lancet*, pp. 1152–1154.

HORN, J. S. and SEVITT, S. S. (1951). Ischaemic necrosis and regeneration of the tibialis anterior muscle after rupture of the popliteal artery. *J. Bone Jt. Surg.*, **33B,** 348–358.

MARMOR, LEONARD. (1963). Repair of peripheral nerves by irradiated homografts. *J. Bone Jt. Surg.*, **45A,** 1542.

SHOREY, W. D., et al. (1965). *Bull. de la Soc. Int. de Chir.*, **24,** 44.

STRANGE, F. G. St. C. (1947). An operation for nerve pedicle grafting. Preliminary communication. *Brit. Journ. Surg.*, **34,** 423.

TS'UI, C. Y., et al. (1966). Microvascular anastomosis and transplantation; experimental studies and clinical application. *Chinese Med. Journ.*, **85,** 610–617.

Chapter 4

COMPRESSION AS AN AID IN ORTHOPAEDIC SURGERY

MAURICE E. MÜLLER

Krompecher (1935) and Trueta (1966) have shown that osteoblasts and osteocytes can develop only in an absolutely undisturbed environment, and only when adequate cell nutrition is available. In 1965 Cameron, investigating the relationship between movement at a fracture and bone healing, attempted to demonstrate that non-union develops only when rotational stresses are present at the fracture site.

In 1949, however, Charnley proved with biopsy studies that a knee arthrodesis healed rapidly when the cancellous surfaces were brought under high compression and thus rigidly immobilized.

Since then, the Charnley compression device (consisting of two Steinmann pins and external clamps) has gained wide acceptance as a method of knee and ankle arthrodesis. Subsequently, Charnley and other investigators, employing the same device, attempted to obtain accelerated union of osteotomies in cortical bone. Their attempts failed but, at about the same time, Danis demonstrated clinically that with more rigid fixation (he used a special tension plate) cortical union of forearm fractures was unquestionably aided and un-united fractures made to join. Unfortunately, Danis failed to support his clinical results with histological proof.

In 1958 a group of Swiss general and orthopaedic surgeons founded an association for the study of osteosynthesis (AO). With their development of new instruments and methods, which allowed absolute immobilization of bone fragments by means of compression, the problem of stable internal fixation appeared to be almost solved from the technical standpoint. It was not until 1960, however, that Schenk from Basle, a coworker of the AO, succeeded in explaining the clinical success of AO techniques, and also provided histological proof of this success. Schenk used dogs for his experimental studies and established histologically the sequence of cortical bone healing with rigid immobilization by means of compression. As long as the bone fragments were not detached from their blood supply no surface resorption at the interface took place, and thus no loss of axial compression occurred. At the osteotomy interface bone osteoclasis and osteogenesis progressed simultaneously. Schenk was also able to show that in man the pattern of healing of cortical fractures was identical. He demonstrated this by autopsy studies of two patients whose tibial fractures had been treated by osteosynthesis and who had died of unrelated causes one month later and three months later respectively.

At the same time Perren (1967) in Davos, another co-worker of the AO, showed by means of strain-gauges applied to a tension plate which held an experimental metatarsal osteotomy (in a sheep) rigidly immobilized under compression, that the tension in the plate dissipated very slowly over a period of 12 to 16 weeks, and that some tension was still present after sound union had occurred. Thus he demonstrated that it is possible to maintain axial compression in cortical bone for a period of time longer than that usually necessary for cortical union.

The AO principles of compression-internal fixation are based on the histological findings of Schenk, the biomechanical experiments of Perren with strain-gauges, and on the enormous experience gained from thorough documentation and evaluation in over 12,000 fractures, 500 non-unions, 2,500 osteotomies and 500 arthrodeses. The AO armamentarium allows one to apply compression to the fragments in nearly all bone operations and fractures. This method affords such great stability that in adults post-operative plaster immobilization has been almost totally abandoned. This fundamental change in post-operative management allowed us to extend our operative indications much more widely; patients whose obesity, precarious cardiac status or other constitutional disorder did not permit post-operative plaster immobilization could now be operated on. We have also spectacularly lowered the hospitalization time to a few days or at the most a few weeks. This in turn has permitted a much greater patient turnover and a statistically more significant follow-up of results. As our patients are able to begin pain-free joint motion on the first post-operative day, thorough joint mobilization and physiotherapy have become feasible. Our physiotherapists are now able to concentrate on the prophylaxis of thrombophlebitis through early motion. This has resulted in thromboembolic phenomena being a very rare complication in our clinics.

We have learned through experience that there are three basic methods of internal fixation by means of compression. These are:

(1) Compression osteosynthesis by means of screws alone, or by screws combined with a neutralization or support plate.
(2) Compression osteosynthesis by means of the application of the "tension band" principle; either by using a suitably placed cerclage wire, or by means of straight or right-angled plates to which tension can be applied with a special device.
(3) Compression osteosynthesis by means of Charnley clamps or dual plates under tension.

All these three techniques are most suitable for the handling of cancellous bone. Experience with diaphyseal fractures has taught us, however, that the first two methods are equally applicable to cortical bone: one prerequisite for success with cortical bone is that the fragments must be viable.

Principle 1: Compression by Means of Screws, or Screws Combined with a Neutralization Plate

CANCELLOUS BONE

If a screw is employed to fix a fracture near the end of a bone, then the screw must have a thread only at its distal end; for the fracture can be compressed only if the entire thread is embedded in the distal fragment. The illustrations (see Fig. 1) indicate how such a cancellous lag screw is employed in different types of cancellous fractures.

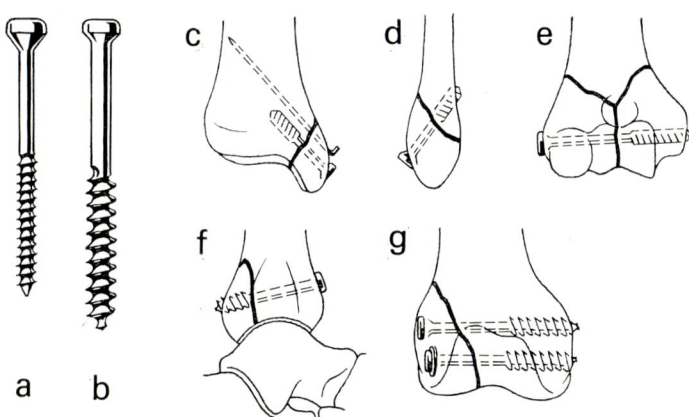

FIG. 1. When using cancellous bone screws the thread must not cross the fracture line.

(a) Malleolar screw with a 4·5 mm. thread.
(b) Lag screw with a 7 mm. thread.
(c) Fracture of the medial malleolus: two screws or a lag screw and a Kirschner wire may be used.
(d) Fractured lateral malleolus fixed with one oblique screw.
(e) Distal humeral fracture: the first step is the restoration of the joint surface.
(f) Posterior triangle of Volkmann: fixed with one screw from front to back.
(g) Fracture of the lateral condyle of the femur: two large cancellous bone screws are used.

CORTICAL BONE

To obtain fixation of cortical bone the screws must have a thread extending the full length of their shaft; for, if a screw with only a distal thread is used, at removal an inevitable fracture of the screw shaft results when high torque is applied, because the screw thread cannot cut its way in reverse through cortical bone.

In order to obtain a lag effect with cortical screws, the proximal bone cortex must be drilled to such a size that the thread of the screw does not engage (Fig. 2).

When the principle of compression osteosynthesis by means of screws combined with a neutralization or support plate is considered, other factors also must be taken into account. If one attempts to immobilize a diaphyseal fracture (e.g. of a tibial shaft) with screws alone, then rigid and secure compression osteosynthesis is only possible in those cases where the fracture line is at least twice as long as the diameter of the shaft (see Fig. 3).

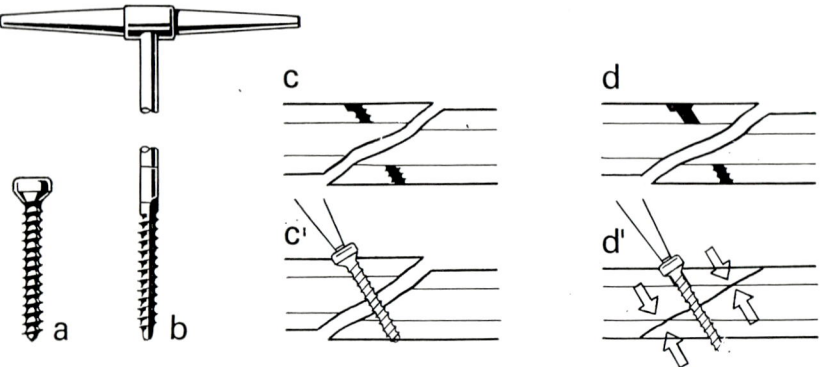

FIG. 2. The principle of applying compression with a cortical screw.
  (a) AO cortical bone screw with an outer diameter of 4·5 mm. The stress bearing surface of the thread is at a right angle to the axis of the screw. The thread in the bone for this screw must be cut with a tap. In this way the drill hole in the bone can be made slightly larger than the stem of the screw. The diameter of the stem is 3 mm. The diameter of the drill hole is 3·2 mm. This screw has a hexagonal recess in the head. In this way the screw is firmly held by the screwdriver without any special holding device which is a considerable advantage when it comes to removing the screw.
  (b) The tap is very sharp.
  (c) When the drill hole traversing both fragments has the same size and if the thread is tapped in both fragments (or if a self-tapping screw is used) then the fragments can never come together. The screw will break before the slightest approximation of the fragments is possible (c').
  (d) If on the other hand the drill hole in the first cortex is of the same width as the thread of the screw, the thread of the screw does not engage the proximal cortex; it gains a purchase only on the distal cortex and as soon as the screw is tightened the fragments are approximated and brought under compression (d').

If the fracture line is shorter, screw fixation must be supplemented with a neutralization plate which bridges the fracture and is fixed to both main fragments. The fixation must be such that at least $2\frac{1}{2}$ screws grip each of the main fragments (Fig. 4). In the tibia the neutralization plate must be placed on the medial aspect.

Principle 2: Compression by Means of a Tension Band

The principle of the tension band is such that all tensile stresses are neutralized by means of a cerclage wire or a plate, and in this way the fragments are strongly compressed. The proper position of the wire or plate is of the utmost importance.

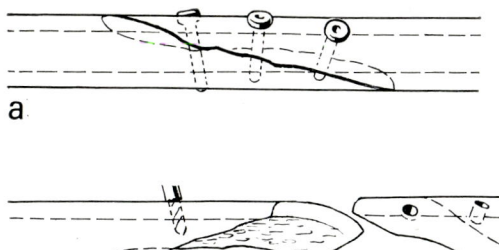

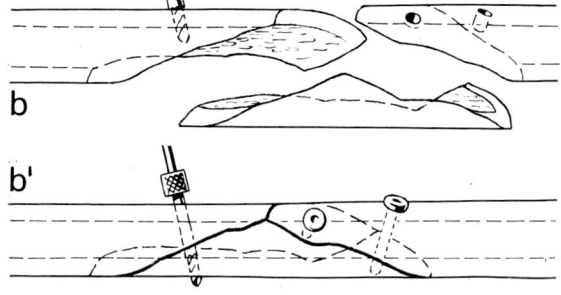

Fig. 3. Diaphyseal fractures of the tibia fixed by means of screw alone. The facture lines are at least twice as long as the diameter of the bone. Positioning of the screws:
(a) In a long spiral or oblique fracture one screw must always be introduced at right angles to the long axis of the bone. The other two screws are placed so that one is more anterior and the other more posterior.
(b) Usually the 4·5 mm. holes in the first cortex are drilled in the correct position before reduction.
(b') A simple torsion wedge: one screw immobilizes the main fragments, the other screws are inserted in such a way that they bisect the angle formed between lines dropped perpendicularly to the plane of the fracture and to the long axis of the bone. All these screws should be tightened only when they are well seated and only when the reduction is perfect.

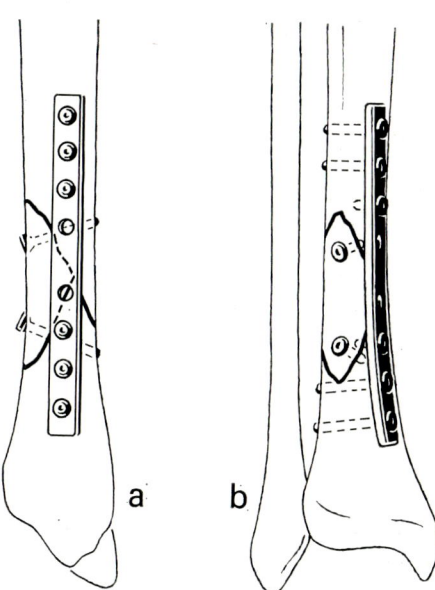

Fig. 4. The principle of the neutralizing plate used for torsion fractures with a short wedge fragment.

(a and b) After applying compression to the butterfly fragment by means of three screws the plate is applied across the fracture in order to fix the two main fragments. Two to three screws at each end are usually sufficient. It is quite obvious that in the region of the fracture line one must not introduce any screws through the holes in the plate.

TENSION CERCLAGE

It is common knowledge that if a patellar fracture is treated by cerclage with the wire in the middle (coronal plane) the fragments always open up anteriorly. If on the other hand the cerclage is placed anteriorly, all the distracting forces are transformed into compressive stresses and immediate joint mobilization is possible (see Fig. 5). The reduction is

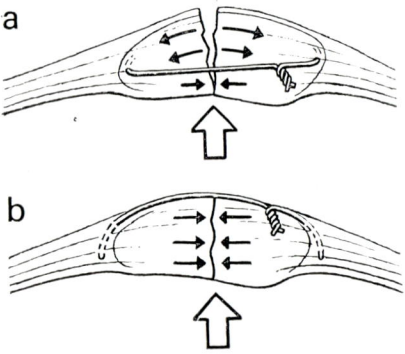

FIG. 5. Application of the tension band principle in fractures of the patella.

(a) If the wire is placed in the centre of the patella, then the fragments must open up anteriorly, a fact which can be observed in simple wire cerclage.
(b) If on the other hand the wire is placed anteriorly, as was originally suggested by Steinmann in 1919, then all the tension stresses are converted into compressive stresses. Active movements can be started immediately after operation.

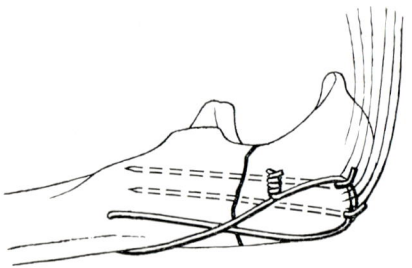

FIG. 6. The tension band principle in fractures of the olecranon.

After accurate reduction and stabilization of the fragments with two Kirschner wires the tension band is applied in such a way that the wire passes under the triceps tendon, is crossed, and passed through a hole in the ulna.

stable and no displacement occurs. It is even possible to treat communited fractures of the patella in this way. If in addition to the distracting forces rotational stresses are present, as in a fracture of the olecranon (see Fig. 6), then the tension band should be combined with two or three Kirschner wires which are used only to neutralize the rotational stresses.

TENSION PLATE

Whenever a plate is used as a tension band, compression is applied with the special tension device: the three varieties are a straight plate, a right-angled blade plate, or a cross-plate (see Fig. 7). The main indication for using a straight tension plate is non-union of the humerus, or of the forearm. In the lower extremity, the straight tension plate can be used for non-union of the tibia (see Fig. 8). If the tibia is varus, which is the common deformity, then the plate must be applied to the lateral aspect of the tibia, as this is the tension side of the bone, and only on this side can the tensile stresses be neutralized. With valgus deformity, the plate has to be placed on the medial side; and with posterior bowing, the plate

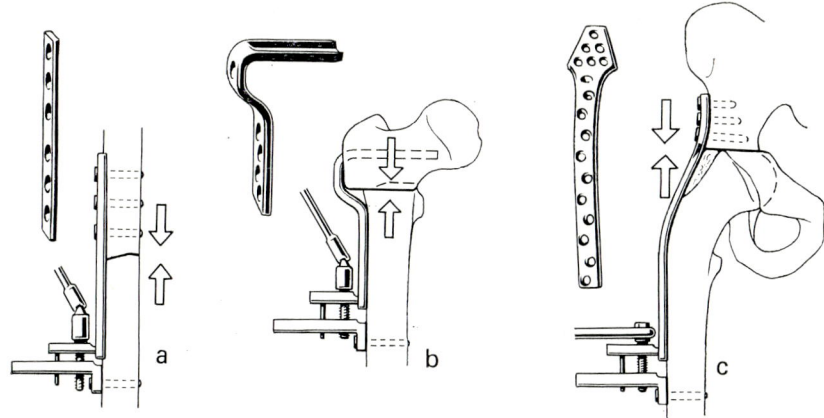

FIG. 7. Tension band principle using a plate and a tension device.
(a) Straight plate: the plate is first fixed to one fragment of the reduced fracture or non-union. The tension device is then screwed 18 mm. from the plate on the other fragment with its hook inserted in the end hole of the plate. With a cardan-key the screw of the tension device is turned, which brings the plate under tension and the fragments under compression. After the screws have been put through the remaining holes of the plates, the tension device is removed.
(b) Right-angled plate in an intertrochanteric osteotomy.
(c) The special cross plate used in hip arthrodesis is brought under tension after the proximal portion of the plate is fixed to the pelvis.

is placed posteriorly. Other indications for straight plates employed as tension bands are for fractures of the forearm (see Fig. 9) and in arthrodesis of the wrist. The cross plate is used as a tension band for arthrodesis of the hip (Fig. 7c). An arthrodesis with such a plate is so stable that after 10 days the patient can be up and about without any plaster fixation and is able to walk quite freely with partial weight-bearing. When such a hip arthrodesis is performed, it is combined with a pelvic osteotomy at which the lower or inferior fragment is displaced medially. The right-angled blade plate has found tremendous use in hip surgery. It is particu-

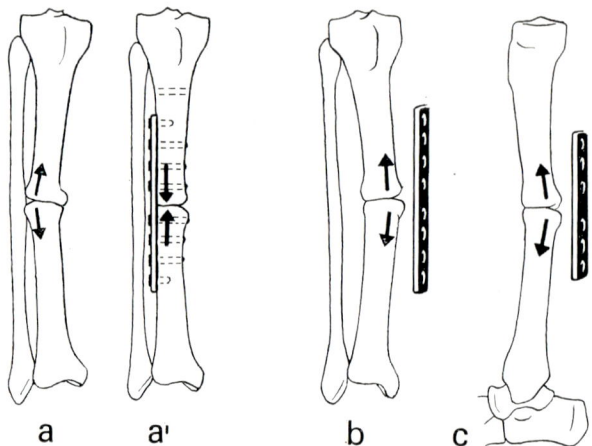

Fig. 8. In a pseudarthrosis of the tibia, the deformity clearly indicates on which side the tension forces are acting: it is on that side that the plate must be applied.

(a) Most often there is a varus deformity. The plate must then be applied to the lateral side. The plate is placed under very high tension which not only corrects the deformity, but at the same time places the fragments under compression (a′).

(b) With a valgus deformity the plate must be applied on the medial aspect of the tibia.

(c) With posterior bowing at the non-union the plate must be applied on the posterior surface of the tibia.

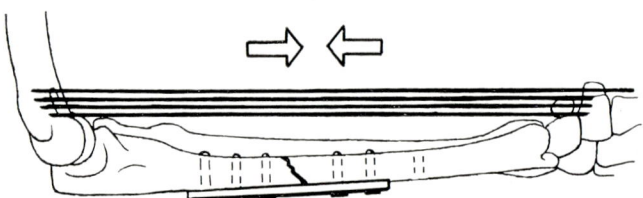

Fig. 9. In the forearm the dorsal side is under tensile stress, which explains why bowing with a gap on that side occurs. The plate must therefore be placed on the dorsal aspect.

larly useful in intertrochanteric osteotomies. The stability obtained with such a plate is so great that nearly all patients can be mobilized within a few days and non-union is virtually unknown (see Fig. 7b and Figs. 10, 11 and 12).

When the right-angled blade plate is used, it is of the utmost importance to appreciate that the blade of the plate must be properly oriented in three planes. There is a very simple method to determine the position of the blade, but the surgeon must calculate the correction very accurately in all three planes before operation. It is best to prepare a drawing before the operation is begun. The frontal plane is that of the A-P X-ray and gives the valgus or the varus angle between the shaft and blade of the plate. The horizontal plane or the axial direction of the blade is given by the direction of the long axis of the femoral neck. In order to place the blade of the plate in the long axis of the neck, it suffices simply to place a Kirschner wire along the anterior surface of the femoral neck, and this serves as a guide.

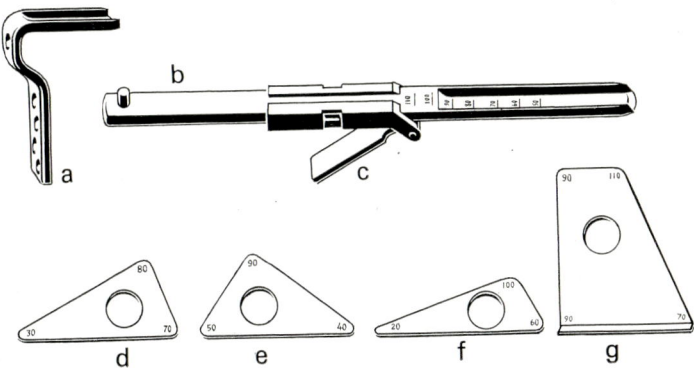

FIG. 10. Instruments for application of the right-angle blade plate.
(a) The standard right-angle blade plate for intertrochanteric osteotomy.
(b) The special chisel, with the same profile as the blade of the plate, is of equal width from the tip to its end, and is graduated on both sides.
(c) On to this chisel one can fix a directional side plate which enables one to determine flexion and extension.
(d, e, f and g) Triangles used to determine the angle between the femoral diaphysis and the directional chisel for the blade.

The sagittal plane is determined from the lateral aspect, and equals the flexion or the extension at the osteotomy. In the treatment of osteoarthritis of the hip, one must almost always perform an extension osteotomy, i.e. the proximal fragment must be allowed to flex. A direction device clamped to the special chisel which cuts the groove for the blade of the plate allows one to determine the angle between the long axis of the shaft and the blade of the plate, and in this way one can determine the extension or flexion which will be produced at the osteotomy site.

Principle 3: Bilateral Compression

One can apply bilateral compression either with two plates or with Charnley clamps. This technique is used in arthrodesis of the knee, the ankle and the shoulder and in osteotomies of the proximal and distal tibia.

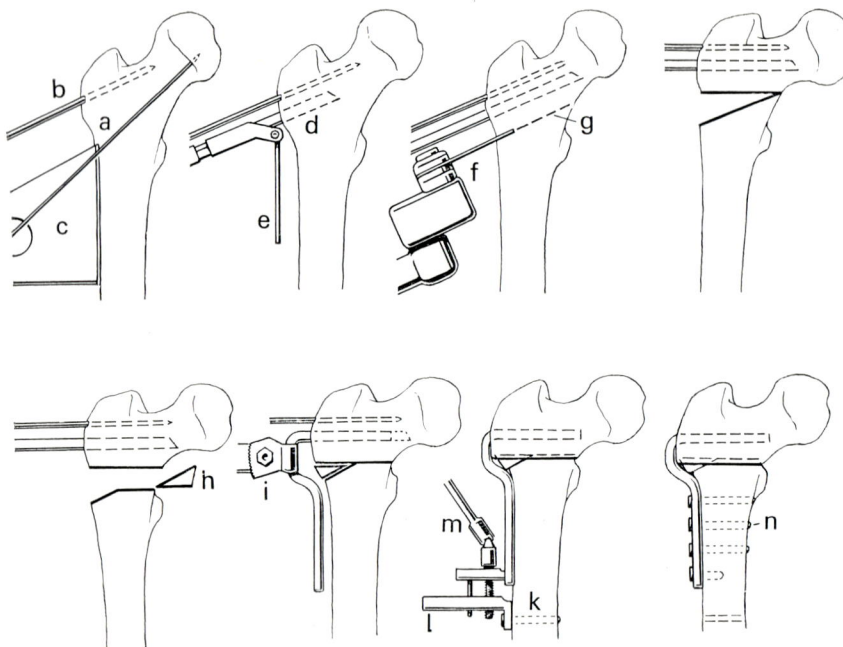

FIG. 11. Technique of intertrochanteric varus osteotomy for coxa valga luxans. The thin Kirschner wire (a) is placed on the neck of the femur and indicates the anteversion of the neck. The thick Kirschner wire (b) is parallel to the first one in the plane of the femoral neck and indicates in the frontal plane the direction of the blade plate. If a correction of 20° is decided upon prior to operation, this wire must be introduced at 70° to the shaft. Triangle (c) applied on the diaphysis shows this angle.

Underneath and parallel to the wire (b) the special chisel (d) is driven into the neck. The guide (e) indicates the direction of the plate in the sagittal direction. Usually a small amount of extension is necessary. By means of an air powered motor saw (f) the femur is osteotomized in the intertrochanteric region. The osteotomy line (g) is parallel to the chisel. After wide opening of the osteotomy line the triangle (h) is cut by an oscillating saw.

The chisel (d) is then taken out of the neck and the right-angle blade-plate, fixed by means of a holder (i), is driven into the prepared channel in the neck. 15–18 mm. from the end of the plate a hole (k) is drilled in the femoral shaft and tapped. The tension apparatus (l) is screwed on and its hook introduced into the last hole of the plate. By means of the cardan wrench (m) the large screw of the tension device is turned as much as possible to bring both osteotomy surfaces under compression. After fixation of the plate by means of screws (n) the tension apparatus is removed.

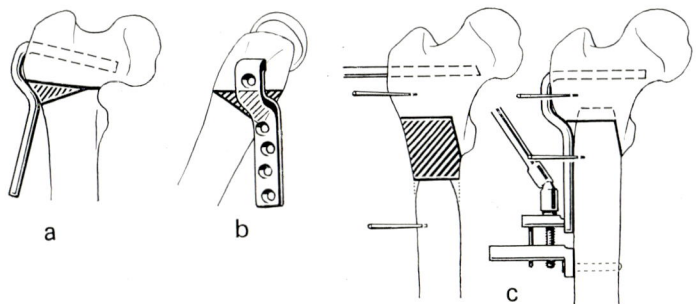

Fig. 12. Application of the right-angle blade-plate and excision of the bone triangle.
(a) For an abduction osteotomy.
(b) For an extension osteotomy.
(c) For shortening the femoral diaphysis in the inter- and subtrochanteric region.

Summary:

For several years now the histological and biomechanical pattern of the healing of bone fragments under compression has been known. Three principles involved in compression techniques have been studied and described.

The technique of intertrochanteric varus osteotomy has been described in greater detail as osteoarthritis of the hip is one of the most common problems in orthopaedics.

All the techniques indicated and many others which could not be discussed in this chapter have been described at length in the latest book on AO techniques.

References

CAMERON, B. (1966). Shaft fractures and pseudarthroses. Springfield: C. Thomas.
CHARNLEY, J. (1953). Compression arthrodesis. Including central dislocation as a principle in hip surgery. Edinburgh: E. & S. Livingstone Ltd.
DANIS, R. (1947). Théorie et pratique de l'ostéosynthèse. Paris: Masson & Cie.
KROMPECHER, S. (1937). Die knochenbildung. Jena: Gustav Fischer.
MÜLLER, M. E. (1963). Internal fixation for fresh fractures and for non-union. Proceedings of the Royal Society of Medicine, Vol. 56, No. 6.
  (1966). Treatment of non-unions by compression. Clinical Orthopaedics, No. 43.
  (1967). Hip Surgery, Twelve Hip Procedures, AO-Bulletin.
MÜLLER, M. E., ALLGÖWER M. and WILLENEGGER H. (1965). Technique of internal fixation of fractures. Springer-Verlag.
  (1969). Manual des osteosynthese. Heidelberg: Springer-Verlag.
PERREN, ST. (1967). AO-course Davos.
SCHENK, R. and H. WILLENEGGER. (1963). Zur Biomechanik der Frakturheilung. Experientia (Basel), **20**, 593.
TRUETA, J. (1963). The role of the vessels in osteogenesis. *J. Bone Jt. Surg.*, **45B**, 402.
  (1966). Congress in Paris. Discussion on bone healing.

Chapter 5

SILICONES IN ORTHOPAEDIC SURGERY

B. HELAL

History. At the turn of the century Frederick Stanley Kipping (Fig. 1) then Professor of Chemistry in the University of Nottingham, discovered and named silicone. His interest in attaching organic radicles to the silicon atom continued for some 45 years of his life and he published over 50 papers on this subject. In 1937 he foresaw no practical application

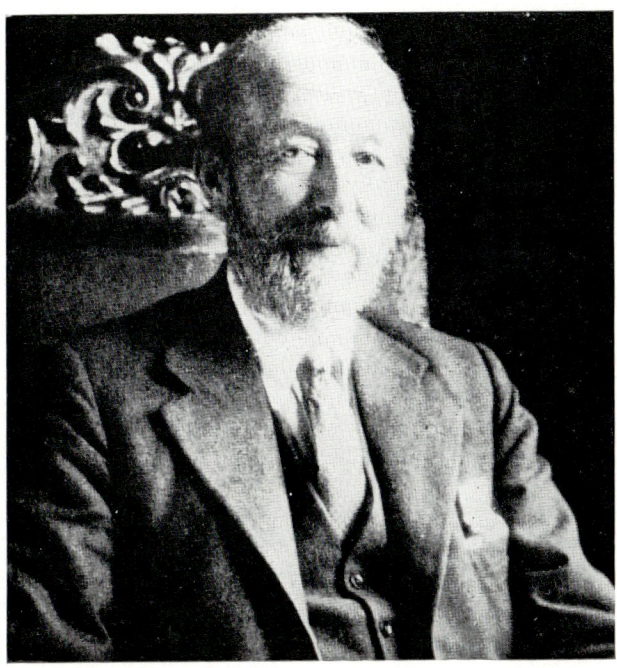

FIG. 1. Frederick Stanley Kipping, the discoverer of silicone. (By kind permission of Dow Corning Co.)

for the compounds he had discovered. By 1942, however, silicone was being used as an ignition seal for fighter aircraft (Levin 1958). Much of the further development of these silicones took place in the United States and in the main by the Dow Corning Corporation of Michigan which was especially interested in their development for medical use.

The synthesis of silicone. The starting point is a sand and carbon mixture which is heated to 1000° Centigrade. Chlorine gas is then introduced; this results in the production of Silicon-tetrachloride, a highly reactive and unstable compound. If one or more of the Chloride radicles is then replaced by an organic radicle a stable substance results. The substitution is achieved by mixing with an organo-magnesium halide, when a polymer is formed whose basic formula is

$$CH_3-\underset{\underset{CH_3}{|}}{\overset{\overset{CH_3}{|}}{Si}}-O-\underset{\underset{CH_3}{|}}{\overset{\overset{CH_3}{|}}{Si}} \text{ etc.}$$

This polymer, the simplest form of silicone, known as Dimethylpolysiloxane, is an oily fluid. The longer the polymer chain is made the more viscous does the fluid become. The measure of viscosity is known as the *Centistoke value*, Centistoke 1 having an equivalent viscosity to water. By the addition of ferric or aluminium chloride, gels are formed; when these are oxidized (using hydrogen peroxide) rubbers are formed which are known as Silastics (Levin 1958).

Physical and chemical properties. Silicone fluids and silastics are heat stable and chemically non-reactive. They are slippery, non-adhesive, water repellent and have foam-breaking properties. The rubbers do not weather or harden and the soft grades will withstand test bending without fatigue almost indefinitely. These remarkable properties account for the wide industrial application of silicone derivatives.

Physiological properties. The chemical stability of the silicones explains their physiological inertness. They appear to excite little or no inflammatory or immunological reaction in living tissues (Andrews 1966, Ballantyne *et al.* 1965, Cutting 1952, Kern *et al.* 1949, McGregor 1960, Polemann *et al.* 1953, Rowe *et al.* 1948). Oxygen is ten times more soluble in silicone fluid than in water. Fish will survive indefinitely in fluid silicone, and even small mammals immersed in and breathing the liquid can survive for periods up to 6 hours (Clark *et al.* 1966). Membranes made of silastic have the strange ability of facilitating gaseous exchange between fluid and gas and may be the basis for developing an artificial gill for divers, an artificial lung (Bodell *et al.* 1965), a placenta (Sarin *et al.* 1966) and even artificial red blood corpuscles (Chang 1966). The same property has also led to the experimental administration of gas anaesthetics intravenously (Folkman *et al.* 1966).

The fate of parenteral silicone. Silicone fluid introduced into animals is partly taken up by the reticulo-endothelial system (Ballantyne *et al.* 1965, Brown *et al.* 1953, 1960, Hodge *et al.* 1949, McGregor 1954, Rees *et al.* 1967, Rowe *et al.* 1948, 1950, Winer *et al.* 1964), but some is completely excreted. The route of excretion has not been fully established because the only reliable way to trace this is by the use of the silicon isotope which unfortunately has a very short life. The implanted silastics become enveloped by a capsule of endothelial cells and, apart from this, cause no serious reaction.

Toxicity in animals. Silicone has been tested on the skin (Bickmore *et al.* 1951, Von Kennel 1952), implanted into subcutaneous tissues

(Ballantyne *et al.* 1965, Rees *et al.* 1967) and muscle (Paul *et al.* 1960), given by mouth (Largent *et al.* 1950, Rowe *et al.* 1948, 1950), intravenously (Helal 1968), implanted into the eyeball (Armaly *et al.* 1962, Cibis *et al.* 1962, Fedorov *et al.* 1965, Hopping 1965) and into the peritoneal cavity (Aboulafia *et al.* 1967, Del Rosario *et al.* 1966) and inhaled (Clark *et al.* 1966, Nickerson *et al.* 1953, 1954, 1955, Pattle 1956, Princiotto *et al.* 1952, Rosenbluth *et al.* 1952, Treon *et al.* 1951)—all without ill effect.

Toxicity in man. In man reactions have occurred only with the use of impure compounds (Winer *et al.* 1964). Because of its non-reactiveness the fluid tends to drift in the tissues and some workers have deliberately added organic oils hoping to stimulate a fibrotic reaction which might localize the silicone fluid (Kagan 1963). Because it is an oil and viscous there exists the possibility of embolic effects if it is introduced directly into the circulation (vide infra). The silastics are easily contaminated by handling and great care should be taken to cleanse them by boiling in detergent followed by rinsing with distilled water before they are sterilized by autoclaving.

General Uses in Man

SILICONE FLUID

This has been extensively used in many branches of medicine:

(1) To lubricate syringes and other instruments (Levin 1958).
(2) As a pharmaceutical vehicle for drugs (Levin 1958).
(3) On the skin as a protective and a water repellent (Bateman 1956, Berger 1966, Bickmore *et al.* 1951, Brusca 1956, Finnerty 1954, Goodman 1955, Plein *et al.* 1953, Suskind 1955, Talbot *et al.* 1951, Tapline *et al.* 1966, Von Kennel 1952).
(4) As a floating bath for burns (Miller *et al.* 1965, Weeder *et al.* 1967).
(5) It has been injected subcutaneously to effect facial and mammary recontouring (Ashley *et al.* 1967, Brown *et al.* 1953, 1960, Fomon *et al.* 1966, Harris 1964, Hoopes *et al.* 1966, Rees *et al.* 1966) and to eliminate wrinkles (Lebon 1966).
(6) In heart-lung machines and in states of pulmonary oedema it has been used as a defoaming agent (Lillehei 1956, Melrose 1953, Nickerson *et al.* 1953, 1954, 1955, Princiotto *et al.* 1952, Rosenbluth *et al.* 1952).
(7) In the bowel fluid silicones have been used as a protective for peptic ulcers and as an antiflatulant (Cohen *et al.* 1966, Largent *et al.* 1950, Nickerson *et al.* 1953, 1954, 1955, Rowe *et al.* 1948, 1950).
(8) Introduced into peritoneal and pleural cavities it prevents adhesions (Aboulafia *et al.* 1967, Furman *et al.* 1966, Malette *et al.* 1965).
(9) Ophthalmologically it has been used as a lubricant for artificial eyes (Morgan *et al.* 1964) and as a replacement for the vitreous in the treatment of retinal detachment (Cibis *et al.* 1962, Federov *et al.* 1965, Hopping 1965).

SILASTICS

These have been produced in the form of sheets (Fig. 2), sponges and rubbers of varying grades of hardness (Fig. 3). They are in wide use:

(1) For intravenous catheters (Fletcher 1956), urinary catheters (Sankey et al. 1962), surgical drains for hydrocephalus (Carrington 1959) and for wound drainage (Waugh et al. 1961).

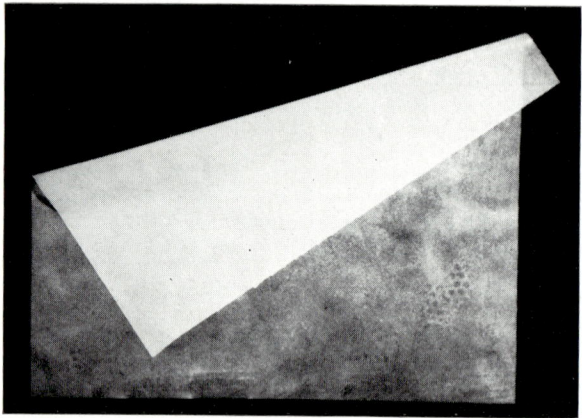

FIG. 2. Silastic sheeting.

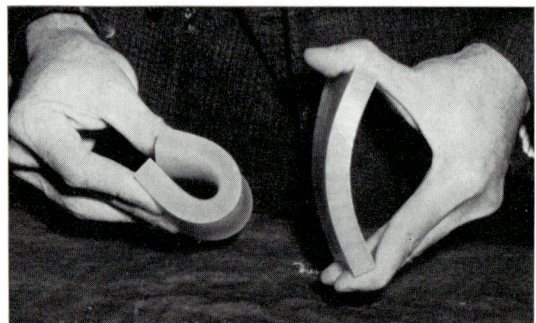

FIG. 3. Silicone rubbers of different grades of hardness.

(2) Reinforced by fabrics they have even been used to replace the ureter (Lewis et al. 1966), the urethra (Sankey et al. 1962), bile duct (Bradley et al. 1967), oesophagus (Fryfogle et al. 1963), and arteries (Crawford et al. 1958, Donovan 1949, Egdahl 1955).
(3) Silastic sheeting has been used as a dural prosthesis (Wallace 1960).
(4) Reinforced with fabrics they have been used as an artificial diaphragm (Folkman 1965) and mechanical heart (Akutsu et al. 1966).
(5) Artificial lenses (Bowen 1962), ear drums (Jaypathy 1960), ears (Cronin 1966), noses (Millard 1967, Patterson 1966), breasts (Fredericks 1966, Taylor 1967) and testes (Prentiss et al. 1963);

even a penile prosthesis (Pearman *et al.* 1967) has been made from silastics.

Orthopaedic Application of Silicone Fluid

My interest in silicone oil began early in 1965. I was anxious that the pre-operative mobilization and muscle rehabilitation of rheumatoid joints destined for arthroplasty should become a less painful process. These arthritic joints are commonly of the dry, grating, 'catching' variety and it was felt that a lubricant would help to make exercises more tolerable and so help to achieve better post-operative results. A bland non-reactive, non-immunogenic oil of suitable viscosity would prove ideal and liquid silicone fulfilled these criteria.

Experiments. Animal experiments were carried out in collaboration with Dr. Murray Brookes of Guy's Hospital to confirm the bland nature

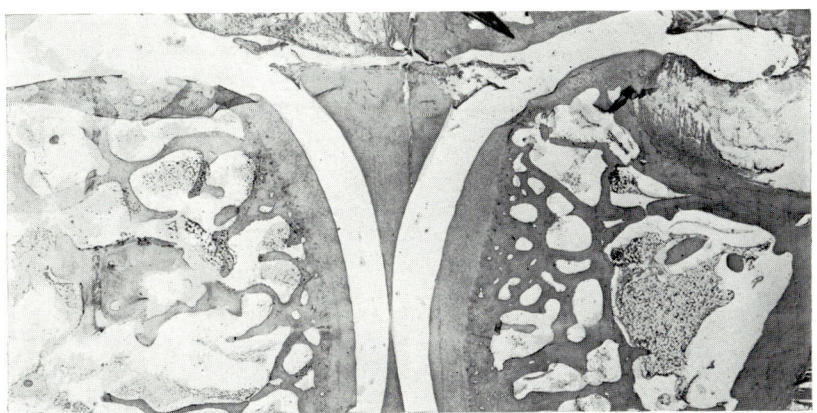

FIG. 4. This rabbit knee joint has contained silicone fluid for 4 months. No abnormality could be detected.

of the fluid, with special regard to its effect on joints. I was conscious of the fact that coating the joint surfaces with oil might interfere with cartilage nutrition. The 200 centistoke pure silicone oil proved the most useful type. Using the rabbit as an experimental animal, joints were injected and examined macroscopically and histologically over a period varying from 1 week to 4 months. No damage of any kind was noted in these joints (Fig. 4). To establish the effect of silicone on the presence of inflammation a chemical acute arthritis was induced by the injection of 10 per cent Phenol into rabbits' knees. One knee was then treated with silicone and there was reduction of adhesion formation in this joint.

The embolic effects were also tested. Amounts rising from 1 ml. to 5 ml. were given intravenously to rabbits. Deaths were constant with 5 ml. and occurred occasionally with 4 ml. There were no deaths with smaller amounts. The fluid mixes easily on very slight agitation with synovial fluids present in various pathological conditions and separates again over a period of 2 to 4 hours. It appears to separate at different rates for different forms of effusion. If this proves constant it may provide the basis for a simple diagnostic test.

An interesting finding was that silicone takes with it the light joint debris as it separates from synovial fluid. The injection of silicone into a joint is followed by a short period of exercise; then the joint is held still in a suitable position for 4 hours after which time the silicone is removed again by aspiration. This has proved a useful way to debride the joint and produces a satisfactory clinical response.

Clinical Trial

Two hundred and forty-two patients have been treated by injection with silicone oil. The first 15 patients to be treated clinically were subjected to extensive testing; they were assessed before treatment and at

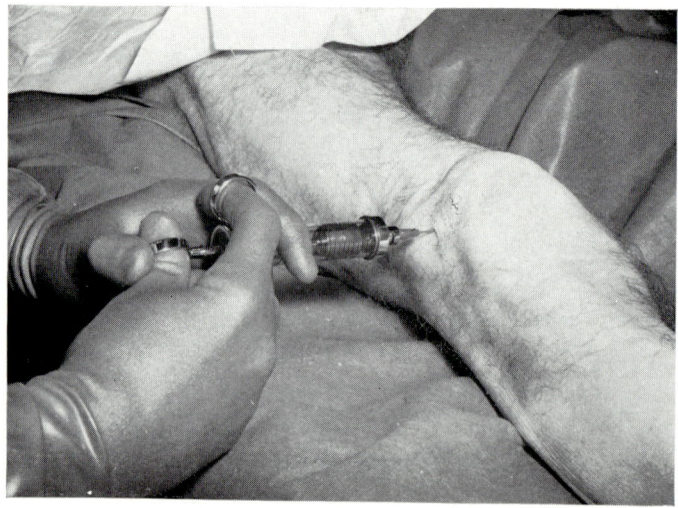

FIG. 5. A three-ring Luer-Lok syringe facilitates injection of the viscid silicone oil through a No. 1 needle.

three-monthly intervals for a year after the injections of silicone. Apart from detailed general physical and orthopaedic examinations, comprehensive blood tests, cardiovascular, respiratory, renal and liver function tests were carried out. No changes in the results of these tests were detected following the silicone injections. The first 31 patients were selected from those awaiting surgery for arthritis and who had already received the full range of conservative treatments. All these patients have been followed up for at least 18 months. Routine mobilizing and muscle strengthening exercises were given to these patients both before and after the injections.

The results of the first 31 patients are detailed (Table 1). Despite the fact that many are elderly there have been no deaths in the total series of 242 patients.

Technique. Silicone fluid of 200 centistoke viscosity is used. It is sterilized by heating to 160° centigrade for one hour and is then stored in sealed sterile bottles ready for use. Under aseptic conditions a number 1 or larger needle on a syringe containing 1 per cent Xylocaine is used to anaesthetize the skin and to ensure that the needle is in the joint. This cannot be done with the syringe charged with oil because the viscosity prevents free suction on the needle. When correctly sited the needle is left in place and a 3 ring Luer-Lok syringe containing the silicone oil is screwed on and the injection is given (Fig. 5). Enough oil is introduced to distend the joint moderately. In a knee, for example, enough is introduced to float the patella off the femoral condyles; usually 10–15 ml. suffices. The shortest period observed before disappearance of the fluid is four months—some patients still retain silicone in the joint at 18 months from the date of injection.

Other Orthopaedic Uses for Silicone Fluid

The damaged hand. Silicone oil has been used as a floating bath for burns and is particularly valuable in the treatment of burns of the hand where it has been used as a medium in which the burnt hand can be exercised. On the analogy of its use in burns it has been employed in dealing with the crushed or degloved hand (Fig. 6).

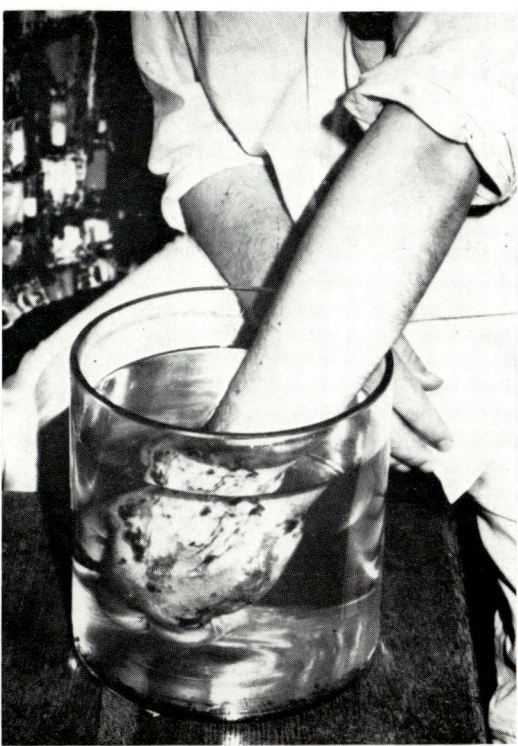

FIG. 6. This patient is exercising his degloved hand in a silicone bath. The process is painless.

TABLE I

Joint	Side	Disease	Sex	Age	Admission for:	Amount injected in ml. × no. of injections	Pain Before	Pain After	Movement Before	Movement After	Crepitus Before	Crepitus After	Other Procedures
1. Shoulder Shoulder	R L	Rh	F	56	Arthrodesis Injection	8×2 8	+++ ++	— 0	Abd. 40 100	80 140	++ ++	— —	
2. Shoulder	R	Rh	F	66	Arthrodesis	10	+++	—	60	90	++	—	
3. Shoulder	R	Rh	M	75	Arthrodesis	12×3	+++	—	50	100	++	0	
4. Elbow	R	Rh	F	55	Excision Arthroplasty	5	+++	0	20–70	10–100	++	0	
5. Elbow	L	Rh	F	61	Excision Arthroplasty	8×2	+++	—	15–70	15–90	+	—	Excision head radius only
6. Elbow	R	Rh	F	52	Excision Arthroplasty	5×2	+++	—	15–50	15–70	+	—	
7. Wrist	R	Rh	F	36	Arthrodesis	4	++	—	Ave ½ range + 10–20 all directions		+	—	
Wrist	L	Rh				6	++	0	Ave ½ range + 10–20 all directions		+	—	
8. Wrist	R	Rh	F	41	Arthrodesis	6	+++	=	Ave ¼ range − ¼ range		+	—	Arthrodesis
9. Wrist	R	Rh	F	44	Arthrodesis	4×3	++	0	Ave ¾ range to full range		+	—	
10. C/MC/Thumb	R	OA	F	56	Excision Trapez.	½	+++	0	No change		+	—	
11. C/MC/Thumb	R	OA	F	63	Excision Trapez.	½	+++	0	No change		—	—	
12. C/MC/Thumb	R	OA	M	44	Fusion	1	+++	0	No change		—	—	
13. C/MC/Thumb	R L	OA OA	F	75	Excision Trapez.	½ ½	+++ +++	0 0	No change		—	—	
14. Prox. I/P	R	Rh	F	66	Silastic Arthroplasties	¼ ¼	+++	=	No change		++	—	Silastic Arthroplasties
15. Hip	R L	Rh	M	56	Arthroplasty Synovectomy	6 6	+++ ++	— —	20–70 15–90	10–100 10–110	++	0	
16. Hip	R	Rh	F	66	Arthroplasty	6	+++	—	15–70	5–90	+	0	
17. Hip	R	Rh	F	72	Arthroplasty	4	+++	—	30–70	20–80	++	—	McKee Farrar Arthroplasty
18. Hip	L	Rh	M	78	Arthroplasty	5×2	+++	—	20–70	10–105	+	0	

							Pain	Crepitus	Range pre-op	Range post-op	Notes	Analgesics
19. Knee	R / L	Rh	F	54	Silastic Arthroplasty	10×2 / 12×2	+++ / +++	0 / –	20–90 / 15–90	10–110 / 5–105		– / –
20. Knee	R	OA	F	77	Trans Fib. Osteotomy	10	+++	–	15–100	5–120		–
21. Knee	R	Rh	F	77	Hinge Arthroplasty	10×2	++	–	10–100	10–110		0
22. Knee	R / L	Rh	M	68	Hinge / Hinge	10×2 / 10×3	+++ / ++	– / –	15–100 / 20–90	5–130 / 5–100		– / –
23. Knee	R / L	OA / OA	F	78	Arthroplasty Ex Patella / Silastic Arthroplasty	10 / 12×2	++ / +++	0 / –	15–80 / 10–80	10–100 / 10–100	Patellectomy	– / –
24. Knee	R / L	Rh / Rh	F	67	Fusion / Hinge Arthroplasty	10 / 10	+++ / +++	– / –	40–80 / 15–100	30–110 / 5–115		– / 0
25. Knee	R / L	Rh / Rh	F	72	Hinge Arthroplasty / Hinge Arthroplasty	10 / 10×2	++ / ++	– / –	15–100 / 30–85	5–120 / 15–105		– / –
26. Knee	R / L	Rh / Rh	F	80	Silastic Arthroplasty / Silastic Arthroplasty	8 / 8×2	+++ / ++	= / –	15–100 / 10–110	5–110 / 10–130	Silastic Arthroplasty	– / 0
27. Knee	R	Rh	F	65	Hinge Arthroplasty	15	+++	0	30–85	20–105		0
28. Knee	L	Rh	F	73	Fusion	10×2	+++	=	20–85	20–85	Arthrodesis	=
29. Knee	L	Rh	F	77	Hinge Arthroplasty	10	+++	0	30–90	30–120		0
30. Knee	R	Rh	M	60	Hinge Arthroplasty	15×2	+++	0	25–85	20–125		0
31. Knee	L	OA	F	58	Previously acrylic plug + patellectomy	10×3	++	0	10–100	5–120		0

Pain   Mild +   Pain free 0   Crepitus   Present +   Rh. Rheumatoid
        Mod. ++   Pain less –   Absent 0   OA. Osteoarthritis
        Severe +++   Pain same =   Less –

        Mild +   0 = No analgesics
        Moderate ++   – = Intermittent use of analgesics
        Severe +++   = Regular use of analgesics

Reproduced by kind permission of The Editor, The Annals of Physical Medicine (August 1968).

Plantar callosities. Balkin (1966) has described a method for treating plantar callosities which I have found remarkably effective: silicone fluid is injected between the callosity and the underlying bone to simulate the fat pad. This can be simply done under local anaesthesia. One patient, a postman, had been visiting a chiropodist twice-weekly for 19 years. After two injections four months apart, his callosities diminished and eventually disappeared (Fig. 7).

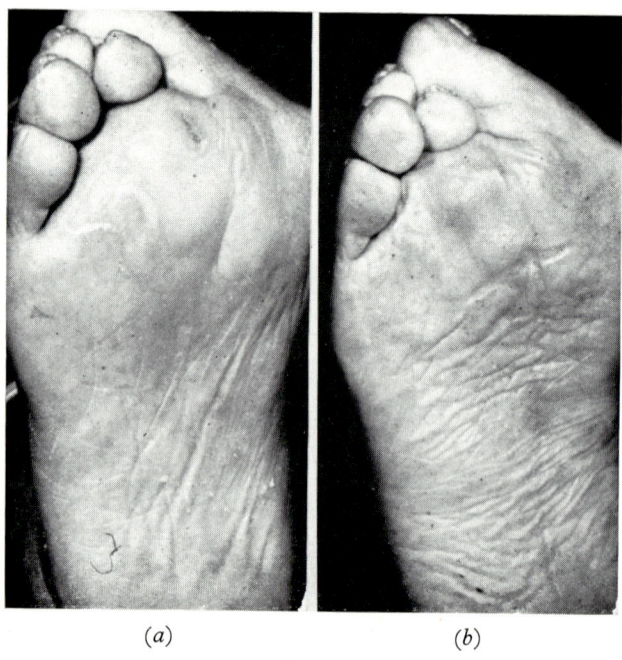

(a) (b)

FIG. 7.

(a) Painful plantar callosities.
(b) Three months after insertion of a liquid silicone cushion between the metatarsal head and the callosity as advocated by Balkin. The callosity and the symptoms have disappeared.

The frozen shoulder. We have used silicone fluid in patients with shoulder adhesions when other forms of conservative treatments have failed. The injection is followed by manipulation of the shoulder and has to date produced a good return of movement which has been maintained.

Protection of articular cartilage. The use of silicone oil as a joint surface protective in acute rheumatoid and haemophylic joints is being explored.

Skin protection. Silicone creams are used as protectives for the skin in chronic discharging sinuses and to protect pressure areas.

Orthopaedic Applications of Silastics

Wound drainage and intravenous infusions. Silastic tubing has been used by orthopaedic surgeons for vacuum wound drainage (Waugh *et al.* 1961) and for intravenous catheters (Fletcher 1956).

Skin loss. Silastic sheeting has been used as a temporary cover for burns (Chardack *et al.* 1961, Hall *et al.* 1966).

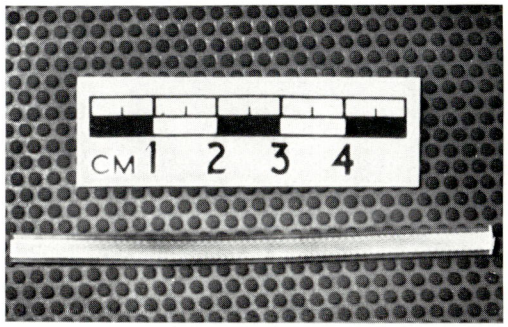

FIG. 8. A manufactured artificial tendon consisting of a woven dacron core encased in silastic.

Leprosy. Intrinsic wasting: an injectable form of self-vulcanizing silastic has been used to mask the intrinsic wasting of leprosy, a factor of considerable social consequence in lands where the disease is endemic (Enna 1966).

Perforating ulcers of the foot. Lennox (1965) has described a method of dealing with these by trimming of the bone underlying the ulcer and

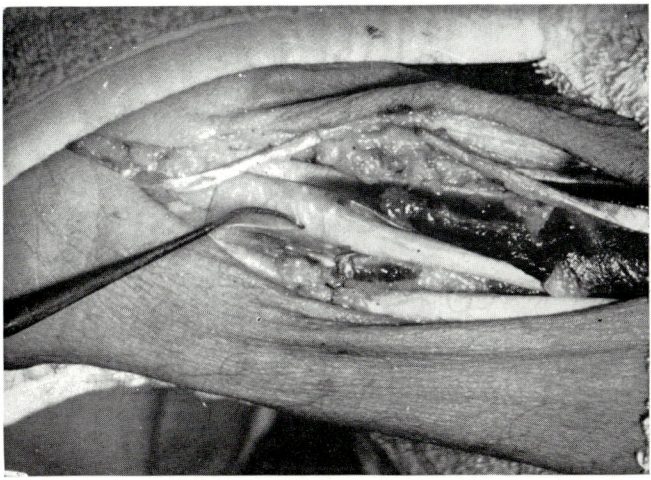

FIG. 9. Silastic membrane wrapped round the site of nerve suture to prevent adhesion between this and repaired adjacent tendons also severed at the same level.

inserting silastic sponge. He has obtained healing in a number of cases resistant to all other forms of treatment.

Tendon repair. Silastic sheeting has been wrapped around the sites of tendon repair to prevent adhesion formation (Ashley *et al.* 1964).

Silastic rods and artificial tendons made of silastic with a central core of dacron have been used as a preliminary to the usual autograft (Fig. 8)

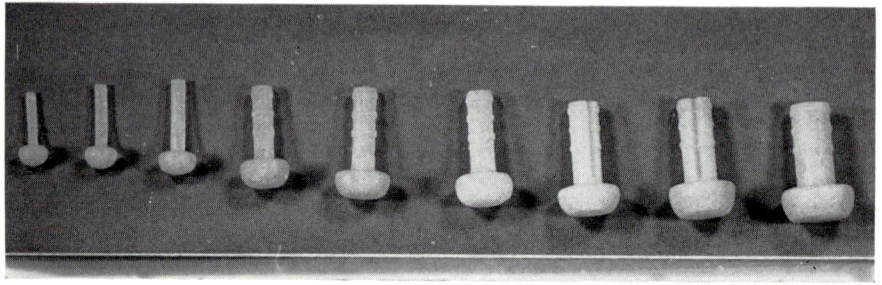

(a)

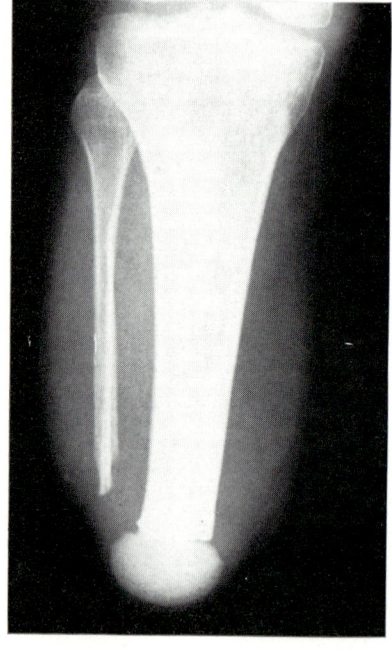

(b)

Fig. 10.
(a) Silastic amputation stump cushions.
(b) Stump cushion in place after a below knee amputation. (By kind permission of Dr. A. B. Swanson.)

particularly in circumstances where the flexor sheath has been obliterated over much of its length. Insertion of an artificial tendon for a few weeks promotes the formation of a smooth fibrous tunnel through which a normal tendon graft will function satisfactorily (Gaisford *et al.* 1966, Hunter 1965, Nicolle 1966).

Nerve repair. Silastic sheeting has been wrapped around the sites of nerve anastomosis to prevent adhesion formation (Campbell *et al.* 1964)

(Fig. 9). Nerve anastomosis without suture at the site of section has been achieved by enclosing the cut ends within silastic tubing and anchoring the nerve sheath to the tubing by stay sutures some way from the cut ends (Ducker et al. 1967). Eight cases of successful ulnar nerve repair by this method in humans are described by Morotomi et al. (1967).

Amputations. To improve the pressure tolerance of end bearing below and above knee stumps silastic pads have been devised by Swanson (1966) to cushion the bone ends. These he reports have greatly enhanced the weight bearing function of these amputated limbs (Swanson et al. 1967) (Fig. 10).

Stump neuromas. This sometimes intractable problem has been dealt with by silicone capping of the neuromas. Tauras et al. (1967) reports favourably on the results of animal experiments and described successes in five out of six patients with painful neuromata of the hand dealt with in this fashion.

A permanently attached artificial limb. Experimental work has been carried out by Hall et al. (1967) to try and create a functional artificial limb which is permanently attached to the amputee. The weight bearing function is a direct extension of the bone and the subject's muscles activate the limb. The only remaining problem to be overcome is the provision of a suitable permanent skin-to-prosthesis interface. Work is going on to find a suitable velour-reinforced silastic to achieve this.

Silastic Prostheses

The hand. In 1963 Brody and White described their experiments with artificial silastic interphalangeal joints of the roller type, i.e. the bone ends were fashioned to take a cylindrical block of silastic which acted as an interposition between the raw bone ends. They had little success with this method. Flatt also in 1963 described the use of a silastic interposition for use in the proximal interphalangeal joints of children since his metal hinge prosthesis was found unsuitable for use in children's finger joints.

Swanson (1966) in the Interclinic Information Bulletin describes a bi-stemmed prosthesis which he inserts after excision of the metacarpophalangeal joints in rheumatoid fingers (Fig. 11(1)). He states that "two years experience with these silastic implants in the hands of 14 patients of all ages have demonstrated that they can be a useful adjunct to the armamentarium of the hand surgeon". In a paper read to the American Academy of Orthopaedic Surgeons Meeting 1968 Swanson and Yamauchi stated that they had operated on 30 hands in 20 patients with rheumatoid arthritis. They have inserted a total of 114 implants. "Three patients have been re-operated for fracture of early designed implants. All patients have subsequently had greatly improved functional and cosmetic appearance with apparent good acceptance of the implant to host tissues. It is felt that the results are far superior to our previous experience with other techniques . . . with up to 75 per cent of normal motion with good stability."

The carpal bones. Silastic replacements of the trapezium, lunate and scaphoid bones have been carried out by Swanson and Yamauchi

(1968) but insufficient time has elapsed for assessment of results (Fig. 11(2)(3)(4)).

The elbow joint. Swanson and Yamauchi (1968) described the use of a bi-stemmed silastic elbow prosthesis. No assessment of the results has yet been made. A replacement for the head of the radius is also described by the same authors (Fig. 11(5)).

The spine. Hjalmar Reitz of Johannesburg, South Africa, has been using a disc-shaped silastic prosthesis to replace the intervertebral discs in the cervical and lumbar spine. The aim is to retain some movement at

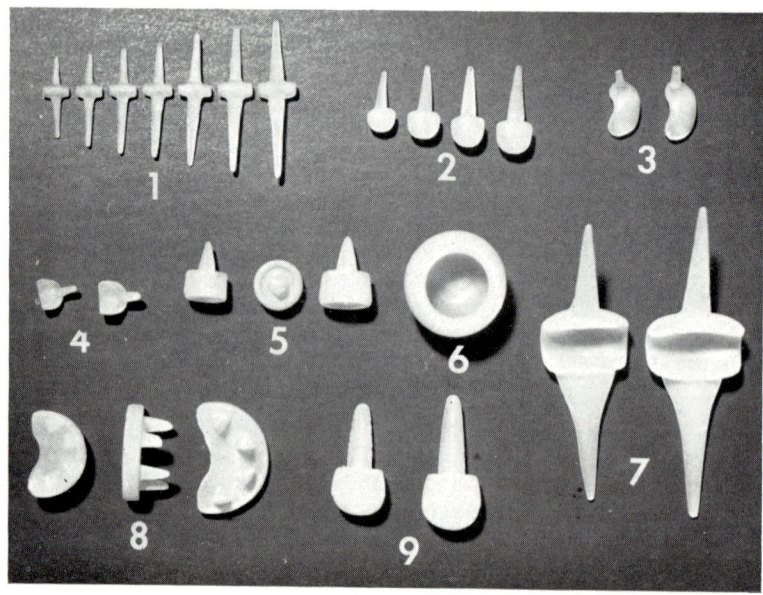

FIG. 11. The range of silastic implants in use and under trial by Dr. A. B. Swanson and his colleagues.

(1) Finger joint prosthesis.
(2) Trapezium replacements.
(3) Scaphoid replacements.
(4) Lunate replacements.
(5) Radius head-prosthesis.
(6) Femoral cup.
(7) Elbow joints.
(8) Knee prosthesis.
(9) First metatarsal head prosthesis.

the site of the excised disc and so avoid undue stress on the adjacent discs. His results in the cervical spine have been moderate but in the lumbar spine excellent. This assessment is based on experience of 300 cases (Fig. 12).

The hip. The late Professor Miki of Tokyo used a silastic cup arthroplasty for treatment of arthritis of the hip. He was to read a paper on this subject at the S.I.C.O.T. meeting in Paris in September 1966 but his untimely death prevented this and no further information regarding this prosthesis is available.

Swanson and Yamauchi have also devised a silastic cup but this, at the time of writing, had not been used clinically (Fig. 11(6)).

The knee. Quadriceps adhesion: Breck (1966) describes the successful use of silastic sheeting to prevent readhesion of the quadriceps expansion in the suprapatellar pouch after this has been surgically freed. Tibial Plateau Fractures: Breck (1966) describes the use of silastic sponge to smooth the articular surfaces of the tibia. He describes good results achieved by its use in six clinical cases. Arthroplasty: Swanson and Yamauchi have described a tibial plateau prosthesis but do not describe its clinical use (Fig. 11(8)).

The foot. Harris (1967) has been using a silastic rubber interposition after Keller's arthroplasty which improves the foot cosmetically by

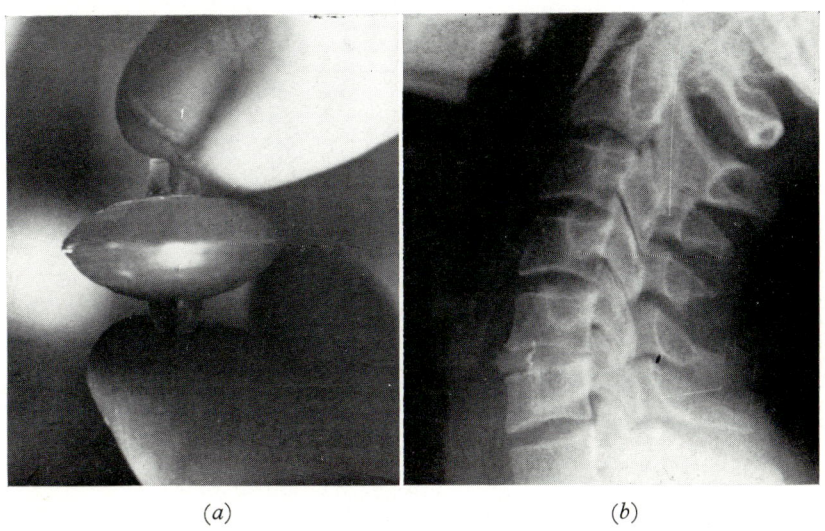

(a) (b)

FIG. 12.

(a) A silastic intervertebral disc.
(b) Inserted into the interspace between 5th and 6th cervical vertebrae.
(By kind permission of Dr. Hjalmar Reitz.)

keeping the great toe out to length and he feels that the function of the great toe is also enhanced.

Swanson and Yamauchi have devised a silastic first metatarsal head but there is no comment as yet upon its clinical use (Fig. 11(9)).

Experience with Silastics in the Enfield Orthopaedic Unit

JOINTS

The hand. Owing to dissatisfaction with the results of metal hinge prostheses for proximal interphalangeal joint arthritis I devised a bi-stemmed soft silastic prosthesis (Fig. 13). After being subjected to exhaustive test bending it has been used in 11 hands to date.

In the first four patients both the base of the middle phalanx and the head of the proximal phalanx were trimmed with only moderate results. Better results were achieved when the base of the middle phalanx was not interfered with.

In the subsequent patients since June 1966 the following technique was employed. Through a mid-lateral incision on the ulnar side of the finger the ulnar collateral ligament is divided and the proximal interphalangeal joint dislocated. The head of the proximal phalanx is cut off distal to the attachment of the radial collateral ligament. The shafts of the proximal and middle phalanx are reamed and the prosthesis is inserted. The joint is reduced and the skin sutured. This procedure leaves the joint with a satisfactory degree of collateral stability, especially in

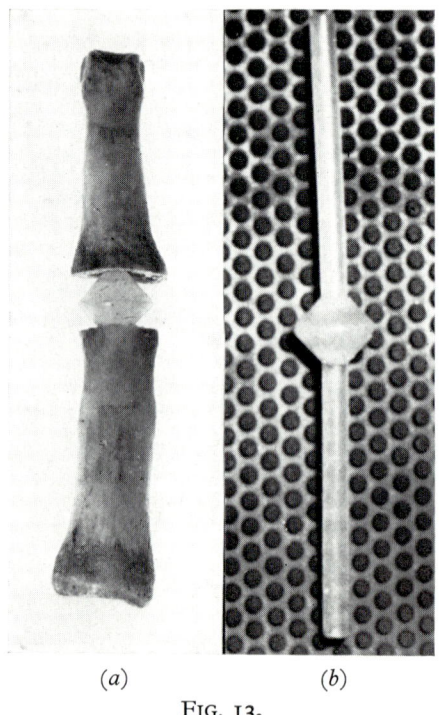

(a) (b)
FIG. 13.
(a) Silastic proximal interphalangeal finger joint.
(b) This is effective in maintaining a good mobile joint space between the proximal and middle phalanges.

normal use when pressures tend to be on the radial aspect of the fingers (Figs. 14, 15). Four patients have 90° of active flexion and three patients have movement beyond this range (Fig. 16). There have been no cases of dislocation of either the proximal interphalangeal joint or the prosthesis. After excision of the heads of the metacarpals the same prosthesis has been used to enhance the cosmetic appearance of the hand.

The knee. In the arthritic knee a hard grade stemmed silastic prosthesis as a tibial plateau replacement similar to the McKintosh device has been employed (Fig. 17). Three patients have had this procedure, two in one compartment, and one in both compartments. The two patients with single compartment prostheses have no symptoms and full control of the

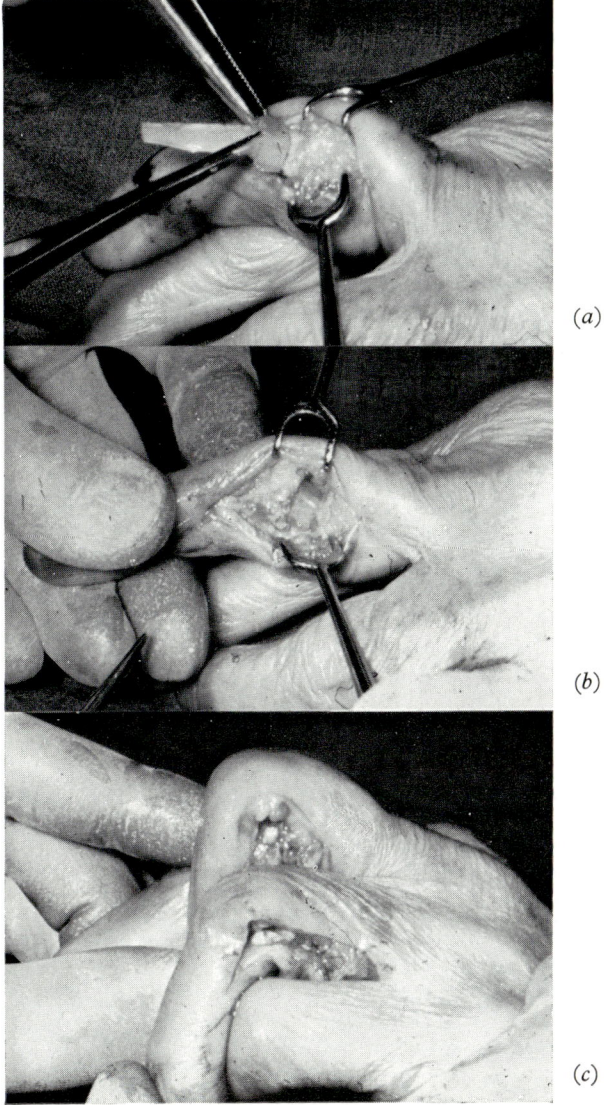

Fig. 14. A bi-stemmed soft silastic finger prosthesis.
(a) Being inserted through an ulnar side approach.
(b) In situ.
(c) Permitting free flexion whilst retaining excellent stability.

knee with movement from 0–90° and from 0–100° respectively after six months. The patient with the prosthesis in both compartments has pain on forcing extension and a 10° fixed flexion deformity. Movement is from 10–90° after six months.

The hallux. I have been using soft silastic as a filler for the gap left by

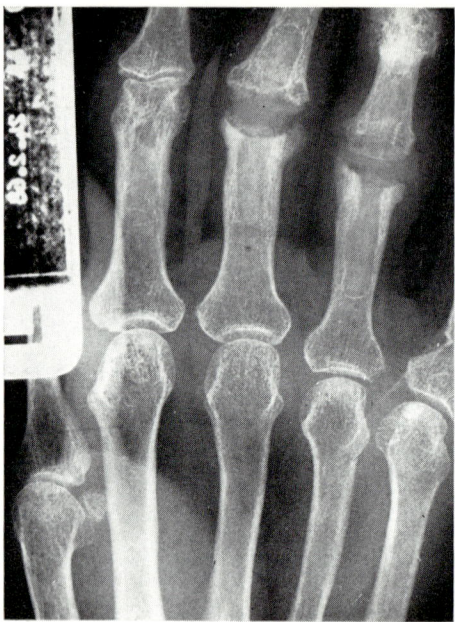

Fig. 15. The proximal interphalangeal joints of the middle and ring fingers were replaced by silastic joints one year before. They now function well.

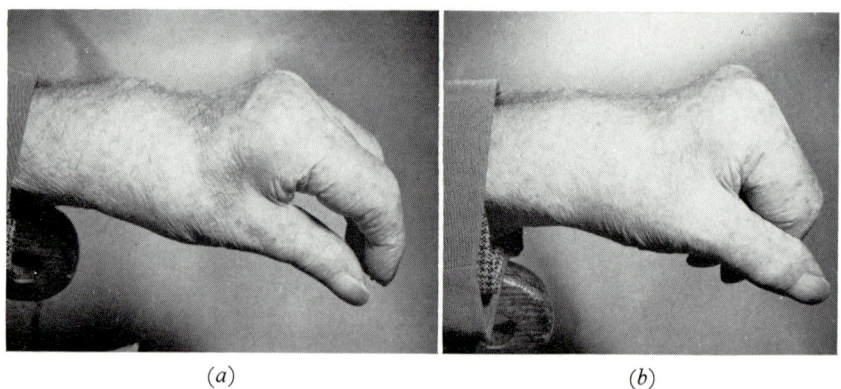

(a) (b)

Fig. 16.

(a) Maximum flexion before silastic replacement of proximal interphalangeal joints.
(b) After silastic arthroplasty of proximal interphalangeal joints and synovectomies of metacarpo-phalangeal joints.

excision arthroplasty of the metatarsophalangeal joint of the great toe (Fig. 18). The cosmetic results are enhanced but there seems to be the same subjective satisfaction with inconstancy of functional results as with the simple excision arthroplasty.

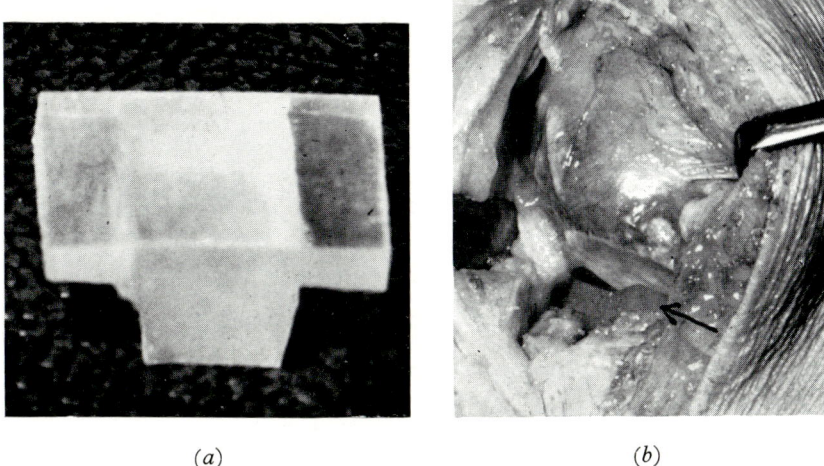

FIG. 17.
(a) A stemmed tibial plateau prosthesis made of hard grade silastic.
(b) Prosthesis in situ arrowed.

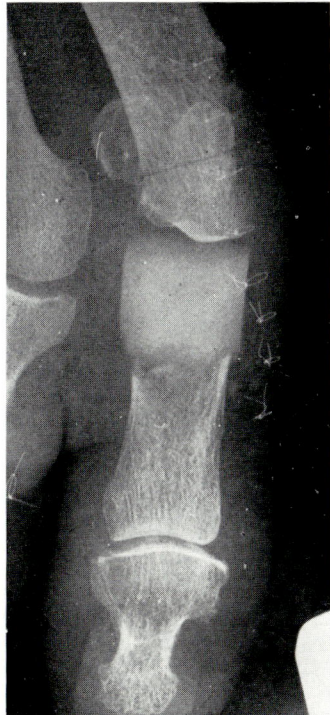

FIG. 18. A silastic 'filler' for the first metatarso-phalangeal joint after a Keller procedure improves the cosmetic appearance, and sometimes this results in a great toe joint indistinguishable from a normal joint.

TENDONS

In the summer of 1966 silastic tendons were devised in this clinic for two patients (Fig. 19). The first patient had had all the flexors of the fingers cut by a knife. The wounds became infected. He presented six weeks after the incident. At operation the tendons were unidentifiable in a mass of scar tissue in the line of the flexor sheath. This was excised and the silastic tendons were inserted. Six weeks later it proved easy to insert a homograft by railroading this on the silastic tendon along what appeared to be a perfect tendon sheath. The result was a hand with good function (Fig. 20).

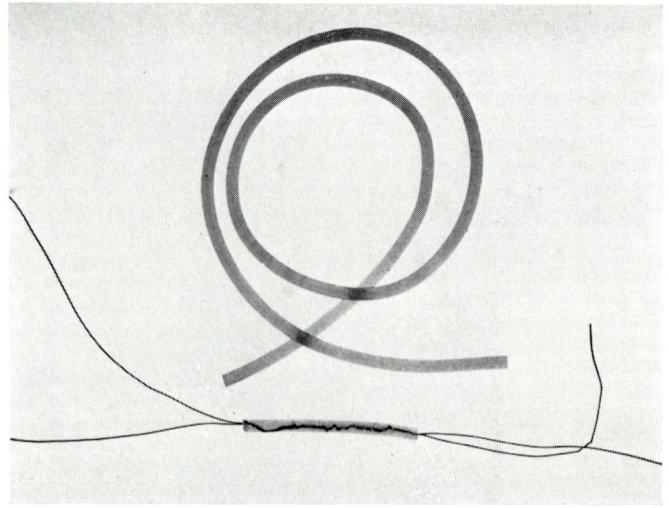

FIG. 19. Artificial tendon made by threading a silk suture through a silastic rod.

The second patient presented with a stiff index finger—the aftermath of a septic tenosynovitis, and was treated in a similar manner, again with a very satisfactory result.

The tendons used were made by threading a silk suture material through soft silastic rods, the silk being used to anchor these to the patient's tendon at both ends of the rod.

DIABETIC ULCERS

Using the same technique as described by Lennox (1965) for leprosy, we have been trimming the bone lying under diabetic ulcers of the foot, inserting a piece of silastic sponge and closing the skin over this (Fig. 21).

In one patient with such an intractable ulcer that had not responded to all other forms of treatment, amputation was being considered, this form of treatment solved his problem and saved his limb.

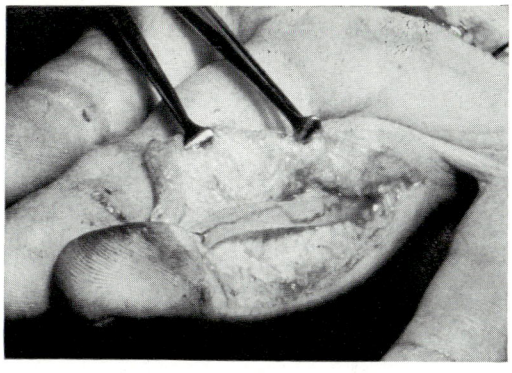

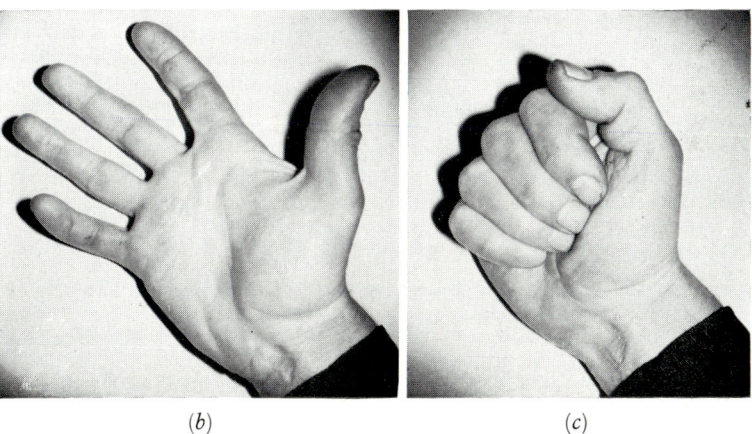

FIG. 20. This patient severed all the flexors to the fingers of his right hand. (*a*) Shows the home-made silastic tendons used. (*b* and *c*) The range of movements six months later.

Conclusions

Silicone oils and silastics have been in clinical use for over a decade. No significant morbidity or mortality has resulted from their use. Their introduction has been properly cautious and based on numerous preliminary animal experiments. The non-reactive bland nature of this material makes it an ideal implant and opens up seemingly endless possibilities for replacement surgery. The silicones may prove to be the most useful implant material of our age. Although silicones have not been in clinical use over a whole human life span and no one can predict with certainty the effect of their presence in human tissues over a period of several decades, this can equally be said of most of the prosthetic implants in use. I believe that their actual and potential value justifies their clinical use. In the field of orthopaedic surgery the clinical applications of the silicones are already wide and growing rapidly. The material is providing answers to many problems that previously seemed insoluble. One can only hope that the initial promise of the silicones will be fulfilled in the long term.

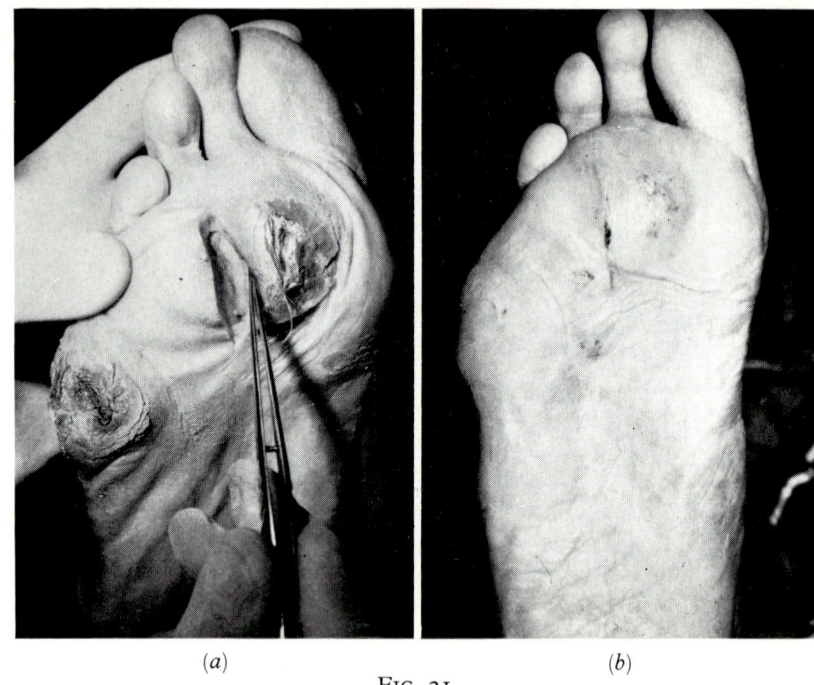

FIG. 21.

(a) A pad of silastic sponge has been inserted deep to the base of this diabetic ulcer, cushioning it from the underlying bone. This healed without complication. (b) The same foot 6 weeks later.

ACKNOWLEDGEMENTS

It gives me pleasure to acknowledge the great help given me by Dr. Murray Brookes of Guy's Hospital with the animal experimental work.

I am grateful to Dr. Hume Kendall, the Editor of The Annals of Physical Medicine for permission to reproduce some of the material from the article "Artificial Lubrication of Joints" published in that journal in November 1968.

I wish to thank the Dow Corning Company and Messrs. S. A. Braley and M. S. Newash for the kind co-operation they have given me.

References

ABOULAFIA, Y. and POLISHUK, W. (1967). *Arch. Surg.*, **94**, 384.
AKUTSU, T., OKURA, T., FREED, P. and KANTROWITZ, A. (1966). *Surg. Forum*, **17**, 103.
ANDREWS, J. M. (1966). *Plast. & Reconstruct. Surg.*, **38**, 58.
ARMALY, M. F. (1962). *Arch. Ophthal.*, **68**, 390.
ASHLEY, F., BRALEY, S., REES, T., GOULIAN, D. and BALLANTYNE, D. JR. (1967). *Plast. & Reconstruct. Surg.*, **39**, 411.
ASHLEY, F L., MCCONNELL, D., POLAK, T., STONE, R. and MARMOR, L. (1964). *Plast. & Reconstruct. Surg.*, **33**, 522.
BALKIN, S. G. (1966). *J. Amer. Podiat. Ass.*, **56**, 1.
BALLANTYNE, D. L. JR., REES, T. and SEIDMAN, I. (1965). *Plast. & Reconstruct. Surg.*, **36**, 3.
BATEMAN, F. J. A. (1956). *Brit. Med. J.*, 554.
BERGER, R. (1966). *New York State J. Med.*, **66**, 2523.
BICKMORE, J. and PLEIN, E. M. (1951). Masters Thesis University of Washington.
BODELL, B., HEAD, J., HEAD, L. and FORMOLO, A. *Jama* 191 (4) 301.

Bowen, S., Dyer, J., Ogle, K. and Neault, R. (1962). *Surv. Ophthal.*, **7**, 378–9.
Bradley, B., Kneyard, A., Defalco, A., Lawson, D. and Hayes, J. (1967). *Amer. J. Surg.*, **113**, 501.
Breck, X. (1966). *The Bull. Dow Corning*, Vol. 9, No. 2, p. 6.
Brody, S. G. and White, W. L. (1963). *Plast. & Reconstr. Surg.*, **32**, 11–18.
Brown, J. B., Fryer, M. P., Randol, P. and Lu, M. (1953). *Plast. & Reconstruct. Surg.*, **12**, 374.
Brown, J. B., Ohlwiler, D. A. and Fryer, M. P. (1960). *Ann. Surg.*, **152**, 534.
Brusca, Donald D. (1956). *New York State J. Med.*, **56**, 894.
Campbell, J. B. and Luzio, J. (1964). *Trans. Amer. Acad. Ophthal. Oto-laryng.*, 1068.
Carrington, R. W. (1959). *J. Mich. State Med. Soc.*, 373–83.
Chang, T. (1966). *Trans. Amer. Soc. Artif. Intern. Organs.*, **12**, 13.
Chardack, W. M., Dayce, Fazekas G. and Minsley, N. (1961). *J. Trauma*, **1**, 54–68.
Cibis, D. A., Becker, B., Okun, E. and Canaan (1962). *The Bull. Dow Corning Center for Aid to Medical Research*, **4**, 13.
Clark, J., Jr. and Gollan, F. (1966). *Science*, **152**, 1755.
Crawford, E. S., De Bakey, M. E. and Cooley, D. A. (1958). *Meeting Arch. Surg.*, **76**, 261–70.
Cronin, T. (1966). *Plast. & Reconstr. Surg.*, **37**, 399.
Cutting, W. C. (1952). *Stanf. Med. Bull.* 10, No. 1, **23**, 26.
Del Rosario, V., Prater, G. and Garvey, J. (1966). *Amer. Surg.*, **32**, 638.
Donovan, T. J. (1949). *Ann. Surg.*, **130**, 1024–43.
Ducker, T. and Hayes, G. (1967). Forum of Amer. Coll. Surg.
Egdahl, R. H. (1955). *Arch. Surg.*, **71**, 694–6.
Enna, C. (1966). *Int. J. Leprosy*, **34**, 30.
Fedorov, S., Bedilo, V. and Zakharov, V. (1965). *Oftal. Zh.*, **20**, 527.
Finnerty, E. F. (1954). *Ind. Med. & Surg.*, **23**, 156.
Flatt, A. E. (1963). Third Int. Cong. Plast. Surg., Washington.
Fletcher, R. F. (1956). *Lancet*, **270**, 509–10.
Folkman, J., Long, D. and Rosenbaum, R. (1966). *Science*, **154**, 148.
Folkman, M. J. (1965). *The Bull. Dow Corning*, Vol. 7, No. 4.
Fomon, S. and Bell, J. (1966). *Arch. Otolaryng.*, **84**, 514.
Fredericks, S. (1966). Paper, *Amer. Soc. Plast. reconstr. Surg.*, Nevada.
Fryfogle, J. D., Cyrowski, G., Rothwell, D., Rheault, G. and Clarke, T. (1963). *Dis. of the Chest*, **43**, 464–75.
Furman, S. and Denize, A. (1966). *Surgery*, **60**, 733.
Gaisford, J., Hanna, D. and Richardson, G. (1966). *Plast. & Reconstr. Surg.*, **38**, 302.
Goodman, H. (1955). *Am. Prof. Pharmacist.*, **21** (2) 129, 172.
Hall, C. W., Eppright, R., Engen, T. and Liotta, D. (1967). *Trans. Amer. Soc. Artif. int. Org.*, **13**, 329.
Harris, H. B. (1964). *Plast. & Reconstruct. Surg.*, **34**, 419.
Harris, N. (1967). Personal communication.
Helal, B. and Karadi, B. S. (1968). "Annals of Physical Medicine", Nov. 1968.
Hodge, H. C. and Sterner, J. H. (1949). *Ind. Hyg. Assoc. Quarterly*, **10**, 93.
Hoopes, J., Edgeston, M., Jr. and Shelley, W. (1966). Presented at Annual Meeting of American Society of Plastic and Reconstruction Surgery. Las Vegas. Oct. 6, 1966.
Hopping, W. (1965). *Deutsch. Orhthal. Ges. Ber.*, **66**, 336.
Hunter, J. (1965). *Amer. J. Surg.*, **109**, 325.
Jaypathy, B. (1960). *The Bull. Dow Corning*, Vol. 2, No. 3.
Kagan, H. D. (1963). *Arch. Otolaryg.*, **78**, 663.
Kern, S. F., Anderson, R. C. and Harris, D. N. (1949). *J. Amer. Pharm. Assoc. Sci. Ed.*, **38**, 575.
Largent, E., Blackstone, M. and Roth, J. (1950). *U.S. Air Force Med. Service*, I.P.
Lebon, P. (1966). *World Med. Dec.*, **13**.
Lennox, W. M. (1965). *Leprosy Rev.*, **36**, 109.

Levin, R. (1958). "The Pharmacy of Silicone and their Uses in Medicine." London: The Chemist and Druggist.
Lewis, H., Sherwood, N. and Pierce, J. (1966). *J. Urol.*, **95,** 700.
Lillehei, C. W., De Wall, R. A., Read, R. C., Warden, H. E. and Varco, R. L. (Jan. 1956). *Dis. Chest*, **29,** 1.
McGregor, R. R. (1954). "Silicones and their Uses." New York: McGraw-Hill Co.
McGregor, R. R. (1957). "Silicones in Medicine and Surgery." Dow Corning Corp.
McGregor, R. R. (1960). (B) Annual Report Aug. 16. Dow Corning.
Melrose, D. G. (1953). *Brit. Med. J.*, **57,** 62.
Miki (1966). Obituary. *J. Bone Jt. Surg.*, **48A,** 1459.
Millard, R. (1967). *Plast. & Reconstr. Surg.*, **40,** 337.
Miller, J. and Hardy, S. (1965). *J. Bone Jt. Surg.*, **47,** 38.
Morgan, J. F. and Hill, J. C. (1964). *Amer. J. Ophth.*, **58,** 767.
Morotomi, T., Okazaki, S. and Mizuta, S. (1967). *Internat. Surg.*, **48,** 164.
Nickerson, M. and Curry, C. T. (1953). *Fed. Proc. Am. Soc. Exp. Biol.*, **12,** 357. No. 1168.
Nickerson, M. and Curry, C. T. (1955). *J. Pharm. Exptl. Therap.*, **114,** 138.
Nickerson, M., Bolt, R. J., Hirshcowitz, B. I. and Curry, C. T. (1954). *Fed. Prox. Am. Soc. Exp. Biol.*, **13,** 391. No. 1282.
Nicolle, F. V. (1966). Canadian Soc. Plast. Surgeons.
Patterson, C. (1966). *Arch. Otolaryng.*, **84,** 457.
Pattle, R. E. (1956). *Pathol. Bacteriol.*, **72,** 203.
Paul, J. and Pover, W. F. R. (1960). *Brit. J. Industr. Med.*, **17,** 149.
Pearman, R. (1967). Western Section Amer. Urol. Assoc., Honolulu.
Plein, J. B. and Plein, E. M. (1953). *J. Am. Pharm. Assoc.*, **42,** 79.
Polemann, G. and Froitzheim, G. (1953). *Arzneimittel–Forschung*, **3,** 457.
Prentiss, R., Boatwright, D., Pennington, R., Hohn, W. and Schwartz, M. (1963). *J. Urol.*, **90,** 208–10.
Princiotto, J. V., Howell, W. L. and Morgan, C. F. (1952). *Am. J. Physiol.*, **171,** 758.
Rees, T. D. (1967). *World Med.* May 2.
Rees, T. and Ashley (1966). *Amer. J. Surg.*, **3,** 531.
Reitz, H. (1968). Personal communication.
Rosenbluth, M. B., Epstein, F. H. and Feldman, D. J. (1952). *Proc. Soc. Exper. Med.*, **80,** 691.
Rowe, V. K., Spencer, H. C. and Bass, S. L. (1948). *J. Ind. Hyg. Toxicol.* **30,** 332.
Rowe, V. K., Spencer, H. C. and Bass, S. L. (1950) *Arch. Ind. Hyg. & Occup. Med.*, **1,** 539.
Sankey, N. and Heller, E. (1967). *J. Urol.*, **97,** 309.
Sarin, C., Sen-Gupta, H., Taylor, H. and Kolf (1966). *Surgery*, **60,** 754.
Suskind, R. R. (1955). *Ind. Med. Surg.*, **24,** 413.
Swanson, A. B. (1966). *Inter Clinic Information Bull.*, **5,** 1.
Swanson, A. B. (1966). *Inter Clinic Information Bull.*, **6,** 16.
Swanson, A. B. and Yamauch, Y. (1968). Personal communication.
Talbot, J. R., McGregor, J. K. and Crowe, F. W. (1951). *J. Invest. Derm.*, **17,** 125.
Tapline, T. and Zaias, N. (1966). *Mil. Med.* **131,** 814.
Tauras, K. and Frackelton, W. (1967). Surg. Forum Amer. Coll. Surgeons.
Taylor, B. (1967). Fourth Internat. Congress Plast. Surg., Rome.
Treon, J. F., Dutra, F. R., Shaffer, F. E., Cappel, J. and Cahegan, T. (1951). U.S. Air Force Med. Service 18 pp.
Von Kennel, J. (1952). *Kosmehische Monatscertschoft*, **1** (18), 7.
Wallace, W. E. (1960). *The Bull. Dow Corning*, Vol. 2, No. 1.
Waugh, T. R. and Stinchfield (1961). *J. Bone Jt. Surg.*, **43A,** 939–46.
Weeder, R., Brooks, H., and Boyer, A. (1967). *Plast. & Reconstruct. Surg.*, **39,** 256.
Winer, L. H., Sternberg, T. H., Lehman, R. and Ashley, F. (1964). *Arch. Derm.*, **90,** 588.

Chapter 6

THE FATE OF BONE GRAFTS

R. GEOFFREY BURWELL

This chapter is divided into two parts: Part I deals with the fate of bone autografts; and Part II with the fate of foreign bone grafts.

The surgical techniques of bone autografting are now established. The current problems of the bone autograft relate less to technique and more to the cellular changes which occur in it *after* grafting. A knowledge of such processes and the mechanisms which control them is of importance to the surgeon because they clearly determine the clinical result. Most of the recent work on bone autografting discussed in Part I of this chapter concerns its cellular biology. Some of this research is academic, but in it there are several lessons for the surgeon.

The use of foreign bone as grafting material obviously has greater convenience both for the surgeon and for the patient. Unfortunately, however, the clinical results using foreign bone have been, in general, less consistent than those obtained by using the patients' own bone as the grafting material. *Fresh* foreign bone is unsuitable for clinical use because of the immunological reactions which it evokes in the host. *Treated* foreign bone (e.g. frozen or freeze-dried bone) is, for practical purposes, dead. Current research in this field is being directed towards finding a treated-bone graft which (*a*) facilitates osteogenesis from the tissues of the host which invade it, and which (*b*) incorporates rapidly into the skeleton at the site of grafting. Only future research can establish whether or not it will be possible to provide a foreign bone which is as consistent in clinical use as the bone autograft.

PART I: THE FATE OF BONE AUTOGRAFTS

"... osteogenesis in general is a problem of which we have relatively little understanding" (Hellstadius, 1955).

The anatomy of bone grafting has evolved greatly since its general introduction into surgical practice 50 years ago (Albee 1915). Since the 1930s the advance of metallurgy has ensured that a bone graft need no longer provide for internal fixation as well as for osteogenesis.

The next great advance occurred during World War II when the myriads of injured led surgeons to a greater use of cancellous bone, at first in facio-maxillary surgery (Mowlem 1941) and later in orthopaedic surgery (Mowlem 1944, Abbott 1944); and from this has stemmed a greater understanding of repair in bone.

In the patient, the fate of a bone graft is followed radiologically and clinically. Only when it fails to establish the desired end-result is the technique questioned; and the complexity realized of the variables, many known, some unknown, which must interact during its healing.

To understand the repair of a bone graft more fully, the approach must be made at the cellular level. But due to the limitations of human biopsy specimens (Abbott et al. 1947, Peer 1951) a sequential analysis of the process is possible only in the animal, and in which the variables can be reduced to a minimum. As with all such work, however, the question remains: how much can be applied to Man?

Clinical Uses and Functions of a Bone Graft

A bone graft is used clinically to provide a bridge of osteogenic tissue, either in a part of the skeleton which is deficient, or to establish the bony fusion of a diseased joint.

The conditions which surgeons are called upon to treat by bone grafting include: (1) the delayed and non-union of fractures; (2) the arthrodesis and arthroreisis of joints; (3) the filling of cavities in bone; (4) the replacement of bone and joint loss; (5) the augmentation of skeletal deficiency in the forehead, nose, maxilla and mandible; and (6) the fusion of growth-plate cartilages.

Rarely, nowadays, is a bone graft called upon to provide for its own internal fixation. Its functions are to establish an additional source of osteogenesis and to act as a scaffold, or trellis, for the ingrowth of new bone.

This 'trellis role' of a bone graft may operate in three ways: *passively*, to permit vascular and cellular invasions from the contiguous living bone (to which the name 'osteoconduction' is applied); *actively*, to induce osteogenesis both by stimulating mitosis and by a process known as 'osteogenic induction'; and *protectively* to allow the delicate newly-forming bone to *maturate* unhindered into cortical and cancellous bone.

The Anatomy of Bone Grafting in the Limbs

It is proposed in this section to give a brief general account of the anatomy and scope of bone grafting as applied to the limbs, but excluding from it a consideration of arthrodeses and arthroreises (bone-block operations).

In the grafting of limb bones, cortical or cancellous bone cut from another site in the patient is most often used. Less commonly the segment of a long bone, such as the fibula or a rib, is utilized. Occasionally in children, a bone graft containing a growth-cartilage is transplanted in the hope that it might continue to grow; but these attempts have been mainly unsuccessful.

In the last few years the free transplantation of joints and the transposition of digits is being re-evaluated particularly in the hand. Such composite tissue, or organ, grafts need a good blood supply for maintenance, which is supplied in the case of digital transpositions by means of a vascular pedicle.

Cortical and Cancellous Bone

Cortical bone is used less commonly for the treatment of delayed union of fractures than it was 20 years ago. The graft may be inserted as an inlay, onlay, double onlay (see Boyd *et al.* 1960), chips, or as osteoperiosteal strips (Fig. 1). More recently, shaped segments of cortical bone inserted into the medulla have been tried clinically and

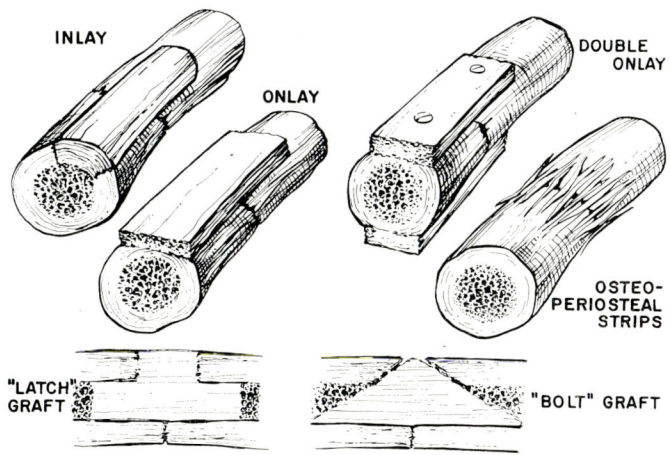

FIG. 1. Some surgical techniques of autografting with cortical bone.

recommended; these are the 'latch graft' (Rizzo and Lehmann 1947) and the 'bolt graft' (McFarland 1951, Corkery 1965).

Cancellous bone is used in the treatment of delayed union as chips (Lawson Dick 1946, see Phemister 1947), as a block (Nicoll 1956, Spira 1963, Sevastikoglou 1965), or as strips (Fig. 2). The 'Phemister principle', to be referred to later in the text, means the surgical treatment

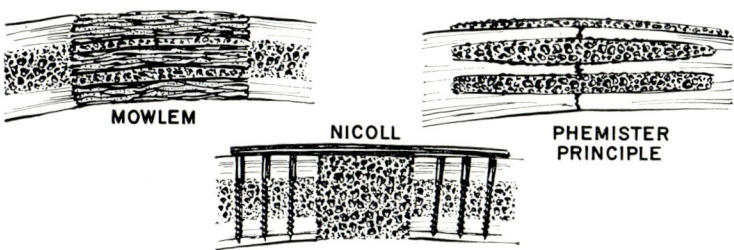

FIG. 2. Some surgical techniques of autografting with cancellous bone.

of delayed union by bone grafting without disturbing the pre-existing callus (Phemister 1931, 1947, Boyd *et al.* 1960). A similar method had previously been used but not reported by Elmslie (Burrows 1940).

The place of cortical and cancellous bone grafting in the treatment of non-union has been questioned again recently by Müller (1963, 1966). Müller, following Judet and Judet (1960), distinguishes two types of non-union, namely: (*a*) a hypervascular ('elephant's foot') non-union (hypertrophic types); and (*b*) a non-union with inert bone ends (atrophic type). He has found that rigid internal fixation *without bone grafting* achieved bony union in 97 of 100 patients with the hypertrophic type of non-union. Müller is of the opinion that bone grafting is needed only for the atrophic type of non-union. Boyd *et al.* (1966) examined the value of compression plates combined with bone grafting in the treatment of non-union and reported union in 88 per cent.

Clearly the indication for bone grafting in the treatment of non-union requires further clinical evaluation.

Segments of Long Bones

Short or long segments of limb bones (with or without the articular surface) are occasionally used as grafting material. The donor bone may be the fibula, a rib, a metatarsal or a metacarpal.

Fibula. The fibula may be used as: (*a*) pedicle grafts for the two-stage replacement of the tibial shaft in children (Huntington); or (*b*) free grafts for the treatment of: femoral neck fractures (Henderson); the Brittain-Howard arthrodesis of the hip (Crawford Adams 1966); replacement of the upper humerus (Clark 1959, Burrows and Lettin 1964), the shafts of the radius and ulna (Miller and Phalen 1947), the lower end of the radius and ulna (Parrish 1966) and the first metatarsal.

Though usually successful in children, fibular grafts in the adult if unsupported by intramedullary fixation, occasionally fracture.

Rib. Split grafts of rib were advocated by Eloesser (1920) for the treatment of delayed union. Recently, whole segments of rib have been used for this purpose (Dineen and Gresham 1962, Lagrot *et al.* 1966).

Metatarsal or metacarpal. To replace a metacarpal lost through injury, both the fifth metatarsal (Graham and Riordan 1948) and a metacarpal (Berg and Trevaskis 1967) have been utilized. In each of these procedures the articular surface of the bone is included in the graft.

Segments of Long Bones Containing a Cartilage Growth-plate

Attempts have been made to transplant bones containing a growth-cartilage plate, principally for the radius and for the lower end of the tibia. The best results, however, have been achieved incidental to the transplantation of digits in young children.

In the treatment of congenital hypoplasia (or aplasia) of the radius (club hand), Riordan (1955), using the upper end of the fibula as the autograft (Starr), did not find any evidence of continued growth from the cartilage plate. This finding has been supported by Carroll (1966) and by Wilson (1966), but recently denied by Blockey (1967).

At the lower end of the tibia, the partial replacement of a growth-cartilage (Straub) previously destroyed by osteomyelitis, was not successful (Spira and Farin 1964).

In the child's hand, the transplantation from the foot of small digital bones for congenital deficiency, or after trauma, has been observed to be followed by continued growth in length of the bone (Graham 1954, Wilson 1966) and this was particularly so if the part had been transplanted by a multiple-stage flap procedure rather than by free-grafting (Freeman 1965)

The Entire Transplantation of Long Bones

The complete length of a bone as an autograft is rarely used in surgery. But it may occasionally find application as: (*a*) the 'turn-up' operation of the tibia and fibula to replace the femur excised for tumour (van Nes 1948); and (*b*) the digital transplants (or transpositions) used in hand surgery to be discussed below (Section 6).

Joint Transplants

The autotransplantation of joints was explored extensively in the first quarter of this century (Lexer 1925). It is again being re-evaluated as the free transplantation of half-joints and whole-joints.

Half-joint transplants. The simplest form of joint transplant is the reattachment of an osteochondral plaque created by trauma or osteochondritis dissecans. The more extensive 'cartilaginous cup arthroplasty' (Moore 1948) may still have a place in the treatment of severe injuries at the upper end of the humerus (Dewar and Yabsley 1967). The use of the fibula to replace the upper humerus and the lower radius has already been mentioned. In the hand, metacarpal heads may be replaced using as donor a metatarsal or an adjacent metacarpal (Graham and Riordan 1948, Berg and Trevaskis 1967).

Whole-joint transplants. Also in the hand various joints (metacarpophalangeal, interphalangeal and carpo-metacarpal) have been replaced using joints freely transplanted from the foot or from amputated fingers (Graham 1954, Entin *et al.* 1962, Conway 1962, Erdélyi 1963, Buncke *et al.* 1967).

Many of these transplanted joints undergo a slow degeneration. Why this should happen is not clear: it might be due to an impaired blood supply, or have resulted from denervation. In discussing this work Riordan (1962) concluded that clinical experience should continue to be gained, but confining the transplants to small autologous non-weight-bearing joints in very young patients in whom the bone is small and readily revascularized.

Digital Transplants (or Transpositions)

Entire bones and intervening joints are occasionally transplanted together with other tissues in the hand as digital transpositions and as the rare toe-to-hand transplantations. The survival of these organ (or composite tissue) grafts is ensured by a vascular bundle or a skin flap.

Digital transpositions in the hand. The successful transplantation from a finger of one hand to the thumb of the other hand was described 50 years ago (Joyce 1918). Today, digital transfers are performed within the same hand as pollicization (Littler 1953, Kaplan 1967) and as transpositions of other digital rays (Graham *et al.* 1947, Peacock 1962). The blood supply and innervation of the digits are maintained through the intact neuro-vascular bundles. Joint degeneration does not occur.

Toe-to-hand transplantation (Pedochirodactyloplasty). Clarkson (1955) described his experience of transplanting toes to the hand using a multiple-stage dorsal-flap method. He transplanted 15 digits in 6 patients and lost only half a digit. Successful toe-to-hand transplants have been reported recently by other surgeons (Byars 1952, Freeman 1956, Davis 1964); but it is a procedure not to be undertaken lightly (Reid 1960, Clarkson 1962).

A new blood supply is created by the use of a skin pedicle. Sensation may be gradually acquired, particularly in the child (Byars 1952, Freeman 1956); though nerve suture has been performed (Chandler and Clarkson 1958, Davis 1964). Joint degeneration does not seem to occur, suggesting therefore that ischaemia rather than denervation is the cause of the slow degeneration of the freely-transplanted entire joint. 'Cartilaginous cup arthroplasty' might therefore find application in the hand (see Chesterman 1965).

It is of interest to note that new techniques are now being developed experimentally for hallux-to-hand transplantations, using a microsurgical method for vascular anastomoses (Buncke *et al.* 1966, 1967).

Pedicle Transplants of Bone and Digits

The digital transplants just mentioned require a blood supply to be provided through either a vascular bundle or a skin pedicle; a muscle pedicle may also be used to support the survival of a bone graft.

Skin-pedicle. Toe-to-hand transplants require a multiple-stage flap procedure. Skin-pedicles have also been used to transplant bone from one site to another. An attempt to use a composite bone-skin cross-leg flap for the treatment of congenital pseudarthrosis of the tibia failed in three children (Farmer 1952). MacGregor and Simonetta (1964), however, have succeeded in reconstructing the thumb using a composite bone-skin flap in which the donor site is the clavicle.

Neuro-vascular pedicle. Digital ray transpositions require a vascular pedicle which is provided by the neuro-vascular bundle. The popliteal neuro-vascular bundle is used to supply the tibia and fibula in the 'turn-up' operation for replacement of the femur (van Nes 1948).

Muscle-pedicle. The transplantation of bone with muscle (or tendon) attached has application in many sites, *viz.*: skull (Watson-Jones 1933); mandible; scapula (to the humerus); the spine (Curran and McGaw 1968); hip joint; femoral neck (Movin 1963); and fibula (to the tibia) (Baadsgaard and Medgyesi 1965).

Experimentally, it has been found that whereas cortical bone transferred by muscle-pedicle largely dies, most of cancellous bone similarly transplanted survives (Baadsgaard and Medgyesi 1965, Medgyesi 1965).

CONCLUSIONS CONCERNING THE ANATOMY OF BONE GRAFTING

In the limbs, bone grafts are employed anatomically in many different ways. Most commonly are cancellous and cortical bone grafts freely transplanted. Occasionally a segment of a long bone (fibula or rib) is utilized, but in the treatment of extensive skeletal loss, the results of bone autografts will need to be evaluated against the use of prosthetic replacement and the massive bone homograft. Joint autotransplantation, explored extensively in the early years of this century, may ultimately find application, particularly in the treatment of joint deficiency in the child's hand.

The viability of a cancellous bone graft is greatly increased if its blood supply is maintained through a muscle pedicle. Vascular pedicles are obligatory for transposing digital rays in the hand (neuro-vascular bundle) and in the occasional toe-to-hand transplantation (skin pedicle). Microsurgical techniques are being developed experimentally for hallux-to-hand transplantation.

Before reviewing the fate of bone autografts and the experimental methods used to assess them, it may be convenient for the reader if knowledge and modern concepts concerning the cellular biology of bone in repair are briefly discussed.

Cellular Biology of Bone with Particular Reference to Grafting

The Periosteum

The periosteum consists of two layers: a fibrous limiting membrane and a cellular osteogenic layer (synonyms: cambium layer and epiosteum —Hey Groves 1917).

In the young, the cambium layer is composed of several layers of cells (predominantly osteoblasts) (Fig. 3) and contributes to the growth of bone in three directions: (a) the cortical bone of the diaphysis; (b) the cartilage growth-plate and (c) the articular cartilage (Tonna and Cronkite 1963).

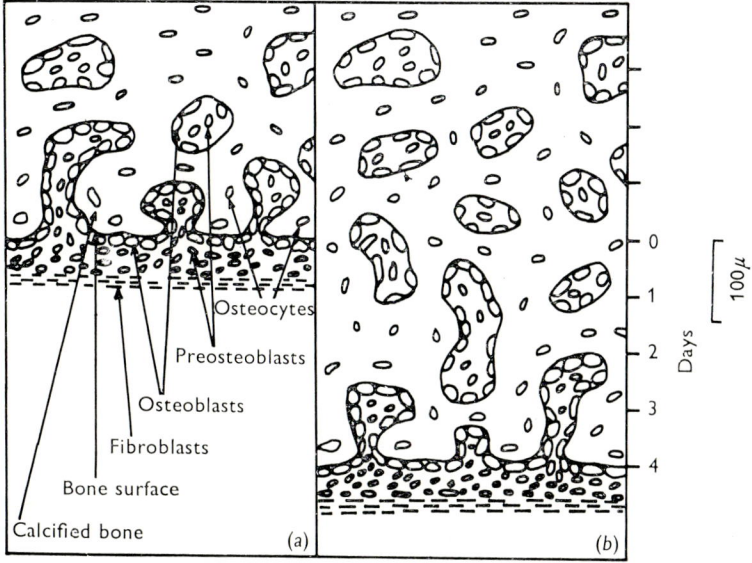

FIG. 3. Diagrammatic representation of the periosteal surface of the shaft of a long bone of a rabbit aged 1–2 weeks, illustrating: (a) the various layers of cells on the bone surface; and (b) the position of the bone surface after 4 days' growth. (Reproduced by kind permission of Dr. Maureen Owen and the Editor, *J. Cell Sci.*)

When growth is over, the cambium layer becomes less noticeable and in the bones of the old it may consist of so few cells that it cannot be identified as a separate entity (Ham and Harris 1956).

Mature Bone

The cortical bone of adult Man (but not all laboratory animals—Enlow 1963), consists largely of Haversian systems (secondary osteons). Each Haversian system consists of lamellae of osteocytes arranged circumferentially around a central canal containing blood vessels which provide for the metabolic requirements of the osteocytes (Fig. 4a). The intercellular matrix of bone consists of collagen, mucopolysaccharides and hydroxyapatite crystals; and the diffusion of substances through bone is greatly facilitated by the lacunar and canalicular spaces in which the osteocytes and their processes are housed. No osteocyte is further than 0·1 mm. from its blood supply (Ham 1952).

In the trabeculae, or spongework, of cancellous bone, the osteocytes are similarly contained in lacunae and canaliculi within calcified matrix (Fig. 4b). Blood vessels penetrate the thicker trabeculae (Ham 1952).

The Endosteum

The inner surface of cortical and cancellous bone is lined by a cellular membrane termed the endosteum. Similar cells extend to line the Haversian canals of cortical bone (Ham and Harris 1956).

Until recently it was thought that the endosteum of the shaft of a long bone contributes largely to the internal callus of a fracture. However, the use of a radioactive label (^{3}H-thymidine) to 'pin-point' dividing cells, has revealed that in the adult mouse the endosteum contributes little to the repair of a fractured femur, the internal callus being largely derived from cells of the marrow (Tonna and Cronkite 1961). In contrast, *cancellous* endosteal cells do proliferate after fracture.

The Marrow and Blood Supply of Bone

Marrow and bone are linked not only in their contiguity, but also in their blood supply and interrelations in repair. While in normal adult Man, red marrow is situated in the axial skeleton, the bones of the limb girdles and proximal parts of the limb bones, in young laboratory animals the red marrow extends throughout the skeleton.

The medullary arterial system supplies the marrow, cortical and cancellous bone and during growth, the cartilage growth-plate. The direction of blood flow in compact bone is centrifugal from the endosteal to the periosteal surface of the bone (Brookes 1964): but some blood flowing through the deeper parts of the cortex returns through the venous sinusoids of the medulla which are lined by reticulo-endothelial (RE) cells (Brånemark 1959). These RE cells of the marrow probably differentiate into osteoblasts after transplantation (Burwell 1964a).

The functional interrelationship which may exist between bone and red marrow is difficult to detect in the intact animal. But certain experimental procedures reveal what may be an occult interdependence. Thus: (a) devitalized bone grafts which form ectopic bone are frequently colonized

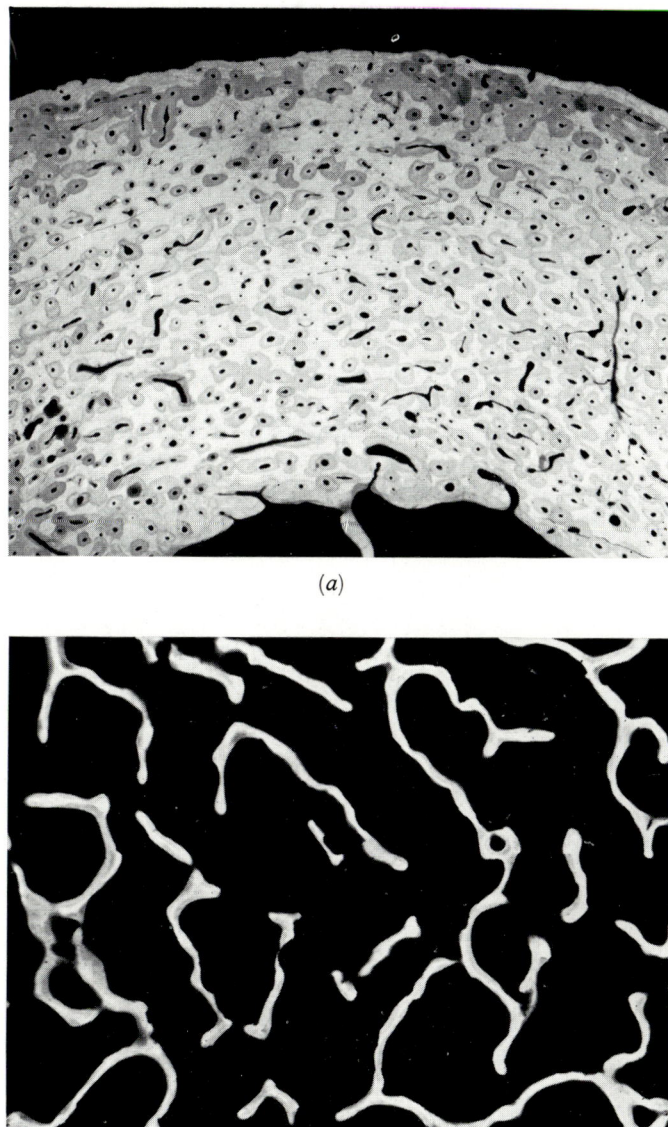

Fig. 4. (a) Microradiograph of normal cortical bone of the femur of a woman aged 20 years. × 21.
(b) Microradiograph of normal cancellous bone of the iliac crest of a woman aged 45 years. × 21.
(Reproduced by kind permission of Dr. H. A. Sissons.)

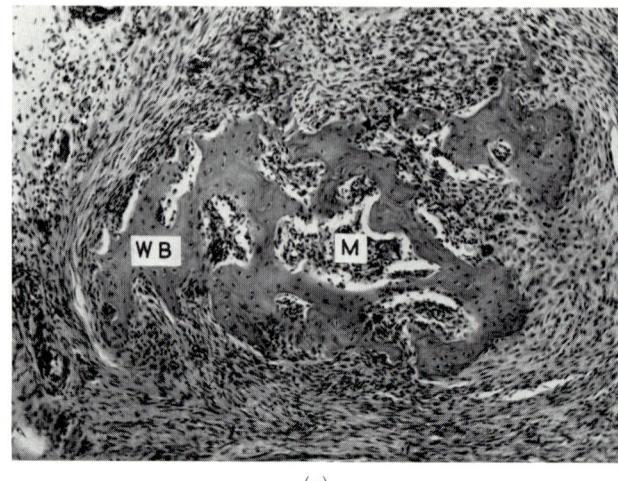

(a)

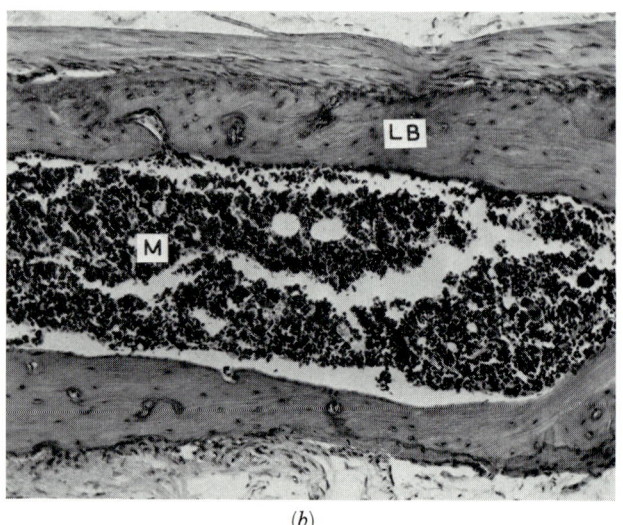

(b)

Fig. 5. Photomicrographs of marrow autografts implanted intramuscularly into rats and removed (a) 2 weeks later and (b) 12 weeks later. Note the formation of woven bone (WB) at 2 weeks and of lamellar bone (LB) at 12 weeks. (M = marrow). Haematoxylin and eosin. × 165.

by haemopoietic cells (Holub 1958, Urist 1965); (b) after irradiation, the regeneration of marrow is associated with the appearance of osteoblasts in it (Tsesarskaya 1960); (c) in pigeons and chickens during their egg-laying cycles, reticular cells of the marrow differentiate into osteoblasts (Bloom *et al.* 1958) and a similar change occurs in animals which have received large doses of parathyroid extract (Heller *et al.* 1950); and (d) red marrow carefully freed from bone particles and endosteal cells forms new bone after transplantation (Fig. 5) (Pfeiffer 1948, Urist and McLean 1952, Bloom 1960).

Such interrelations revealed by experiment may have a considerable bearing upon the changes which occur after transplantation in marrow-containing cancellous bone grafts (e.g. from the ilium) (Burwell 1964a).

The Osteogenesis of Repair

Microscopical types of bone. The repair of bone after fracture, or transplantation, is largely a function of the osteogenic cells of the periosteum, endosteum (of cancellous bone only in trauma) and marrow.

The first formed bone is *woven bone* (Fig. 5a). It consists of a network of bony trabeculae in which the arrangement of cells and fibres in the trabeculae is chaotic; the formation of woven bone as a network may be determined by the selective aggregation of osteoblasts (Burwell 1964a). Later, the woven bone is replaced by *lamellar bone* which exists as a succession of bony trabeculae deposited with the utmost regularity (Fig. 5b). When arranged concentrically in cortical bone it forms the osteons (primary and secondary) (Pritchard 1961) (Fig. 4a).

The dividing cells in bone—osteoprogenitor cells, pre-osteoblasts and pre-osteoclasts. The use of the radioactive label tritiated-thymidine (^{3}H-thymidine) has enabled dividing cells to be localized in normal bone, in fractures and after the grafting of skeletal tissues (Tonna and Cronkite 1961, 1962, 1963, Young 1963, Ray and Sabet 1963, Urist *et al.* 1965, Scott 1967).*

In normal bone, neither osteocytes nor osteoclasts incorporate ^{3}H-thymidine; and osteoblasts are rarely labelled in the periosteum and endosteum of adult animals. The cells which are labelled on the periosteum are of unspecialized morphology. A name for them was necessary and they have been called '*osteoprogenitor cells*' (Young) and 'pre-osteoblasts' (Tonna).

Osteoprogenitor cells (which are believed to be derived from primitive connective tissue cells) give rise to osteoblasts, osteocytes and osteoclasts. Moreover, there is evidence that osteoblasts and osteoclasts can rejoin the osteoprogenitor population as dividing cells. More recent work (Scott 1967) has shown that primitive connective tissue cells give rise to osteoblasts through an intermediary stage—the *pre-osteoblast*; and to osteoclasts through a *pre-osteoclast*.† These cellular interrelationships can be summarized as follows:

Primitive connective tissue cells ⟨ Pre-osteoblasts⇌Osteoblasts→Osteocytes
Pre-osteoclasts⇌Osteoclasts

The osteoblasts synthesize collagen and probably mucopolysaccharide into the micro-environment of the cell as *osteoid*. Calcification usually,

---

* ^{3}H-thymidine is incorporated into the DNA of the nuclei of cells shortly before mitotic division and is rapidly removed (in 10 minutes) from the extra-cellular fluids of the animal and is hence shown as 'flash labelling'. When a 'tagged' cell divides, the radioactive thymidine is passed into the daughter cells. Hence it is possible to label a cell and follow its evolution.

† The term osteoprogenitor cell should then be applied collectively to pre-osteoblasts and pre-osteoclasts as defined by Scott (1967). However, because a definitive terminology in this field must await the results of further ultrastructural research, it is proposed in this Chapter to use the term osteoprogenitor cell as defined by Young (1963).

but not always, lags behind the formation of matrix, after which the osteoblasts become housed as osteocytes (see Bassett 1962a, Hancox and Boothroyd 1964).

In this chapter, pre-osteoblasts and osteoblast cells will be termed *'osteogenic cells'* (Tonna and Cronkite 1961); and for the convenience of discussion the osteogenic cells of the periosteum and endosteum will be referred to, collectively, as *'littoral osteogenic cells'*.

The natural stimulation of osteogenesis. In repair, osteogenesis may be stimulated in two ways: (a) by mitotic stimulation of osteogenic cells; and (b) by osteogenic induction of primitive connective tissue cells.

(a) **Mitotic stimulus to repair.** Trauma (and to a less extent infections and tumours) causes periosteal proliferation, but the precise way in which this happens is unknown.

Lexer thought that necrotic bone released a growth stimulus which worked upon the osteoblasts; but equally, in the light of more recent work (Bullough 1962), could proliferation be initiated by a release from a normal mitotic inhibition (Burwell 1965).

Leaving aside the biochemical mechanism, there is considerable evidence to support the view that necrosis of bone is the stimulus to repair. Thus in the femur, periosteal proliferation follows necrosis of the underlying cortex caused by sucking out the marrow (Richany et al. 1965) or by freezing the bone (Gage et al. 1966); furthermore, the placing of bone which necroses in contact with periosteum causes it to proliferate (Puranen 1966). Even more potent evidence is the finding that in muscle-pedicle bone grafts, osteogenesis is inversely related to the death of bone (Baadsgaard and Medgyesi 1965).

In a fracture, however, the problem seems to be even more complex; for after a closed fracture of the femoral shaft in the mouse the periosteal proliferation during the first 48 hours is not limited to the fracture site but generally extends along the *entire* length of the shaft (Tonna and Cronkite 1962). This surprising finding clearly requires further study.

(b) **Osteogenic induction.** The term osteogenic induction is used to define the process whereby one tissue, or products derived from it, causes a second tissue to differentiate into bone. In repair, therefore, bone tissue may induce osteogenic differentiation in either: (i) marrow; or (ii) extra-skeletal tissues.

The first mechanism (bone→marrow) has been studied by using composite, or recombinant, grafts of bone and marrow in rats (Burwell 1964a, 1966).* It was concluded from these experiments that cancellous bone, after transplantation, has the property to induce and promote osteogenesis in marrow. Moreover, that this property is contained in the organic components of bone.

The second mechanism (bone→extra-skeletal tissue) has been demonstrated by transplanting bone into extra-skeletal (or heterotopic) sites in the same animal (see Bridges 1959). In this connection it has been

---

* An analogous experiment has recently been reported using recombinant grafts of epidermis and dermis procured from different sites on the body of guinea-pigs (Billingham and Silvers 1967). They concluded that in the normal animal *inductive* stimuli from the *dermis* determine the regional specificity of the overlying epidermis. This knowledge may find application in plastic surgery.

shown that *immature* bone carries the property of inducing osteogenesis in extra-skeletal connective tissues (Urist and McClean 1952, Hellstadius 1955, Goldhaber 1961, Ray and Sabet 1963, Post *et al.* 1966); and recent work has suggested that osteogenic induction is also a property of *mature* bone (fresh, frozen or freeze-dried) (Burwell 1964b, 1966, Heiple *et al.* 1967, 1968). The property of osteogenic induction is even more developed in HCl-decalcified bone, which has been found to be intensely inductive in a variety of mammals (Urist 1965, van de Putte and Urist 1966, Büring and Urist 1967, Urist *et al.* 1967, 1968a).

The mechanism of osteogenic induction is unknown. Levander (1938) thought that the phenomenon might be due to a soluble substance passing from bone and evoking osteogenesis in susceptible tissues. Lacroix (1951) coined the name 'osteogenin' for this substance, but attempts to extract it from bone has not been consistently successful (Bridges 1959). Recent work in this field has been reviewed by Burwell (1966) (see also Post *et al.* 1966).

Most recently, Urist *et al.* (1967, 1968a) have examined the effect of a variety of physical and chemical procedures upon the inductive capacity of HCl-decalcified bone. They have concluded that protein is an essential constituent of the inductive agent, but further investigations are necessary to elucidate its composition and structural relationships to bone collagen.

Urist (1965) has proposed that the inductive agent may operate only after an interaction between cells. His scheme assumes that macrophages which have resorbed bone then induce primitive connective tissue cells to become osteoprogenitor cells and ultimately osteoblasts. Urist's *theory of autoinduction* may be outlined as follows:

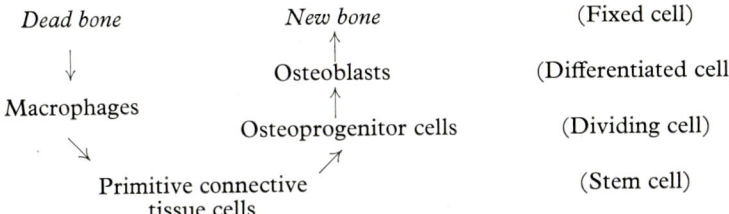

Should Urist's theory be substantiated by modern cytochemical techniques it might shed considerable light upon the process of creeping substitution and also perhaps on the condition of 'essential osteolysis' (Lagier and Rutihauser 1965). Urist has discussed the theoretical aspects of his work more fully in a recent publication (Urist *et al.* 1968a).

The artificial stimulation of osteogenesis. The foregoing discussion suggests that osteogenesis may be artificially stimulated in one of two ways, *viz.*:

(1) Primitive connective tissue cell —inductive effect→ osteoprogenitor cell (Osteogenic induction)

(2) Osteoprogenitor cell —mitogenic effect→ osteoblasts (mitotic stimulation)

In the last 30 years, attempts have been made to stimulate osteogenesis by means of inorganic and organic substances. Bisgaard (1936) reported that the synthetic inorganic salts of bone have no influence on osteogenesis. Calcium hydroxide has been claimed (Mitchell and Shankwalker 1958) and refuted (Rönning and Koski 1966) as an osteogenic inducing substance.

However, with organic substances, successful results have been achieved. Such agents include: amniotic fluid (Morrison et al. 1937); a commercial calf bone paste (Moss 1958, 1960; Anderson et al. 1960); chondroitin sulphate (Burger et al. 1962, Moss et al. 1965); β-aminopropionitrile* (Gardner 1964, 1966); oestradiol (Suzuki 1959, but see Ross 1966); and ground-egg-shell (Tarsoly and Tomory 1966, 1967).

The mechanism of action of most of these substances is unknown. They could act, as their originators believed, by being osteogenic inductors; but some such substances may act as mitotic stimulants. Further work in this important field is urgently needed. Some of the substances might find application in providing an additional osteogenic stimulus to bank bone.

THE RESORPTION OF BONE

It is generally considered that bone is resorbed largely by osteoclasts (Hancox 1956, Irving and Migliore 1965).

Recent work has indicated that macrophages (Anderson and Parker, 1966, Eger and Kammerer 1967) and perhaps endothelial cells (Cameron 1961) may play a role in the removal of bone. In the present work this group will be referred to as '*osteoclastic cells*'.

The osteocytes themselves may also, under certain conditions, resorb the bone around them (perilacunar osteolysis), which may contribute, along with remodelling, to calcium homoeostasis (Belangér et al. 1966).

Remodelling

Normal cortical bone in most mammals is undergoing internal (Haversian) remodelling throughout the life of the individual. In the process, resorption equally matches accretion.

Resorption is a continuous tunnelling operation, producing *resorption cavities* after which there is a reversal of cellular activity: the place of osteoclastic cells is taken by osteogenic cells which fill in the resorption cavities with concentric lamellae of new bone (McLean 1965). In cancellous bone, resorption takes the form of *resorption lacunae* (Howship's lacunae).

The mechanism of the 'switch-over' from bone resorption to accretion is unknown. It could involve osteoclastic cells redifferentiating as osteoblasts (Hattner et al. 1965); or the autoinduction of stem cells by osteoclastic cells (Urist 1965).

To this complex process of remodelling, which occurs in a more exaggerated manner in bone grafts, Phemister (1914) gave the name *creeping substitution* (from 'schleichender Ersatz'—Barth 1893).

*β-aminopropionitrile is the active principle contained in the seeds of the sweet-pea (*Lathyrus odoratus*) which causes *lathyrism* in rodents, chicks and frogs (Ponseti and Shepard 1954, Ponseti 1957, Bélanger 1959, Bottcher 1962).

Growth-control

After growth has ceased, many factors interact to maintain the skeleton in its mature state. In basic terms the problems relate to the factors which control *mass* and those which control the *shape* of bone.

The *mass* of the skeleton is determined by genetic, dietary, endocrine and mechanical factors (Sissons 1956); and there may be an additional central mechanism of growth-control (Burwell 1965). Bassett (1966) has recently concluded that the relation in bone between architectural and mechanical principles (Wolff's Law, Jansen 1920, Evans 1957) may be mediated through bioelectric phenomena, i.e., the deforming force causes electrical signals which stimulate osteoblasts to lay down bone to resist the force.

The *shape* of bones in the embryo is largely determined by intrinsic factors (Fell 1956, Felts 1961, Chalmers and Ray 1962). In the normal mature skeleton, though it is generally considered that shape is fixed, studies of bone grafts have indicated that the internal (Haversian) organization of cortical bone is also influenced by intrinsic mechanisms (Holmstrand 1957). In contrast the pattern of cancellous trabeculae is generally considered to be determined by mechanical forces.

CONCLUSIONS CONCERNING THE CELLULAR BIOLOGY OF BONE

In the last few years it has been confirmed that the specialized cells of bone (osteocytes, osteoblasts and osteoclasts) are different morphological and functional states of the same cell. These reversible changes have been termed modulations.

The basic cell-type in normal bone is found in the periosteum and endosteum. It is of unspecialized morphology and is called the *osteoprogenitor cell*; from it are derived all the specialized cells of bone; and to it return the osteoblasts and osteoclasts for cell division. In this chapter, for the purposes of discussion, the osteoblasts and osteoprogenitor cells of the periosteum and endosteum will be referred to as '*osteogenic cells*' (Tonna and Cronkite 1961).

The stimulus to the repair of bone after fracture, or after transplantation, is still unknown. However, there is increasing evidence that it is the necrosis of bone which leads, in some way, to the *proliferation* of osteogenic cells in the periosteum of a long bone after injury. There is an additional way in which wounded bone may stimulate osteogenesis: that is by *osteogenic induction*. Osteogenic induction is the process whereby bone (or other tissue such as urinary mucosa) may cause extra-skeletal tissue to differentiate into bone. Tissues which are susceptible to osteogenic induction are red marrow and, to a less extent, connective tissues at other sites in the body. Recently, successful attempts have been reported to stimulate artificially osteogenesis in animals. This work has not yet been applied to Man.

Remodelling is a complex process of resorption followed by accretion (creeping substitution). The resorption is undertaken by a group, termed *osteoclastic cells*; their place is then taken by osteogenic cells which lay down the lamellae of new bone. Such remodelling is the instrument by which the *mass* of the skeleton is controlled by metabolic, endocrine and mechanical factors. There is evidence that the *internal organization* of cortical bone in adults, as in embryos, is determined by mechanisms intrinsic to the bone.

Experimental Methods Used to Study Bone Grafts

If there are restrictions in studying the fate of bone grafts in patients, there are limitations perhaps equally as great when studying the process in animals. This is due not only to the question of applicability to man, but also because of: species variations; the difference between animals of the same species; the effect of age; the difference between the same tissue procured from different sites of the same animal; and differences in adjacent areas of the same graft.

Moreover, in attempting to review the fate of bone grafts, the problem is made even more complex by the fact that over 60 variables in experimental design have been used (Bassett 1962b).

Animals and Surgical Technique*

Dogs, rabbits, rats and to a less extent sheep, guinea pigs, cats and mice have been used for experimental work in bone grafting. Unless a special study is being made of the influence of age, adult (and not aged) animals are utilized in order to exclude the high osteogenic capacity of youthful bone.

The operative techniques available by which to compare one type of bone with that of another, as already stated, are numerous (Fig. 6). Those most commonly used are as follows:

Cortical site. The graft is inserted as an onlay (Campbell *et al.* 1953) or as an inlay (Reynolds and Oliver 1950) into the radius, ulna or tibia, and less frequently the humerus or femur.

Cancellous site. The graft is inserted into a defect (drill hole or core) prepared usually at the end of a long bone (Maatz *et al.* 1954, Bauermeister 1958, Fuchs 1966) or in the ilium (Bush and Garber 1948, Kingma and Hampe 1964).

Complete defects of the shaft of a long bone. A complete segment of the shaft is removed either subperiosteally or as a complete osteoperiosteal defect (Key 1934, Heiple *et al.* 1967, Zadek and Robinson 1967) of the radius, ulna or femur.

Paraskeletal site. The grafts are inserted alongside, and occasionally into, a long bone (Puranen 1966).

Spine. The spinous processes are split and the graft inserted into the prepared bed (Abbott *et al.* 1947).

Heterotopic site. The term heterotopic is used to mean the insertion of a graft into a different tissue in the same animal, e.g. skeletal muscle, subcutaneous tissue or the anterior chamber of the eye. The method is

---

* One of the major disadvantages of the many comparative studies of bone grafts is that the experimental situation bears no resemblance to any clinical procedure. Moreover, the largest defects that can be created in the skeleton of small animals are small by clinical standards; only large defects in large experimental animals are comparable to the human situation and unfortunately there have, as yet, been few studies of this kind (Chalmers 1967).

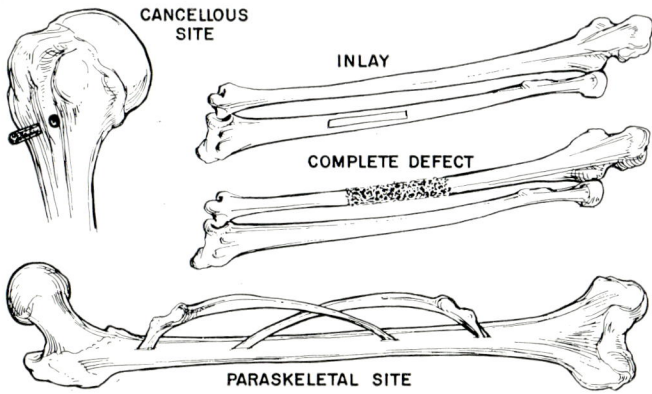

FIG. 6. Some surgical techniques used to study bone grafts experimentally.

used for studying ectopic (or heterotopic) bone formation (Bridges 1959).

Transparent chambers. The revascularization of bone grafts has been studied *in vivo* using transparent chambers: either naturally in the anterior chamber of the eye (Mosiman 1950); artificially in the rabbits' ear (Sandison 1928); or on the dorsum of the body of the rat (Kiehn *et al.* 1952); or mouse (Nishimura *et al.* 1962).

Types of Bone Graft Studied

Bone has been grafted experimentally in an almost infinite number of ways, both in the fresh state and after treatment by various physical methods, e.g. fragmentation, freezing, boiling, decalcification and deproteinization.

In the last few years there have been few reports on the fate of transplants of segments of long bones. More work in this field is needed. Firstly, because fibular grafts still have a place in orthopaedic surgery—and they still fracture!; and secondly, because of the recent attempted renaissance of massive frozen bone homografts.

Radiological and Histological Techniques

During the life of the animal the bone graft may be studied by X-ray examination and by scanning after injection of a radioactive isotope (e.g. ^{18}F; Sako and Marchetta 1966). Bone grafts in transparent chambers are examined microscopically.

After retrieval of the graft, the methods which have been used for its examination include: X-ray examination; conventional histological techniques; histochemistry, vascular perfusion; fluorescent microscopy; polarized light microscopy; radioactivity and autoradiography; microradiography; electron microscopy; and X-ray diffraction.

Alizarin, which was formerly used in studies of bone growth, has been found to inhibit osteogenesis (Harris *et al.* 1964, 1968).

Quantitative Analyses

In an attempt to overcome 'biological variability', several workers have recently made a quantitative assessment of bone grafts obtained at different time intervals after transplantation.

The methods used include: (1) a planimetric technique measuring the residual grafted bone and newly-forming bone in histological sections (Chalmers *et al.* 1960, Fuchs *et al.* 1963, Anderson *et al.* 1965, Chalmers 1966, Fuchs 1966); and (2) an arbitrary scale of measurement (Bush and Garber 1948, Kreuz *et al.* 1951, Turner *et al.* 1955, 1956, Heiple *et al.* 1963, 1967, Ecke *et al.* 1964*a,b*, Burwell 1966).

Such analyses have made possible a statistical comparison between different types of bone-grafting materials.

CONCLUSIONS CONCERNING THE EXPERIMENTAL METHODS USED TO STUDY BONE GRAFTS

The practical worth of a bone graft is determined by the rate at which it is remodelled and incorporates into the skeleton of the host.

In the experimental assessment of a cortical bone graft the inlay, or the onlay technique is the most suitable, because these are the ways in which it is used clinically. But for a cancellous graft, the complete skeletal defect of a limb bone is preferred, because in a cancellous site the high osteogenic activity of the bed will tend to cloud any differences which may exist between the various grafts. A heterotopic site is particularly useful for establishing the contribution of the graft itself to osteogenesis.

After retrieval of the graft, the examination most commonly used has been the histological method. In recent years, this has been supplemented by more sophisticated microscopical techniques; but of paramount importance is the quantitative analyses which have made possible statistical comparisons between different bone grafting materials.

The Cellular Changes Occurring in Bone Autografts

It is proposed to deal with these changes in two parts. Firstly, to give a 'bird's eye view' of the changes which occur in a bone autograft after its transplantation; and then to deal more fully with these changes and the factors which influence them.

A General Narrative

The changes which occur in a cortical or cancellous bone autograft after transplantation are of two broad types: *degenerative* and *proliferative*.

Cortical bone. Inserted as an inlay, cortical bone is rapidly surrounded by a haematoma which lies principally deep to it in the medullary cavity. The mature bone of the graft largely dies, though a few osteocytes lying near the surface may survive (Fig. 7).

Proliferation in such a skeletal site is mainly a function of the graft bed, which occurs first from the endosteal and medullary tissues. This vascular and cellular proliferation invades the haematoma and organizes it. Woven bone then appears mainly in the medullary cavity and to a less extent on the periosteal surfaces of both shaft and graft. The Haversian canals are invaded, leading to resorption of the grafted bone after which new bone is laid down as lamellae, which together constitute creeping substitution, or remodelling; such remodelling occurs in a much more exaggerated manner than in normal bone (Abbott et al. 1947, Reynolds and Oliver 1950, Ham 1952).

Finally, the graft is incorporated into the skeleton and is then subjected to the mechanisms which normally control the mass of bone tissue in the body.

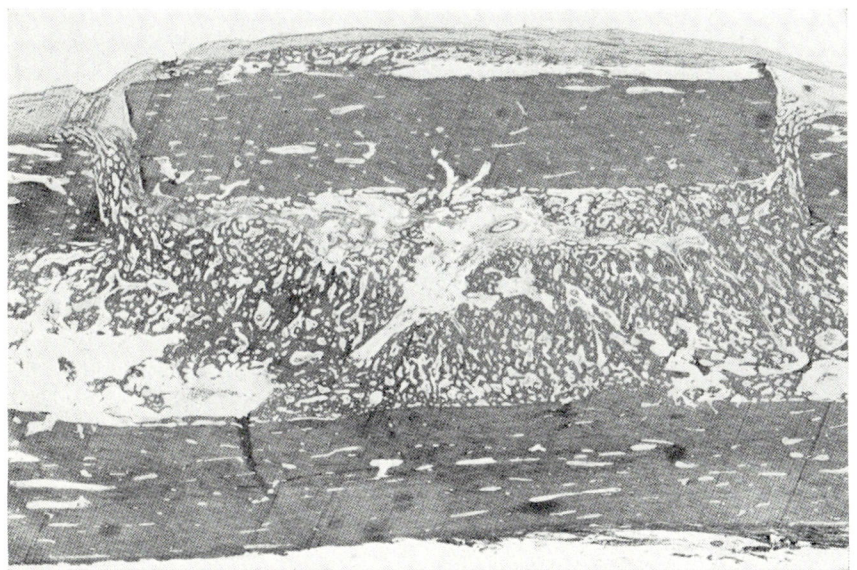

FIG. 7. An autograft of cortical bone inserted as an inlay into the tibia of the dog and removed for study 3 weeks later. Note, the graft, the considerable proliferation of new bone in the medullary cavity and the small amount of new bone on the periosteal surface of the graft. (Reproduced by kind permission of Dr. F. C. Reynolds and the Editor, *J. Bone Jt. Surg.*)

Cancellous bone. Mowlem (1944) argued that the rapidity with which his cancellous autografts adapted structurally in the human, implied their early revascularization and cellular activity (see Abbott 1944).

Experimentally it has been shown that cancellous bone, like cortical bone largely dies after transplantation, but given a good blood supply its peripheral portions survive to provide a lively source of osteogenesis (Abbott et al. 1947, Ham and Gordon 1952, Hutchinson 1952, Siffert 1955).

The central necrotic tissue is rapidly invaded by a young vascular connective tissue derived from the peripheral portions of the graft and from the tissues of the bed (Fig. 8). Thus within a few days of transplanting a small cancellous bone graft, its spaces are filled with a

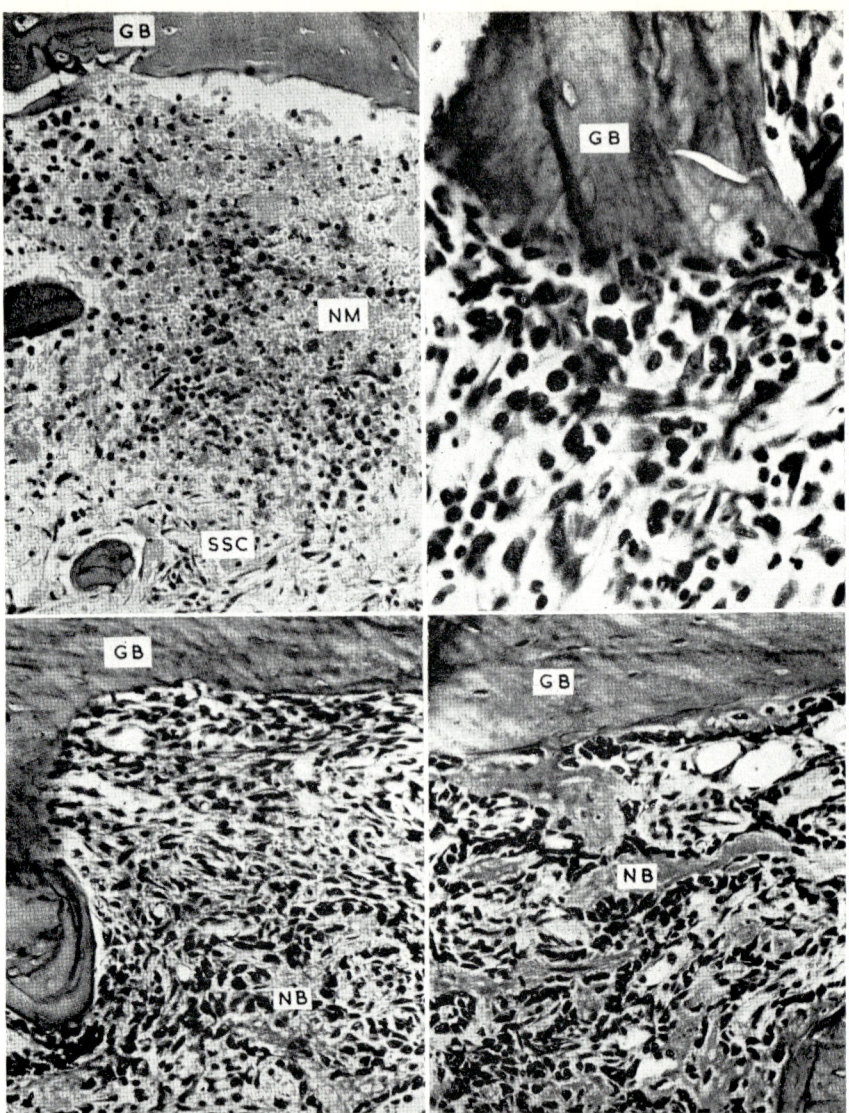

Fig. 8. Autografts of fresh marrow-containing iliac bone, removed 3, 5 and 7 days after transplantation (Hematoxylin and eosin). (*Top, left*): Three days. Note the grafted bone (GB), the necrotic marrow (NM) and the spindle-shaped cells (SSC) in the superficial (lower) part of the marrow ($\times$ 230). (*Top, right*): Five days. Note the grafted bone (GB) and the cells occupying the intertrabecular space, namely, spindle-shaped cells, round and ovoid cells with prominent nucleoli, small round cells and polymorphonuclear leukocytes ($\times$ 400). (*Bottom, left*): Seven days. Note the grafted bone (GB), the young cellular tissue occupying the intertrabecular space and the small amount of new woven bone (NB) ($\times$ 230). (*Bottom, right*): Seven days. Note the grafted bone (GB) and the new woven bone (NB) occupying the intertrabecular space. Healthy osteoblasts are seen on the surfaces of this new bone ($\times$ 230). (From Burwell, R. G., *Clin. Orthop. and Related Res.*, **40**, 35, 1965.)

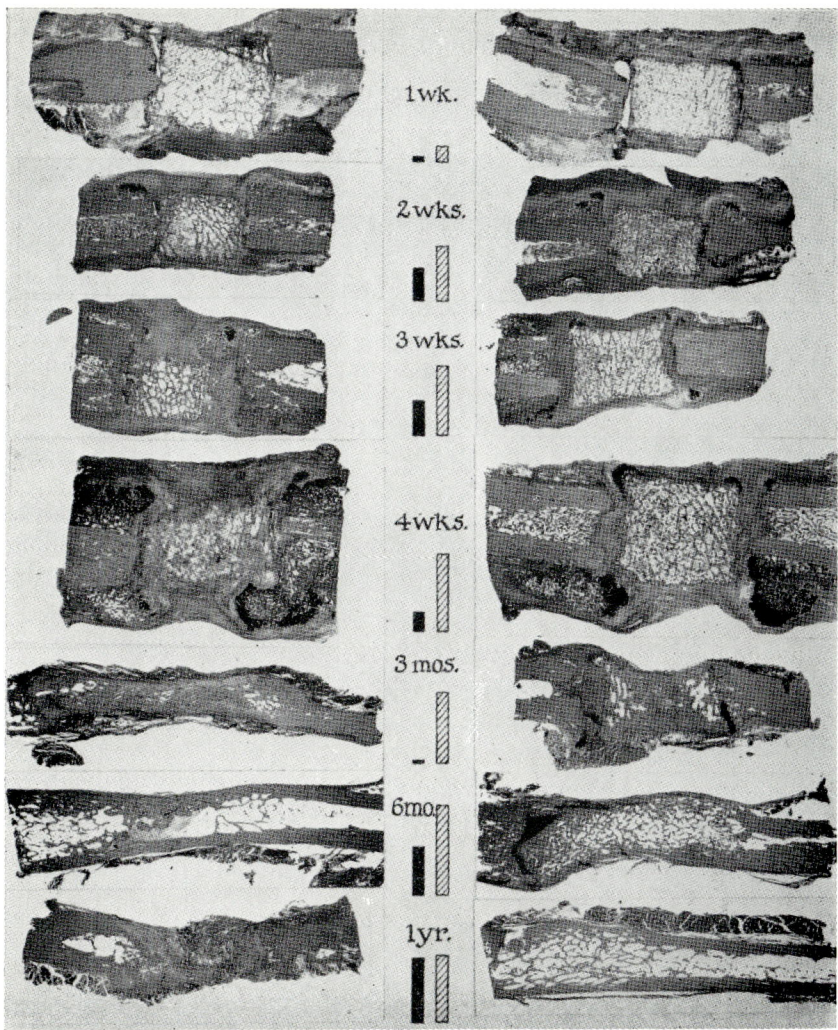

Fig. 9. Representative sections on the right of *autografts* of fresh cancellous bone and on the left of *homografts* of fresh cancellous bone inserted into complete defects of the ulnae of dogs and removed for study at intervals from 1 week to 1 year. Note the incorporation and remodelling of the grafted area in both the homografts and the autografts. (Reproduced by kind permission of Dr. K. G. Heiple and the Editor, *J. Bone Jt. Surg.*)

proliferating complex composed of several cell types derived from endosteum, marrow and the tissues of the graft bed.

From the proliferating cellular complex, pattern and order are re-established with the production of a scaffolding of woven bone, a scattering of myeloid cells and blood vessels which permeate the burgeon of newly-forming tissues. In the ensuing weeks, the woven bone is replaced by lamellar bone and the graft either incorporates into the skeleton (Fig. 9) or in a heterotopic site, forms an ossicle.

The above account refers to a small cancellous bone graft transplanted under optimal conditions into a bed with a good blood supply. However, it is the experience of many clinicians that a block of cancellous bone may fail to be replaced by normal bone or may even disappear. In this connection it is of interest to note that in a recent experimental series of cancellous autografts inserted into prepared defects of the ulna in dogs after one year, complete resorption of the graft had occurred in 30 per cent (5/17 grafts) leaving the bony gap bridged only by connective tissue, fat or muscle (Heiple et al. 1963).

Cortical-versus-cancellous bone as grafting material. For osteogenic purposes, cancellous bone is vastly superior to cortical bone because: (1) the endosteal surface of cancellous bone is large (Abbott et al. 1947); (2) iliac cancellous bone contains red marrow which is itself osteogenic (Burwell 1964a); and (3) the spongework of cancellous bone is usually readily invaded by living cells.

Cancellous bone does not of course provide rigidity. This is why Albee (1915) chose cortical bone for grafting. But rigid internal fixation is now provided by inert metals. Hence the use of cortical bone in surgery has declined.

A Detailed Narrative

The fate of a bone autograft—be it to create the desired bridge of osteogenic tissue, to remain inert, or to be erased and leave no mark, is controlled by many interacting factors.

Fundamentally, these factors relate to: the graft; the bed in which it lies; the host; and whether or not it becomes infected. For purposes of review, it is convenient to discuss the factors as they may operate during the natural history of a bone graft under the following headings:

    Necrosis
    Mitosis
    Revascularization
    Osteogenesis
    Remodelling
    Growth

Necrosis

Although it is now established that most of a cortical bone graft dies after transplantation, until recently one question remained: but how much survives?

Nisbet and his colleagues (Heslop et al. 1960) have critically re-examined this question quantitatively in rats, studying, for this purpose, tubular sections of the tibia transplanted supra-pannicularly (i.e. between the *panniculus carnosus* and the skin). They confirmed that most of a cortical bone autograft dies, but they found a strip of cells survive in the outermost portion of the graft. The survival of this band of cells (which never exceeded 0·3 mm. in depth from the surface of the transplant) was attributed to a plasmatic circulation passing through bone canaliculi supplemented later by the development of a new blood supply.

More recently other workers, also using a quantitative technique, have confirmed that considerable numbers of osteocytes survive in mature autologous bone after its transplantation (Nishimura et al. 1962).

The effect of fragmentation. Fragmentation of bone is frequently performed in surgical grafting to provide for: (a) more prolific new bone formation; (b) speedier reconstruction; and (c) greater resistance to infection. The particular value of cancellous bone chips for certain procedures in surgical practice is now well-substantiated. However there are experimental observations showing that if bone is broken up too finely, then it is no longer osteogenic and may even act as a foreign body.

Cortical shavings. Osteoperiosteal shavings are widely used in (a) spinal fusion operations, supplemented at times by joint excision and grafting; and (b) in myoplastic amputations. But cortical shavings prepared from the shaft of a long bone (previously freed from its periosteum) are of little value as grafting material. For it has been shown in adult animals that such shavings not only die, but excite a strong foreign-body reaction and play no part in osteogenesis (Keith 1934, Siffert 1955).

Cortical chips. Likewise, it has been found that small cortical bone chips die and contribute little to osteogenesis (Hey Groves 1917, Anderson 1961).

Anderson (1961) studied the fate of two sizes of cortical chips: the smaller being 0·3–0·7 mm. diameter; the larger averaging $2·8 \times 1 \times 1$ mm. The chips were inserted into the anterior chamber of the eye in rats. Surprisingly it was found that the smaller fragments underwent complete necrosis; they did not form new bone, probably because they incited an inflammatory response. In the larger fragments, osteocytes did survive but only a small amount of appositional new bone was formed.

Cancellous chips. Anderson (1961) found again that tiny fragments of cancellous bone (0·3–0·7 mm.) died completely without any new bone being formed. In the larger cancellous chips, however, while the major portion still died at the periphery a few cells survived to form new bone which extended vigorously into both graft and surrounding tissues.

Segments of long bones. The fate of segments of whole rib after transplantation has been studied in a paraskeletal site (Campbell et al. 1953, Puranen 1966) and in the spine (Abbott et al. 1947).

The graft again largely dies, being revascularized by vessels growing down into the necrotic medullary canal from both ends; but the medulla may become fibrotic (Owen et al. 1958). If the rib is first split to expose its medullary surface more rapid revascularization and greater survival occurs (Eloesser 1920, Campbell et al. 1953).

CONCLUSIONS

Most of a bone graft (cortical and cancellous) dies after grafting; only the most superficial parts survive to be a source of osteogenesis. It is fallacious to fragment a bone graft more than is necessary for the technique of the operation, since minute fragmentation not only lowers its osteogenic function, but also kills the bone. Further work is required to establish the optimum size of cancellous chips and the optimum thickness for strips of cancellous bone.

Mitosis

Relatively little is known about the mitotic proliferation in grafts of mature bone. Two studies using ^{3}H-thymidine related to neonatal bone (Ray and Sabet 1963) and fracture callus (Urist et al. 1965).

Conventional histological methods, however, have shown that proliferation occurs first in the region of the endosteum and to a lesser extent in the periosteum of the graft (Abbott et al. 1947, Reynolds and Oliver 1950).

By analogy with the recent studies of fracture healing (Tonna and Cronkite 1963, Young 1963), it might be expected that the elements which are first stimulated to divide are the osteoprogenitor cells. The mechanism which triggers mitosis in such cells is unknown, but, as discussed previously, it may be due to the necrosis of the adjacent bone.

Revascularization

The 'take' of a bone graft, like that of a skin graft, is a race between impending death and the struggle to survive.

Whereas a full-thickness skin autograft usually survives, a bone autograft largely dies. This difference is due to the inability of the vessels of the graft bed to gain a ready access to bone. In cortical grafts only the periosteum and certain osteocytes survive; the contents of most of the Haversian canals die before the new capillary sprouts can support them. In iliac cancellous bone, death of the deeper-lying tissues occur probably because of the delicacy of the medullary vessels and the failure of diffusion alone to support the high metabolic needs of red marrow.

In recent years, several workers have studied experimentally the revascularization of bone autografts inserted into skeletal and heterotopic sites (Ham 1952, Stringa 1957, Hammack and Enneking 1960, Zeiss et al. 1960, Kingma and Hampe 1964, Deleu and Trueta 1965).

Cortical bone. The periosteal proliferations of a cortical bone graft (transplanted with its periosteum intact) are rapidly revascularized and is followed by invasion of the underlying cortex (Hammack and Enneking 1960). In periosteal-free cortical transplants, most of the revascularization occurs along necrotic Haversian canals (Fig. 10a) (Ham 1952, Zeiss et al. 1960, Kingma and Hampe 1964).

Revascularization is essential for the next stage of bone repair, namely its resorption. But even in the relatively small cortical bone grafts inserted into animals, revascularization may still be incomplete eight months after grafting (Zeiss et al. 1960).

A problem of some practical importance is: does an intact periosteum hinder or facilitate the revascularization of a cortical bone graft? An attempt has been made to answer this question using the uptake of a radioactive isotope (^{32}P) as an indicator of revascularization. The findings showed that an intact periosteum hinders revascularization of the underlying bone of the graft (Ferguson et al. 1959).

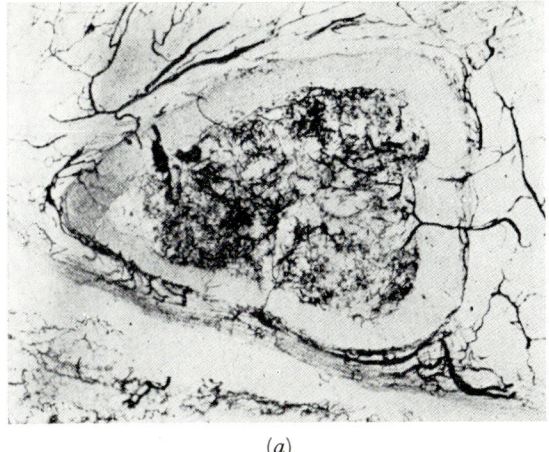

(a)

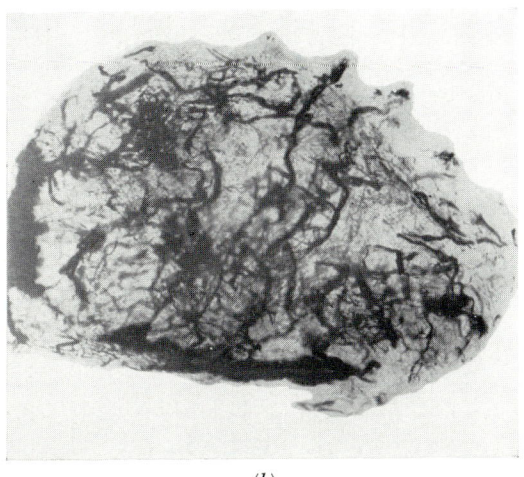

(b)

FIG. 10. (a) A cortical tibial autograft removed 5 weeks after its insertion suprapannicularly into a rat. Note the medullary vessels (filled with Berlin blue) and the moderate revascularization of the cortex. (Reproduced by kind permission of Mr. N. W. Nisbet and the Editor, *Brit. J. Exp. Path.*)
(b) A cancellous autograft removed 8 days after its insertion into the anterior chamber of the eye of a guinea-pig. Note the complete revascularization of the graft. (Reproduced by kind permission of Professor J. Trueta and the Editor, *J. Bone Jt. Surg.*)

Cancellous bone. After an initial delay (due to necrosis of the central tissues of the graft), cancellous transplants are revascularized quickly in one to three weeks, depending upon their size (Fig. 10b) (Stringa 1957, Deleu and Trueta 1965). Clinical experience suggests that blocks of cancellous bone, under certain circumstances, are revascularized poorly if at all. This may be linked to the vascularity of the bed into which the bone is implanted; thus cancellous bone transplanted to the abdominal fat in Man is said to die completely or be replaced very slowly by fibrous tissue (Peer 1951).

Segments of long bones largely die after transplantation and are revascularized from the periosteal surface and by vessels growing into the medullary canal from both ends (Haldeman 1933, Abbott et al. 1947, Puranen 1966). Further work is required to define which route is the more important and to study the effect of: (a) intra-medullary fixation (see Göthman 1960, 1961, 1962); and (b) multiple perforations of the shaft, upon the process.

CONCLUSIONS

Unlike a skin graft, the circulation in a bone graft is never re-established sufficiently rapidly to enable more than a proportion of its cells to survive. Bone is usually transplanted with its periosteum removed and there is evidence that this may hasten revascularization of the graft. In a long tubular bone graft, it is not known whether the revascularization is predominantly periosteal or medullary; if it be medullary then multiple perforations of the shaft might facilitate the process (Küpperman and Schwier 1964).

In practice, the optimal conditions for survival will be provided by placing the bone graft in the closest contact with a vascular bed of bone and marrow, and with healthy muscle overlying it. In this connection efficient suction drainage of the wound would seem to be essential.

Osteogenesis

The formation of new bone is obligatory in order to achieve union between a bone graft and the part of the skeleton with which it is placed in contact.

The osteogenesis of repair is derived both from the graft and from its bed, but the relative contribution of each depends largely upon the type of bone grafted: while a cancellous bone graft will contribute much to osteogenesis, a cortical graft will give little.

Many factors are known which influence this repair process. In this section it is proposed to discuss firstly, the source of the new bone; and secondly, the factors which influence the osteogenesis of repair in a bone graft.

(a) THE GRAFT

Source of the new bone. A bone transplant is a composite tissue graft, being composed of mature bone, periosteum, endosteum and frequently marrow. Each of these tissues can contribute to osteogenesis.

Periosteum. In transplanting bone, the surgeon needs to know the answer to the question: should a bone graft be transplanted with or without its periosteum?

Experimentally the periosteum has been the butt of discussion since Axhausen (1908) claimed for it an osteogenic role and Macewen (1912) denied it. The argument was resolved with the knowledge that the periosteum is composed of two layers: a fibrous limiting membrane and a cambium layer. The fate of a *free* transplant of periosteum, i.e., whether or not it forms bone, is influenced by many factors including the age of the animal; the species; the bone; the site along the bone from which it is procured; and whether or not the periosteum has been recently 'activated' by a fracture (Fang and Miltner 1934, Lacroix 1951, Axhausen 1956, Zucman et al. 1968a,b).

However, the experimental finding that stripping the periosteum from a limb bone of the adult dog leaves the cambium layer attached to the shaft suggests, from the standpoint of osteogenesis, that cortical bone need not be transplanted with its periosteum (Phemister 1914). In this connection Gallie (1918) wrote: "This view has been corroborated clinically to our satisfaction in a long series of bone transplantations in which we have been unable to detect any difference in the clinical results following transplantations with and without periosteum" (Gallie and Robertson 1918).

Gallie's opinion is now generally accepted in orthopaedic and plastic surgery (Watson-Jones 1946, Peer 1955), though it has not passed unchallenged (Haldeman 1933, Vainio 1950). In the practice of bone grafting, however, the problem may be of little importance because a cortical bone graft (with or without periosteum) contributes poorly to osteogenesis and, in a cancellous graft, the proliferation is largely endosteal (Abbott et al. 1947, Ham and Gordon 1952).

Cortical bone. The mature bone of a cortical graft largely dies. Hence its contribution to osteogenesis must be negligible.

Bassett et al. (1961), however, using a tissue-culture technique found that cortical bone from which the periosteum and endosteum had been removed, showed an initial burst of cell migration (Dobrowolskaja 1916). These migrating cells were probably derived from the surviving cells of the Haversian and Volkmann canals and, it would seem, can under certain circumstances contribute to the repair of bone (Bassett and Rued 1966).

Endosteum. The endosteum is a potent source of new bone when a good blood supply is provided for its survival. This is most clearly seen when living cancellous bone is transplanted to a heterotopic site, e.g. to skeletal muscle or to the anterior chamber of the eye (Ham and Gordon 1952, Hutchinson 1952, Urist and McLean 1952, Siffert 1955).

Under such conditions cancellous grafts form much more new bone than do grafts of cortical bone; this has been attributed to the larger endosteal surface of cancellous, as opposed to cortical, bone (Abbott et al. 1947).

However, iliac cancellous bone grafts contain *red marrow* as well as trabeculae of bone; and red marrow is itself highly osteogenic after transplantation. Hence, a proportion of the new bone formed by iliac cancellous bone grafts is presumably derived from its contained medullary cells (Burwell 1964a, 1966). This may explain why iliac cancellous bone is superior in terms of osteogenesis than say tibial, or tarsal, cancellous bone. An additional factor may be that cancellous bone procured distally in a limb and used as a graft contains fatty marrow which after necrosis will impede revascularization (Abbott et al. 1947).

Red marrow. Grafts of red marrow, carefully freed from bone particles and endosteum and transplanted to a heterotoptic site, form new bone (Pfeiffer 1948, Urist and McLean 1952, Bloom 1960). The reason why red marrow, after transplantation, is osteogenic is unknown (Burwell 1964a).

In the last few years some light has been shed on this change by a study of recombinant grafts of bone and marrow removed for examination at intervals of time after transplantation (Burwell 1964a, 1966).

It was found that while fresh cancellous bone (as well as frozen and freeze-dried bone) will stimulate osteogenesis in marrow, other types of bone (deproteinized) appeared to inhibit it. These effects are shown schematically in the following diagram (Fig. 11):

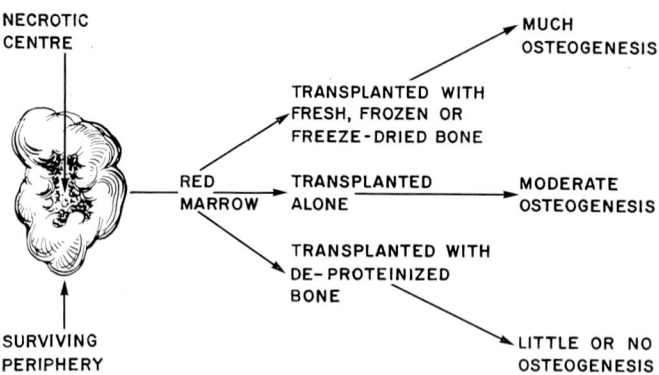

FIG. 11. Diagrammatic representation of the fate of different varieties of bone grafts impregnated with fresh red marrow and implanted intramuscularly into rats.

A theory has been proposed to account for these findings. Briefly this theory states: that the central necrotic marrow stimulates the peripheral surviving marrow to form bone by the process of osteogenic induction (*theory of medullary intrinsic induction*). It will be seen that the presence of bone adds an *extrinsic* element in the form of necrosing, or dead, bone to the theory.

Thus, marrow in repair may have a *dichotomy in differentiation*: under optimal conditions to form new bone; and in adversity to become phagocytic, viz.:

$$\text{Red marrow} \begin{cases} \text{osteogenesis} \\ \text{phagocytosis} \end{cases}$$

This could explain why infection frequently leads to the delayed union of fractures. Clearly further work is needed to substantiate or refute this concept.

(b) THE GRAFT BED

The contribution of the graft bed to the repair of bone transplant is a dual one, namely blood vessels and connective tissue cells. In a skeletal bed the connective tissue cells are osteogenic and require only a mitogenic stimulus to form bone; in a heterotopic site the connective tissue cells must first be induced to become osteoprogenitor cells by the process of osteogenic induction.

Skeletal defect. A complete skeletal defect will provide callus derived from the periosteum, endosteum and marrow to form the so-called periosteal intermediary and medullary callus (Phemister 1914). Cartilage may appear and undergo endochondral ossification, a formation which may result from a limited blood supply (Ham 1930) or more particularly from a low oxygen tension (Bassett and Herrmann 1961). The intermediary callus is the last to undergo ossification and requires months for its completion.

Paraskeletal site. When the Phemister principle of grafting is adopted, osteogenesis will largely be a function of the graft and to a lesser extent, the periosteum. Hence cancellous bone is preferable to cortical bone as grafting material (but see Zucman *et al.* 1968*a*).

Heterotopic site. Experimental observations have shown that connective tissues in heterotopic sites, e.g. subcutis, skeletal muscle, anterior chamber of the eye, can be induced to become osteogenic by the presence of a bone graft; but only after a few weeks, and then only in small amounts. This is known as *late-phase bone* (Axhausen 1956) and is shown most clearly by implanting devitalized bone into an extra-skeletal site (see Bridges 1959).

The mechanism which causes such late-phase bone is probably osteogenic induction.

CONCLUSION

From the standpoint of osteogenesis, the adult patient can provide three orders of bone for grafting purposes: *first order bone* is iliac cancellous bone: it supplies a large trabecular endosteal surface covered with osteogenic cells plus red marrow which is itself osteogenic after transplantation. *Second order bone* is fatty cancellous bone from the tarsus, tibia and lower femur: this bone does not contain red marrow and its fat, after necrosis, probably inhibits revascularization. *Third order bone* is cortical bone whose contribution to osteogenesis is minimal and is much less than that of the skeletal bed into which it is inserted.

The small amount of new bone which may be induced (by osteogenic induction) in the extra-osseous connective tissues surrounding a bone graft, is probably of little importance in clinical practice.

Factors influencing osteogenesis. As stated previously the fate of a bone graft is determined by the interaction of many factors which relate, basically, to the graft, its bed and the host in which it lies; and whether or not it becomes infected.

The complexity of the problem is shown by the following summary of factors which can influence osteogenesis in a bone graft.

(1) THE GRAFT

Type of bone. The superiority of cancellous over cortical bone as grafting material has already been discussed.

Time interval between procurement and transplantation. Puranen (1966) has recently examined the effect of leaving bone exposed to air or lying in saline before it is transplanted. He found that one hour's exposure of the rabbit rib to air reduced its osteogenic ability to that of deep-frozen bone, i.e. virtually nil. Preserved in normal saline the bone retained its viability for two hours. This effect was not prolonged by immersing the bone in blood at 37°C. Bohr et al. (1967, 1968) have confirmed these observations using rabbit iliac bone.

The practical lessons from these observations are two: (*a*) to cut a bone graft immediately before it is needed; and (*b*) if there is a delay, to insert the graft in saline.

Freezing. It is now generally agreed that freezing at −15°C (or below) kills adult bone and prevents osteogenesis developing from it after grafting (Ham and Gordon 1952, De Bruyn and Kabisch 1955, Haas 1957, but see Ray et al. 1954); though frozen autografts of bone do incorporate ^{32}P from the blood stream (Kiehn et al. 1948, 1950). Haas (1957), however, reported that bone stored in citrated whole blood at +5°C for two weeks showed proliferation after transplantation to muscle.

The duration of refrigeration affects the speed of incorporation of a bone autograft. Thus, while two weeks storage has little effect on resorption of a bone graft (Bush and Garber 1948), resorption is delayed if the bone has been refrigerated for four weeks or longer (Maatz et al. 1954). This effect may result from slow denaturation of bone proteins. It might be avoided by storing bone at −70°C.

Boiling and autoclaving. Such heat kills bone, denatures the proteins, impairs revascularization (Deleu and Trueta 1965) and the uptake of ^{32}P from the blood stream (Kiehn et al. 1950); it also markedly retards resorption of bone by the tissues of the host (Curtiss and Wilson 1953, Maatz et al. 1954, Holmstrand 1957). Despite the severe impairment of the biological properties of bone produced by heat there are, of course, occasions in surgery when boiled bone must be used (see Part II: Preserved homografts—boiled bone).

Size of the graft. If a bone graft is large, resorption of it will be prolonged, and, if osteogenesis does not follow in its wake, the graft may fracture. On the other hand, if a bone graft is fragmented into tiny particles even cancellous bone is killed and is no longer osteogenic (Hey Groves 1917, Anderson 1961).

Mowlem (1944) argued that iliac cancellous chips remain viable in Man. This effect of size was shown clearly in a recent series of 137 bone autografts: the failure rate using a full-thickness bone block was 17 per cent; with autograft chips it was only 8 per cent (Carnesale and Spankus 1959).

Bone powder. The fate of bone powder ('blenderized' bone) after implantation depends largely on the site into which it is inserted. In the shaft of a long bone the powder is absorbed and does not promote union (Hey Groves 1917). Williams (1964), however, has used minced boiled iliac bone successfully for the treatment of non-union in the shafts of long bones. At the end of a long bone (i.e. in cancellous bone), the particles are rapidly incorporated into the host; and a successful clinical application has been reported (Rosenberg *et al.* 1955). It has also been claimed that powdered bone mixed with gelatin is a useful matrix for grafting (Swanker and Winfield 1952).

It should be added in this connection that plaster-of-paris has been used experimentally and clinically to fill defects of bone. It is absorbed, neither inhibiting nor encouraging, osteogenesis (Peltier 1961). If plaster-of-paris is mixed with ground egg-shell, the mixture is claimed to have a stimulating effect on osteogenesis (Tarsoly and Tomory 1967).

Previous 'activation' of the graft. The 'activation' of a bone graft by surgical means (saw-cuts) one to two weeks before it is transplanted, has been found to result in accelerated attachment and incorporation of the bone (Brooks 1919, Sako and Marchetta 1966). However, Siffert and Barash (1961) were unable to confirm these findings.

In this connection it should be remembered that Orell (1937, 1938) used specially-prepared tibial callus ('os novum') for the treatment of non-union and for arthrodesis with good results.

Vascular pedicles for bone grafts. Cancellous bone grafts transplanted on a muscular pedicle largely survive, though cortical grafts similarly transplanted mostly die (Davis and Taylor 1952, Baadsgaard and Medgyesi 1965, Medgyesi 1965). A skin flap may be used both to transplant bone (McGregor and Simonetta 1965) and to transplant digits from the foot to the hand (see Section "Anatomy of Bone Grafting"). Neuro-vascular bundles are utilized in the hand for transposing digital rays, and in the lower limb for 'turning-up' the tibia and fibula to replace the femur excised for tumour (van Nes 1948).

(2) THE GRAFT BED

Site of grafting. In a skeletal bed, the resorption and replacement of a bone graft occurs more rapidly at the (cancellous) end of a long bone than at the centre of the shaft (cortical bone). Hence dead (bank) bone can be used to fill a cyst, but living bone is better for grafting of delayed union.

In an experimental heterotopic site the bone may die completely if the blood supply is poor, e.g. iliac cancellous bone implanted into the fat of the anterior abdominal wall in Man (Peer 1951). In a more vascular site, the graft survives, but the amount of new bone formed is said to be less than in an orthotopic (skeletal) site (Hellstadius 1950). Moreover, with increasing time, bone in a heterotopic site slowly wastes and may ultimately be replaced by fibrous tissue (Haas 1921, Klinkerfuss 1924, Peer 1951, Mowlem 1952). These experiments show clearly that unless a bone graft is in contact with the skeleton, it wastes. Hence a functional stimulus (mainly mechanical) is necessary to maintain the mass of the skeleton (Wolff).

Contact between graft and host. Albee (1923) emphasized the importance of accurate contact between a cortical bone graft and its bed. He made this recommendation not only for mechanical but also for biological reasons.

Bone-to-bone contact is equally necessary when the Phemister principle is adopted in the treatment of delayed union; or when a graft is used to fill a skeletal defect.

Insecure fixation. Hey Groves (1917) and Albee (1923, 1944) each stressed the need for rigid immobilization of the part after bone grafting. Difficult delayed unions are frequently fixed internally as well as grafted. It would be rewarding to study experimentally the effect of rigid internal fixation upon the healing of a bone graft, because such fixation has already been shown to modify fracture repair.

Infection. Sepsis is one of the most important causes of non-union of a fracture.

Previously, when cortical bone grafts were in vogue, it was considered tantamount to malpractice to graft bone in the presence of sepsis (Hey Groves 1917). Now, it is known that cancellous chips will occasionally survive in the presence of sepsis (Cleveland and Winant 1952) and particularly, as in the case of chronic osteomyelitis of the tibia, if a 'back-door' approach is used for their insertion (Harmon 1945, Marmor 1964).

Irradiation. A bone graft is occasionally used to replace an excised tumour which is then followed by irradiation therapy. It has been found in dogs that irradiation (2000 rads) of the site of bone grafting, has little effect upon the repair process (Hartman and Rapp 1965).

Previous 'activation' of the graft bed. The surgical preparation of a skeletal bed one to two weeks before a cortical or cancellous graft is transplanted into it, leads to a more rapid attachment and incorporation of the bone than if it is inserted into a freshly-prepared defect (Siffert and Barash 1961, Sako and Marchetta 1966). This method may find a limited clinical application in the treatment of delayed union.

(3) THE HOST

Animal variation. The animal used in experimental work may influence the fate of a bone graft by its species, age and by individual variation (Brooks and Hudson 1920, Heiple *et al.* 1963, Zadek and Robinson 1967).

Steroids. Cortisone administered to dogs (1 mg./lb. body weight) has no apparent effect upon the healing of bone grafts (Curtiss and Wilson 1953). But oestradiol has been found to stimulate endosteal new bone formation in autografts of tibiae transplanted subcutaneously into growing mice (Suzuki 1959). Ross (1966), however, found that neither diethylstilboestrol nor prednisolone influenced the healing of bone grafts inserted into dogs.

Negative calcium balance. Bone autografts inserted into dogs which had received a low calcium diet, were reported to be rapidly revascularized through the widened Haversian canals of cortical bone (Ghormley and Stuck 1934).

Mechanical factors. During the incorporation of a bone graft into the skeleton, it is likely that mechanical forces crossing the site of grafting act to modify both the proliferation of osteoblasts and the orientation of collagen fibres secreted by them.

Ill-understood factors. Finally, there is a group of factors which must operate upon bone after grafting and about which, as yet, little is known. These factors relate to the mechanisms which control: (*a*) mitotic proliferation; (b) the internal organization of woven, lamellar and Haversian bone; and (c) the succession of resorption by osteogenesis.

CONCLUSION

Many factors interact to control osteogenesis in a bone graft. In essence they relate to the graft, its bed and the host in which it lies.

The most important factors are: the type of bone transplanted (cancellous > cortical bone); the site into which it is inserted; the degree of fixation; and whether or not infection occurs.

Factors which sap the vitality from a bone graft include: being left in the air to dry; being cut up into tiny fragments; and, of course, freezing and boiling. The adherence of a bone graft to its bed can be increased by preparing the bed surgically one to two weeks before the bone is inserted into it.

Finally there are a group of factors, or mechanisms, which must operate upon a healing bone graft and which, as yet, little is known. These are the mechanisms which control the growth of tissues; and their action may explain how species, age and individual variation influence repair in bone.

Remodelling

Basically, remodelling consists of two processes, namely resorption followed by accretion. The cellular elements which are essential for these actions are osteoclastic cells, osteogenic cells and blood vessels.

The internal remodelling of a bone graft is similar to the internal remodelling of normal bone in the intact skeleton, but it occurs in a much more exaggerated manner in a bone graft. The remodelling of bone grafts has been studied in numerous experimental sites (orthotopic and heterotopic), using many different types of bone. It is proposed here to restrict the discussion to studies published in recent years relating to the remodelling of cortical bone, cancellous bone and chips of a long bone (rib).

Cortical bone. *Morphological changes.* Several workers have recently described the remodelling of cortical grafts inserted as inlays into the radius of the dog (Reynolds and Oliver 1950, Kreuz *et al.* 1951, Bassett and Creighton 1962, Karges *et al.* 1963).

The bone is invaded by blood vessels which show a preference to travel along the pre-existing Haversian canals. Osteoclastic cells then produce a porosity which is most marked after 4–6 months, and at this time a graft is liable to fracture (Fig. 12). In the resorption cavities, so formed, bone is laid down as concentric lamellae to form new Haversian systems. This process of resorption followed by accretion ('creeping substitution') continues until all the dead cortex is replaced. It may take three months to a year or more for its completion depending upon the size and density of the graft (Phemister 1914).

Mineralization follows in the wake of new osteoid formation. The accretion bone of the new Haversian systems is at first poorly mineralized and only slowly acquires a higher mineral content (Holmstrand 1957).

The mechanism of the 'switch-over' from resorption to accretion. While the morphological changes of remodelling which occur in a cortical bone graft are well-understood, the mechanism which ensures that, in most cases, osteoclastic cells are replaced by osteogenic cells is still problematical. Two theories have been suggested: (*a*) that the osteoclastic cells have a 'built-in' progression to become osteogenic cells (Hattner *et al.* 1965); and (*b*) that the osteoclastic cells induce osteogenic-cell formation in primitive connective tissue cells (autoinduction) (Urist 1965).

This problem is of practical importance, because the failure of this 'switch-over' to occur will lead to complete resorption of the graft. An electron microscopical study of the resorption spaces of HCl-decalcified bone might shed considerable light on the problem.

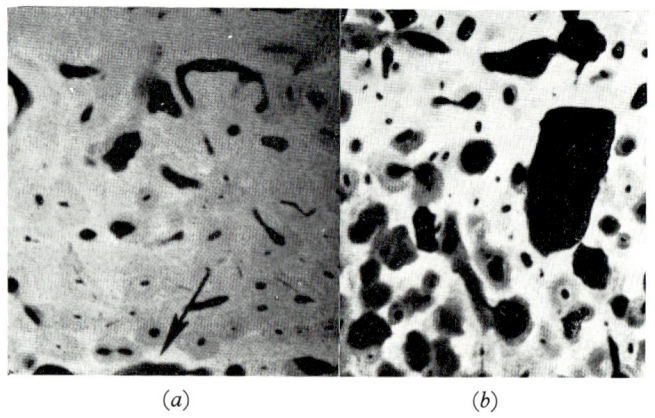

(*a*) (*b*)

FIG. 12. (*a*) A microradiograph of a cortical bone autograft removed 3 months after its insertion as an inlay into a dog.
(*b*) A similar graft removed 6 months after its insertion as an inlay. Note in the microradiograph the large resorption cavities. (Reproduced by kind permission of Dr. D. E. Karges and the Editor, *Clin. Orthops and Related Res.*)

Cancellous bone. A few workers have made a careful and comprehensive study of the remodelling of autografts inserted into prepared defects of the forearm bones in the dog (Fig. 9) (Heiple *et al.* 1963, Karges *et al.* 1963).

The grafts are rapidly invaded in two weeks by woven bone which is laid down upon the trabeculae and within the spaces of the bone. Resorption of the grafted and newly-formed bone then occurs, associated with the development of lamellar bone. By three months, Haversian systems have appeared and by six months the shaft of the bone is reconstituted. Hence the remodelling of cancellous grafts is much more rapid than that of cortical grafts.

Resorption does not always follow accretion, as in the case of cortical bone. This was shown very clearly in a recent series of cancellous bone grafts inserted into complete defects of the ulna in the dog (Heiple *et al.*

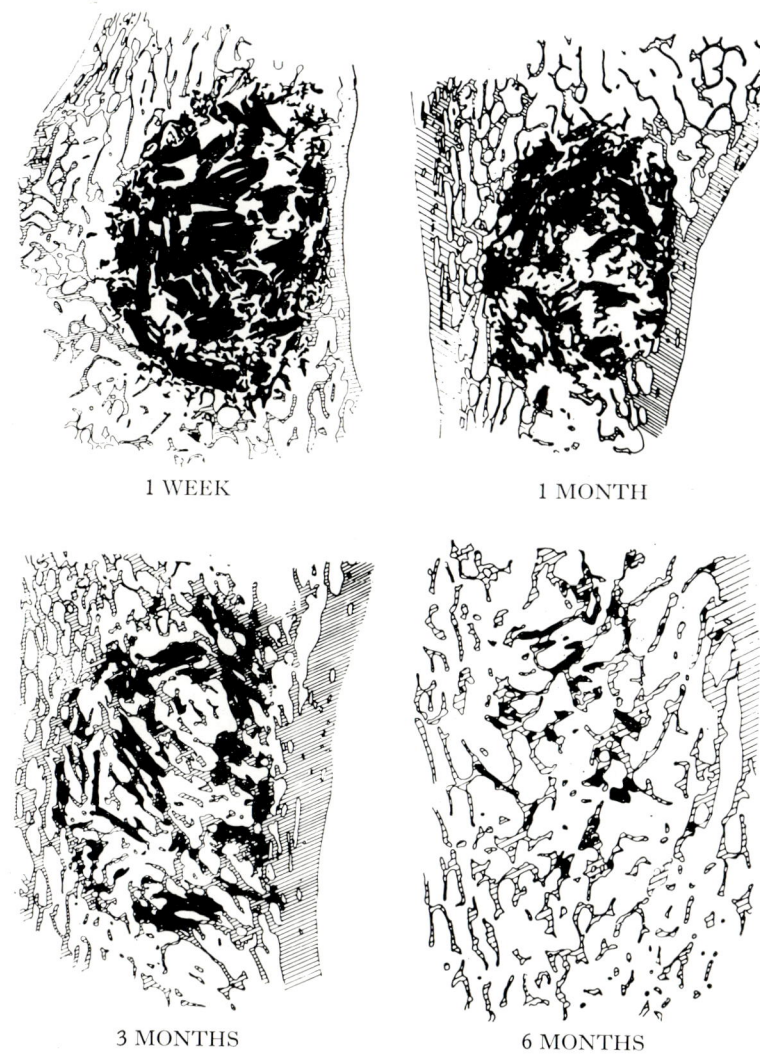

Fig. 13. Camera lucida tracings of the femora of dogs into which autograft chips of rib bone had been inserted previously (1 week to 6 months). Note the gradual removal of the grafted bone (black) with increasing time intervals. (Reproduced by kind permission of Mr. J. Chalmers and the Armour Pharmaceutical Co., Ltd.)

1967); after one year, 30 per cent of the grafts had been replaced by connective tissue, fat or muscle.

Chips of rib. Chalmers and his colleagues have studied the remodelling of chips of rib bone inserted into a prepared defect at the lower end of the femur in dogs (Chalmers *et al.* 1960, Chalmers 1966). They used a quantitative (planimetric) method to assess the removal of dead grafted bone and the formation of new bone (Figs. 13 and 14). New bone formation in this highly osteogenic site occurred rapidly; but resorption took six months or more for its completion.

This method was used to quantitate the remodelling of different varieties of bank bone, and compare one against the other statistically (see Part II: Fate of Preserved Homografts of Bone).

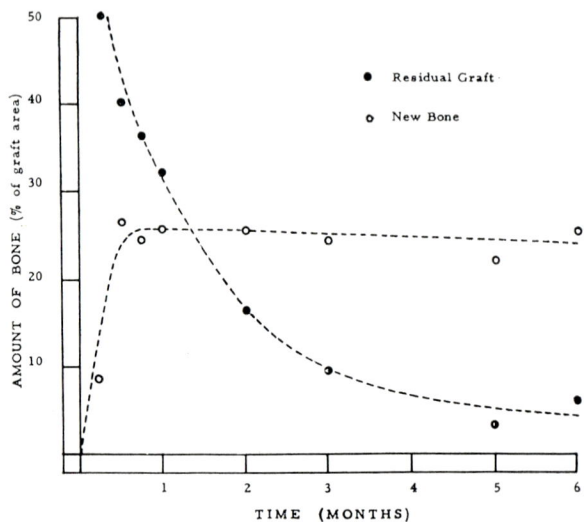

FIG. 14. A graph showing the resorption and new bone formation of chips of autologous rib bone after their insertion into the lower femora of dogs. (Reproduced by kind permission of Mr. J. Chalmers and Blackwell Scientific Publications.)

CONCLUSION

Cancellous bone is much more rapidly remodelled than is cortical bone. Indeed the remodelling and remineralization of a large cortical bone graft may take a year or more. Ultimately, however, the area of grafting, remodels to form bone characteristic of the skeletal site.

Though the morphological changes which occur in bone grafts are well-understood, the cellular mechanisms which ensure that accretion follows resorption is problematical. The problem is of practical importance because, failure to 'switch-over' from osteoclasis to osteogenesis will lead to complete resorption of the graft.

Growth-control

The restitution to normality of a bone graft and its skeletal bed is familiar to all orthopaedic surgeons. The factors which determine this maturation are incompletely understood. The problems relate basically to the mechanisms which control the *mass* of the skeleton; and those which control the *shape* of a bone.

The skeletal *mass* is influenced greatly by mechanical forces, which probably determine the distribution and proportion of cortical to cancellous bone formed at the site of grafting.

The *orientation* of the trabeculae of *cancellous* bone is also determined by mechanical factors (Jansen 1920, Evans 1957). However, there is evidence that in *cortical* bone the orientation of Haversian systems is *intrinsically* determined. Thus, Holmstrand (1957) found that in bone grafts inserted with their Haversian systems at right angles to the shaft, the same orientation was re-established in the remodelled bone removed 16 months later. He concluded that mechanical factors do not determine the reorganization of Haversian systems within a cortical bone graft.

This surprising finding may be due merely to the canals of the cortical graft serving as a template for resorption and accretion. But equally might it express the control which the bone cells themselves exert on the orientation of Haversian systems.

The solution to this fundamental problem of organization in bone might be found in cortical grafts removed for study many years after their transplantation.

CONCLUSIONS

A bone graft is used clinically to provide a bridge of osteogenic tissue either in a part of the skeleton which is deficient or to establish the bony fusion of a diseased joint. Rarely, nowadays, is a bone graft called upon to provide for its own internal fixation. Its functions are: (1) to establish an additional source of osteogenesis; and (2) to act as a scaffold, or trellis, for the ingrowth of new bone.

The place of bone grafting in the treatment of certain types of non-union of limb bones has been questioned recently and requires to be re-evaluated clinically.

Bone grafts are obtained from one of three animal sources: from the patient's own tissues as an autograft; from another individual of the same species, as a homograft (or allograft); or from an animal of a different species, as a heterograft (or xenograft).

An autograft of bone is most usually freely transplanted as a *composite tissue graft* containing bone, periosteum, endosteum and marrow. Rarely is bone transplanted with its cartilage growth plate; with articular cartilage as a half or whole-joint transplant; or as part of an organ graft as in the digital transpositions and in the toe-to-hand transplantations.

In the patient, the fate of a freely-transplanted autograft of bone is followed radiologically and by clinical examination. To understand more fully the fate of a bone graft, the approach must be made at the cellular level. But, owing to the limitations of human biopsy specimens, a sequential analysis is possible only in the animal, and in which the variables are reduced to a minimum. Many different experimental techniques have been used to study the fate of bone grafts; although there are disadvantages of such studies, the cellular changes which occur in bone autografts after transplantation have now been clearly described. However we are still largely ignorant of the mechanisms which initiate and control these changes.

After its transplantation, the changes which occur in a free autograft of bone are of two broad types: *degenerative* and *proliferative*.

Cortical bone largely dies after transplantation, though recent studies have established that a proportion of osteocytes survive in such bone. Revascularization occurs across its periosteal and endosteal surfaces into its necrotic Haversian canals. There is evidence showing that a cortical bone graft is more rapidly revascularized if its periosteum is removed than if it left attached to the bone. The first-formed new bone occurs mainly on the medullary surface of the graft and is derived mainly from the graft bed. After the revascularization of the Haversian canals, osteoclastic cells erode the bone to form resorption cavities; this erosion leads to osteoporosis and hence to a weakening of the mechanical strength of the graft. Subsequently lamellar bone is laid down in these cavities. This combined process of resorption and accretion is termed creeping substitution (Phemister) and with Haversian remodelling leads to the full incorporation of the graft into the skeleton. The grafted area is then subjected to the mechanisms which normally control the mass of bone tissue in the body.

The fate of *cancellous bone* grafts is broadly similar to that of cortical bone grafts. The details, however, differ for several reasons: firstly, the peripheral surviving portions of cancellous bone grafts contain large numbers of osteogenic cells (endosteal and medullary) which invade the deeper-lying necrotic tissues; secondly, the revascularization is facilitated by its open spongy texture of cancellous bone; and thirdly, the first-formed bone is of woven type which only later matures into cortical and cancellous bone. Because red marrow is itself highly osteogenic, iliac bone may be a better osteogenic medium than tarsal or tibial cancellous bone.

Segments of long bones largely die after transplantation and are revascularized by vessels growing down into the necrotic medullary canal from both ends. Further work is required to study the effect of intramedullary fixation and of multiple perforations of the shaft upon the remodelling of such bones.

Many factors influence osteogenesis in and about a bone graft. Basically, these factors relate to the graft, its bed and the host in which it lies; and whether or not it becomes infected. Factors appertaining to *the graft* include: the type of bone, be it cortical or cancellous; the size of the graft—fragmentation can create a material which is no longer osteogenic and may even act as a foreign body; and whether the bone is devitalized by freezing or by boiling. The *graft bed* has an important influence on osteogenesis: a cancellous site (e.g. in the spine or at the end of a long bone) is more osteogenic than the centre of the shaft of a long bone; close contact between the graft and its skeletal bed is essential for osteoconduction; insecure fixation and infection will each militate against the repair of a bone graft. *The patient* himself influences osteogenesis in a bone graft not only by the mechanical forces which cross the site of grafting, but also by the biological mechanisms, as yet ill-understood, which control the mass and shape of bone formation.

The experimental study of bone and bone grafts in recent years has clarified and unmasked many fundamental problems of bone repair.

The use of radioactive isotope (^{3}H-thymidine) has established the interrelationship between the differentiated cells of bone, namely the osteoblast, the osteocyte and the osteoclast. Moreover, it has revealed the presence of a precursor cell as the dividing cell of bone; the name *osteoprogenitor cell* has been given to this cell. Red marrow, itself, has been shown to be intensely osteogenic after transplantation, a change which no doubt accounts, in part, for the great worth of iliac cancellous bone as a grafting material.

The unsolved problems of bone repair relate to: the stimulus which 'triggers' mitosis in repair; the mechanism of osteogenic induction; the mechanism of the 'switch-over' from osteoclasis to osteogenesis in creeping substitution, failure of which may result in the complete resorption of a bone graft without it being replaced by new bone. Finally, the biological mechanisms which control the mass, shape and cellular organization of bone are still incompletely understood.

PART II: THE FATE OF FOREIGN BONE GRAFTS

"... there is still a great deal of work to be done in the proper assessment of bone transplants" (Roaf 1966).

To-day, most authorities are agreed that in clinical surgery the best bone for use as grafting material is that obtained from the patient's own tissues as cortical, but more particularly as cancellous bone.

There are, however, occasions in surgery when it is either desirable or essential to obtain bone from a source other than the patient. This is especially so in the extensive spinal fusions performed in children for scoliosis, when it may be inconvenient, or frankly impossible to procure enough autograft bone to complete the operation. In the filling of cysts it may be unjustifiable to make a second incision, with its attendant risks, to obtain bone for grafting. In the treatment of delayed union of fractures, the replacement of bone loss and in the arthrodesis of joints, the operation could be completed with greater ease by the surgeon and with more comfort and less risk to the patient if *preserved* bone could be used as effectively and as consistently as the patient's own bone as the grafting material.

The need then for an effective bank, or preserved, bone is great. This applies not only to orthopaedic surgery, but also to facio-maxillary surgery, dental surgery and neurosurgery. Such bone, however, has four disadvantages compared with autograft bone. Firstly, it is foreign and may therefore excite an immune response in the patient. Secondly, it is dead and cannot of itself contribute directly to osteogenesis. Thirdly, bank bone may not be inductively as active as fresh autograft bone; and fourthly, it may not remodel as rapidly.

Clearly then bank bone, of all types, needs a careful biological evaluation before it is tried in clinical surgery. Unfortunately, until recently, the approach has been empirical rather than analytical (Ray 1956).

The Clinical Use of Fresh and Preserved Bone Homografts

DEFINITIONS AND PROCUREMENT

A homograft (or allograft) is the term used to denote a graft exchanged between genetically-dissimilar individuals of the same species. The word graft is applicable to both living and dead tissues. In order to distinguish between the latter, *transplant* is used to describe a *living* graft and *implant* to mean a *devitalized* graft.

Bone homografts are procured surgically by resection (e.g. of ribs) or from amputated limbs, but most commonly from the fresh cadaver. Nowadays they are used almost exclusively after preservation by one of a variety of methods. Parental bone, however, is still being transplanted sporadically in the fresh state into children with congenital pseudarthrosis of the tibia.

CLINICAL USE OF FRESH HOMOGRAFTS

Historical. Macewen (1887) in Glasgow, was the first to transplant successfully fresh homologous bone which he used to replace $4\frac{1}{4}$ in. (10·8 cm.) defect of the humeral shaft lost through osteomyelitis. His patient was a boy aged 3 years. The donor bone was procured from patients having corrective wedge resections for 'anterior tibial curves' (presumably rickets) and cut into *minute fragments* before insertion. Two further grafting operations were needed in the next five months to achieve union. Macewen attributed the success of his operation to the proliferation of bone-forming cells contained in the grafts.*

Following this great achievement, a few clinicians reported favourably upon the use of *massive* homografts of fresh bone procured from amputation specimens of the cadaver to replace parts of limb bones (and joints) excised for tumour or tuberculosis (Wade 1920, Ellmer and Schminke 1925, Lexer 1925). But the results of those procedures were not impressive enough to justify their popularization (Chase and Herndon 1955).

Subsequently, homografts of fresh bone usually procured from a parent were utilized mainly in children for the treatment of pseudarthrosis, cysts and tumours (Smith 1937, Boyd 1939, Ghormley 1939, Henry 1948). Alldredge (1948) reported the use of homografts of fresh bone for the treatment of non-union in adults: 10 of 15 cortical grafts were successful.

The present position. In the last 20 years with the growth of knowledge concerning the immunity caused by homografts, the clinical use of fresh bone homografts has virtually ceased. However, parents are still occasionally asked to donate bone to their children for the treatment of congenital pseudarthrosis of the tibia. In the present state of knowledge this method is biologically unsound and particularly so for the treatment of such an intractable condition. But if such bone must be used, then there are certain recommendations that can be made concerning (1) the choice of the donor and (2) the preparation of the bone.

The donor is usually a parent, but, by analogy with renal transplantation, better results might be achieved by using a sibling if such be available (Barnes 1965). In a female recipient, the mother (or a sister)

---

* In the light of subsequent knowledge the success of this operation may be attributed to: (1) the minute fragmentation of the bone would probably have caused death of the grafts; (2) the dead bone fragments would provide a scaffolding for osteoconduction of the patient's bone; (3) the extreme youth of the patient; and (4) functional demand would ensure hypertrophy of the newly-formed bone.

may be a better donor than the father (or a brother) because there is evidence that females can react immunologically against Y-chromosomally-determined antigens (Eichwald and Silmser 1955, Zeiss 1966). In recent years the choice of the donor for renal and cardiac transplantation has been facilitated by the introduction of *tissue typing techniques* which include: (a) the normal lymphocyte transfer test (Brent and Medawar 1963, Ceppelini et al. 1965); (b) the mixed lymphocyte culture test (Bain and Lowenstein 1964, Elves and Israëls 1965, Chalmers et al. 1966); and (c) the use of cytotoxic antisera (Dausset et al. 1965, van Rood et al. 1965, Vredevoe et al. 1965, see Elves and Nisbet 1969).

Having selected the donor for the bone grafting procedure, the red marrow should be washed out of the graft because marrow itself, is strongly antigenic (Burwell and Gowland 1962).

The use of immuno-suppressive therapy (Gabrielson and Good 1967, Calne 1967) in the form of total-body irradiation, chemicals (such as the thiopurines and prednisone) or antilymphocytic sera is not justified at the present time in the transplantation of foreign bones and joints into the human; but experimental work (Reeves 1968) is continuing.

THE CLINICAL USE OF PRESERVED HOMOGRAFTS

Historical. The storage of bone for clinical use was practised by Albee (1912), Hey Groves (1917) and Gallie (1918). But the current widespread use of bank bone is due to a Cuban, Inclán (1942) who re-awakened interest in it during World War II.

Inclán used bone procured at operation and stored it in fluid media (blood or saline solution at $+2$ to $+5°C$) before implanting it, at a later date, into the same or another patient. In 1947, Bush and Wilson working independently in New York City, modified the method by storing the

TABLE I
Varieties of Homologous Bank Bone

Type of bone	Writer	Year
Chilled bone	Albee	1912
Boiled bone	Gallie	1918
Bone stored in fluid media ($+2°$ to $5°C$)	Inclán	1942
Frozen bone	Bush	1947
	Wilson	1947
Merthiolated bone	Reynolds and Oliver	1950
Freeze-dried bone	Kreuz et al.	1951
Deproteinized bone	Williams and Irvine	1954
Frozen-irradiated bone	Cohen	1955
	DeVries et al.	1955
Decalcified bone	Ray	1956
Freeze-dried irradiated bone	Turner et al.	1956
	Berkin et al.	1957
Freeze-dried β-propiolactone-treated bone	LoGrippo et al.	1957

TABLE

Some of the Clinical Results Reported Using Different Varieties Conditions in Ortho

Type of bank bone	Surgeon and year	Shafts of limb bones			Cavities		Meta-physis epiphysis
		Fresh fractures	Osteo-tomy	Delayed and mal-union	Infec-tive	Cyst dysplasia tumour	
Frozen	Bush (1947)		10/12			5/5	
	Weaver (1949)		1/2	17/20	1/2	9/9	
	Lecocq et al. (1950)	1/1		3/3		3/3	
	Stuck and Dandredge (1950)	12/12		30/33		2/2	
	Wilson (1951)			24/28	9/11	25/29	
	Brav (1954)	27/29		17/19		6/6	
	Bürkle de la Camp (1954)						
	Sieber (1954)			14/20			
	Ansari (1966)			287/331	4/7	5/5	
	Kingma (1967)						
Frozen-irradiated	Bassett and Packard (1959)						
Freeze-dried bone	Carr and Hyatt (1955)	17/17		21/25		9/12	
Freeze-dried BPL-treated bone	Berkin et al. (1957)	8/8	4/4	9/11	5/5	6/7	1/1
	Pain (1959)	11/14	7/7	11/15	6/9	6/11	
Merthiolated bone	Reynolds and Oliver (1951)	9/10	4/4	10/25	6/7	6/9	
	Amer. Acad. Orthop. Surg. (1953)						
	Arden (1956)			1/4		6/6	
	Carnesale and Spankus (1959)	22/24		25/34	3/5	10/14	
Boiled bone	Lloyd-Roberts (1952)	2/3		5/6	3/4	1/1	
	Williams (1964)			14/15			

* The figures in the different columns refer either, to the number of bone-grafting operations performed, or to the number of patients. The first figure (in all but the last two columns) refers to the number of successful results; the second figure to the total number of operations or patients. Failure includes both failure due to infection and graft failure.

II

*of Homologous Bank Bone for the Treatment of Various paedic Surgery.**

Arthro-desis	Bone block	Spinal fusion	Miscel-laneous	Overall results No.	Success %	Failure %	Infection† No.	%
5/7		43/43		63/67	94·0	6·0	3/67	4·5
8/8	1/2	6/6		43/49	87·7	12·3	4/49	8·2
6/6		33/41	2/2	48/56	85·7	14·3	1/56	1·8
4/5		8/8		56/60	93·3	6·7	—	—
17/19		134/159	7/7	216/253	85·5	14·5	14/307	4·6
14/14		6/7		70/75	93·3	6·7	7/75	9·3
				258/281	84·7	15·3	12/360	3·3
				14/20	70·0	30·0	—	—
35/35				331/378	87·6	12·4	21/378	4·8
				227/260	87·3	12·7	—	—
				36/44	81·8	18·2	9/1037	0·9
13/16		30/33		90/99	90·1	9·9	6/125	4·8
1/5		3/4	1/1	38/46	82·6	17·4	—	—
5/17		10/13	2/2	58/88	65·9	34·1	—	—
16/17		33/50	5/7	89/129	69·7	30·3	11/129	8·5
				81/630	87·1	12·9	30/630	4·8
8/11		8/17		23/38	60·5	39·5	4/55	7·2
14/22		36/44		110/143	76·9	23·1	—	—
15/20				26/34	76·5	23·5	1/34	2·9
				14/15	93·3	6·7	1/15	6·7

† The incidence of infection is recorded as post-operative infection and includes, in some instances, wounds which were infected before bone-grafting and which continued to be infected after operation.

bone in air in sealed glass containers at temperatures of −10 to −24°C. The use of cadaveric bone for bank purposes was introduced by Weaver (1949).

Dissatisfaction, however, with bone preserved by such methods, in terms of both convenience and clinical results, stimulated other workers to try the use of bone stored by immersion in merthiolate solution, a solution of penicillin and streptomycin, or after treatment by freeze-drying, boiling, autoclaving, removal of the bone protein or of the bone mineral (Table I). Sterilization of bone grafts has been attempted by heat, by chemical means and by high-energy radiation.

The clinical results using bank bone. Some of the clinical results obtained using the different varieties of bank bone for general orthopaedic conditions are shown in Table II.

Clinically, each of the different varieties of bank bone had had their advocates: e.g. frozen bone (Bush 1947, Coley and Higinbotham 1949, Weaver 1949, Wilson 1951, Brav 1954, Bürkle de la Camp 1954, Ehalt 1954, Buser 1959, Ansari 1966); freeze-dried bone (Carr and Hyatt 1955, Berkin 1957, Hyatt 1960); and boiled bone (Lloyd-Roberts 1952, Baumgart 1958, Williams 1964).

Schwier (1960), however, found the clinical value of bank bone decreased progressively from fresh autografts through frozen bone to chemically-preserved homografts. Ritter (1956abcdef) reported unfavourably upon the use of boiled, autoclaved, alcohol-preserved and deproteinized bank bone.

By summating the results shown in Table II for frozen and merthiolated bank bones, the findings shown in Table III are obtained.

TABLE III

A Summation from Table II showing the Percentage Failure of Frozen and Merthiolated Bank Bones Used for the Treatment of Certain Orthopaedic Conditions

Type of bank bone	Percentage of failures				
	Limb bones			Arthrodesis of limb joints	Spinal fusion
	Fresh fractures	Delayed and mal-union	Non-infective cavities		
Frozen	4·8%* (2/42)	14·0% (64/456)	7·4% (4/54)	5·3% (5/94)	12·9% (34/264)
Merthiolated	8·8% (3/34)	42·9% (27/63)	24·5% (7/29)	24·0% (12/50)	30·6% (34/111)

* The number of failures and the total number of procedures is indicated in parentheses below each percentage.

These findings show: firstly, that frozen bone is more effective than merthiolated bank bone; and secondly that bank bone can be used more effectively for filling non-infective cavities in bone than for the grafting of delayed (and mal-union) of fractures. The latter may be due to the cavities being situated mostly towards the cancellous ends of long bones; and cancellous bone is known to have a higher osteogenic capacity than the cortical bone of the diaphysis.

Freeze-dried bone (Carr and Hyatt 1955) would seem to be equally, but no more, effective clinically than frozen bank bone. Freeze-dried β-propiolactone-treated bone (Pain 1959) and boiled bone (Lloyd-Roberts 1952) do not appear to match up to either frozen or freeze-dried bank bones (Table II).

A comparison of bank bone with autograft bone. The clinical results using frozen bone (Table II and III) and freeze-dried bone (Table II) are as good as can be expected from the use of the patient's own bone as the grafting material. However, it is the clinical experience of most authorities that bank bone in many of its variants is, in general, less satisfactory than that obtained by using autograft bone and particularly autologous cancellous bone.

Objective clinical evidence to support this impression is scarce; for there are surprisingly few reports in which a comparison has been made in patients between bank bone and fresh autograft bone. The relevant work is summarized in Table IV.

TABLE IV

A Comparison of Bank Bone with Autograft Bone

Writer	No. of procedures		Percentage of failures	
	Homograft	Autograft	Homograft	Autograft
Sicard and Binet (1950)	100 operations	205 operations	14%	20%
Bosworth et al. (1953)	104 bone grafts	135 bone grafts	32·7%	13·3%
Brav (1954)	75 patients	75 patients	6·7%	8·0%
Hay (1954)	22 patients	33 patients	13·6%	15·2%
Sieber (1954)	20 patients	26 patients	30·0%	0·0%
Carnesale and Spankus (1959)	143 patients	137 patients	23·0%	12·0%
Kingma (1967)	260 operations	599 operations	12·7%	13·9%

In Table IV it can be seen that Sicard and Binet (1950) reported better results with frozen homografts than with autograft bone. Hay (1954) found little difference between his autologous and homologous bone grafts (33 grafts and 22 grafts respectively). But his report was short, full details were not given and he did not state the type of bank bone used. Brav (1954) reported comparable results using frozen homologous bone and autograft bone for treating a variety of orthopaedic conditions. However some selection was practised: he did not use cortical blocks of bone but only cancellous bone either as chips or as slabs; and he did not attempt to bridge large defects of the shafts of long bones. But by analysing the cause of failure (e.g. due to infection, poor skin or subsequent injury), in his two groups, Brav found that where the cause of failure was unknown the failure rate with bank bone was three times as great as with autograft bone.

Sieber (1954) reported that frozen bone homografts were much less effective than fresh autografts for grafting by the Phemister method. The reason for his high incidence of failure with bank bone (30 per cent), may have been due to the utilization of blocks of bone procured from rib or from amputation specimens. Similarly, Carnesale and Spankus (1959) found merthiolate-preserved bone grafts to be about half as effective as fresh autografts of bone and particularly so if blocks of bone rather than chips or bank bone had been used. Kingma (1967), however, reported frozen homografts to be as effective as fresh autografts of bone.

These comparisons, while by no means consistent, do tend to support the impression that autograft bone is superior in clinical use to frozen bone. The difficulty in the *clinical* analysis of bank bone is the numerous variables which can influence the result in the patient. Such differences include (in addition to the method of preservation of the bone): (1) the type of bone used (cortical or cancellous); (2) the physical state of the graft (as blocks or as chips); (3) the clinical condition for which it was inserted; (4) the surgical technique adopted (e.g. Phemister method or inlay); (5) individual variation; and (6) infection.

Bosworth et al. (1953) attempted to overcome some of these difficulties by using a standard operation, namely a Hibbs spinal fusion performed for tuberculosis and by inserting frozen bank bone and fresh autograft bone respectively into different interspaces in each patient in their series. They then assessed radiologically the incidence of pseudarthrosis at each grafted spinal interspace. For primary bone grafting procedures, they reported a failure of 13·3 per cent with autografts and 32·7 per cent with their bank bone. Similarly for secondary bone grafting operations, the failure rate was 11·8 per cent for autografts, but 33·3 per cent for the bank bone. These findings have been confirmed by McElroy (1963) who compared frozen-irradiated with fresh autograft iliac bone. However, such comparisons suffer from the known difficulty of assessing the state of fusion of a spine by radiology. An accurate assessment can only be made by exposing the fusion area at operation (James 1967).

In conclusion then, the clinical evidence suggests that fresh autograft bone is, in general, superior to frozen bank bone which in turn is superior to merthiolate-preserved bone as a grafting material. No report is available in which autograft bone has been compared with freeze-dried bone; but freeze-dried bone would seem to be equally effective as frozen bone. Bank bone (frozen and freeze-dried) may be, at times, as effective clinically as autograft bone, if it be used as chips of cancellous bone and placed in intimate contact with the skeleton at the site of grafting; and especially in sites of cancellous bone, such as the ends of long bones.

The recent re-evaluation of massive frozen homografts. In the last few years several reports have been published from the United States of America, Russia, France and South America relating to the use of

FIG. 15. Some of the skeletal sites in which massive frozen homografts have been used clinically (Modified after Afanassieff, Parrish, Peer, Petrokov and Volkov).

FIGURE 15

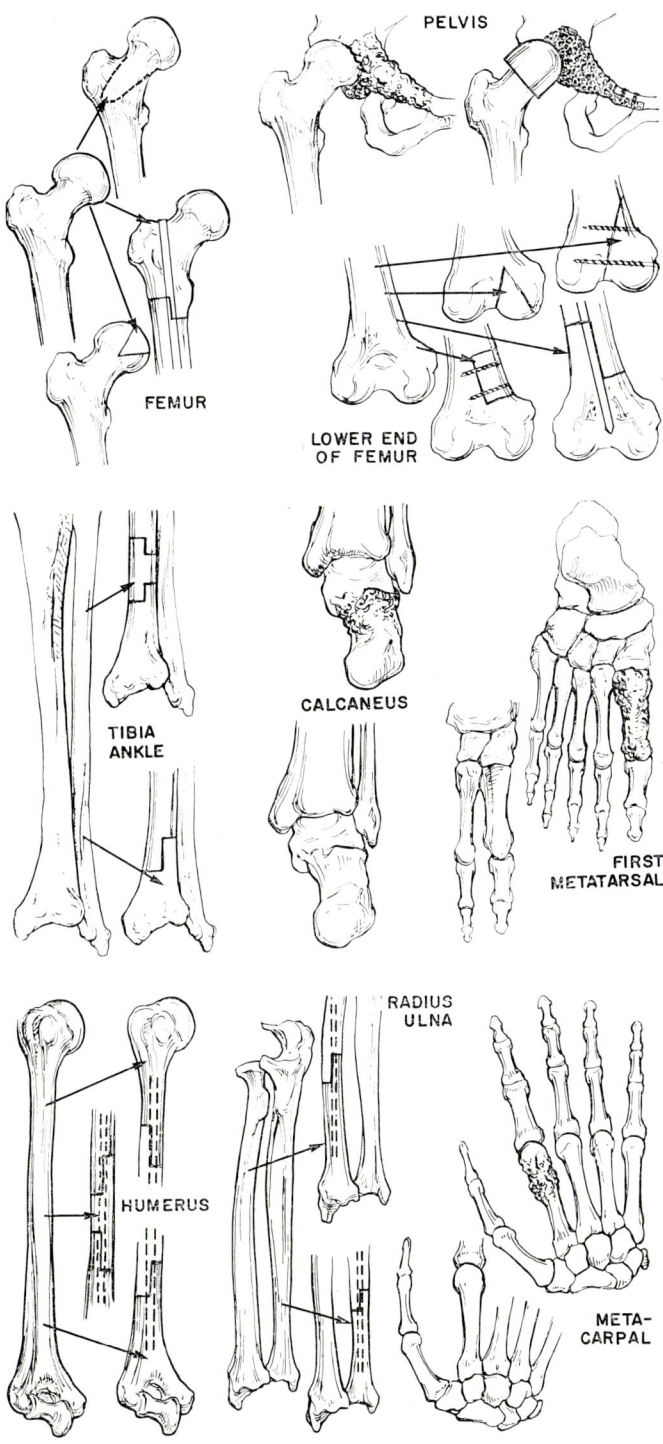

massive frozen homografts to replace surgically-created defects of the shaft and extremities of long bones.

The bone resections are being performed principally for tuberculosis, but also for tumour, osteoarthritis and osteomyelitis. It is not being used for the treatment of highly malignant neoplasms of bone, but only for giant-cell tumour, parosteal osteoma, juxta-cortical sarcoma, chondrosarcoma developing in a cortical chondroma, and for benign lesions which would probably recur if treated by curettage (Parrish 1966).

The donor bone is procured from young adults who died from trauma or from non-infective conditions and is removed aseptically in the operating theatre. It is then stripped carefully of all soft tissue without damaging the articular surface. The graft is then stored in a sterile container at -5 to $-183°C$. Twenty-four hours before operation, the graft is immersed in antibiotic solution until used (Merle D'Aubigné *et al.* 1966, Krupko *et al.* 1966, Kovalenko and Vereshchagin 1966, Ottolenghi 1966, Parrish 1966, Volkov and Imamaliev 1966, Afanassief 1967 and Petrokov *et al.* 1967).

In Fig. 15 is shown some of the permutations of resecting and grafting which are being tried. Internal fixation is usually employed. It is of interest to note that multiple perforations of massive tubular homografts seem to hasten the revascularization and incorporation of the implant (Küppermann and Schwier 1964, Ottolenghi 1966, Petrokov *et al.* 1967).

The clinical results obtained using these massive homografts are encouraging. Ottolenghi (1966) commented that the transplants were well accepted, though there was a varying degree of absorption of bone and necrosis of cartilage; but the functional results were very satisfactory. Merle D'Aubigné *et al.* (1966) after resecting 60 tumours in different sites claimed 82 per cent of successes. Afanassieff (1967) in reviewing the Russian work of 170 patients summarizes the results as follows:

Partial reconstruction of the hip	= 19 operations	— 2 bad
Replacement of the femoral head	= 16 cases	— 2 bad
Total upper femoral replacement	= 39 cases	— 16 bad
Partial reconstruction of the knee	= 101 cases	— 7 bad

Parrish (1966) is more cautious. He writes: "Neither the number of patients treated nor the consistency of the surgical technique will permit any definite conclusions at this time. The eventual fate of massive homografts is undetermined. However, it seems likely that gradual resorption or degeneration or both, may take place."

The trial of massive frozen homografts is a clinical experiment. The results of the method will have to be compared against the use of custom-made prosthetic replacements (Brav *et al.* 1958, Scales *et al.* 1965, Burrows 1968).

The Fate of Fresh Homografts of Bone

In the last 20 years, the fate of fresh bone homografts has been reappraised in the light of knowledge concerning the mechanism by which skin homografts are rejected (Medawar 1944, Billingham *et al.* 1954).

This aspect has been discussed at length elsewhere (Burwell 1964b, Nisbet 1966) and it is intended here to provide only a summary.

The Mechanism of Rejection of a Skin Homograft

Medawar and his colleagues found that fresh skin transplanted as a homograft from one animal to a genetically-dissimilar animal of the same species evokes an actively acquired immunity in the host; this immunity is responsible for rejecting the foreign graft in 9–12 days. Such a sensitivity to donor tissue in a host is termed homograft sensitivity, or, more usually, *transplantation immunity* (Fig. 16).

It has been found that the principal site of the immune response to a skin homograft applied to a subcutaneous bed is in the regional lymph nodes draining the graft. This state of transplantation immunity is distributed by the blood stream throughout the animal, and may be

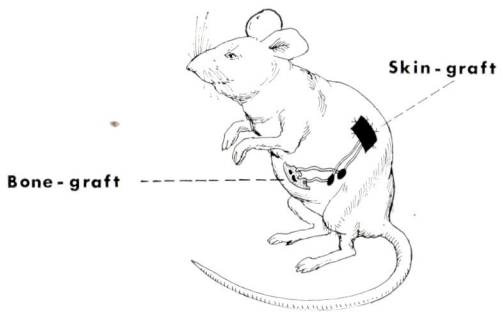

Fig. 16. The skin-graft test system for bone antigens. The skin graft is applied three weeks after a bone graft from the same (or syngeneic) donor.

revealed at a later date by the application to the host of a second-set skin graft from the same donor (or from another donor of the same inbred strain as the first donor). The early rejection of the second graft in 5–6 days indicates the presence of transplantation immunity.

The antibodies are of two kinds: humoral and cell-bound; the main instruments of homograft rejection are thought to be cell-bound antibodies (Medawar 1959).

This immunological concept of graft rejection indicates firstly, that tissue antigens in the graft evoke the formation of antibodies in the lymphoid tissue of the host; and secondly that the rejection of a homograft results from antigen-antibody reactions.

Transplantation Immunity Caused by Bone

It is now known that transplantation immunity can be caused by homografts of iliac cancellous bone (Chalmers 1959, Burwell *et al.* 1963), femoral bone (Brooks *et al.* 1963) and tibial bone (Massé *et al.* 1965a).

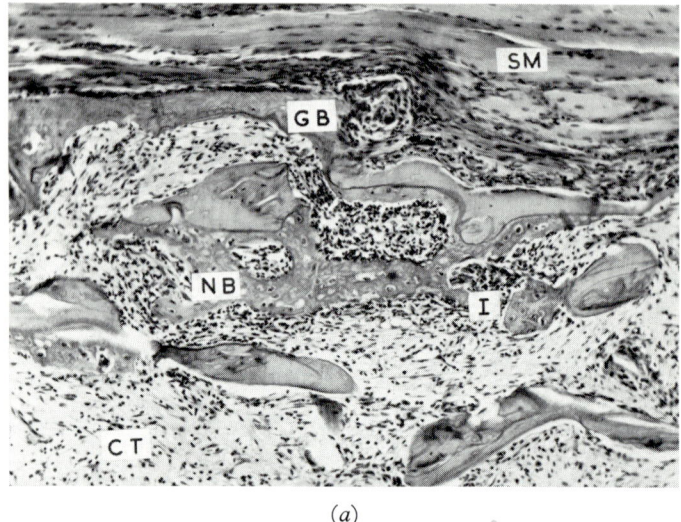

(a)

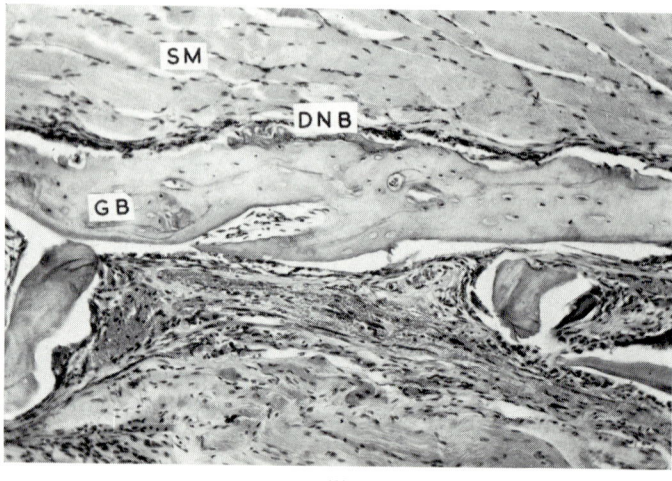

(b)

FIG. 17. Homografts of fresh marrow-containing iliac bone removed two and six weeks after their transplantation.

(a) *Two weeks:* note the grafted bone (GB), the new woven bone (NB) the osteocytes and osteoblasts of which appear abnormal, the inflammatory reaction about this new bone (I), and the loose cellular tissue (CT) highly infiltrated with small round cells occupying the intertrabecular space.

(b) *Six weeks:* note the grafted bone (GB), the small amount of dead periosteal new bone (DNB) and the fibrous tissue lightly infiltrated with small round cells occupying the intertrabecular space. SM = skeletal muscle fibres (H. & E. × 165).

The principal antigenic component of such grafts is the contained red marrow (Burwell *et al.* 1963). Nevertheless, cortical bone carefully freed from red marrow is antigenic. Hence it can be concluded that transplantation antigens are present in fresh adult bone (see Gallinaro *et al.* 1966).

The Inflammatory Response around Bone Homografts

The instruments of transplantation immunity, in terms of graft rejection, are antibodies carried by cells of the lymphoid series, namely small lymphocytes.

The infiltration of small round cells (and other cells) around a bone homograft 6–12 days after transplantation is generally referred to as the 'inflammatory response'. It consists predominantly of small lymphocytes, plasma cells, eosinophils and macrophages (Chalmers 1959, Burwell and Gowland 1961, Massé *et al.* 1965*b*) (Fig. 17).

After the insertion of *first-set* homografts of bone, the inflammatory response is variable in amount and is seen particularly around the newly-forming bone on the periosteal and endosteal surfaces. This infiltration may be replaced by a dense and abnormal connective tissue containing osteoclastic cells (Campbell *et al.* 1953, Heslop *et al.* 1960).

If the host is sensitized previously to donor tissue the inflammatory response about the bone homografts is usually very marked (Bonfiglio *et al.* 1955, Enneking 1957, Chalmers 1959, Bonfiglio and Jeter 1962, Burwell 1962, Massé *et al.* 1965*b*).

It is generally considered that the inflammatory response is the instrument of graft rejection and leads to: (1) death of the newly-forming homologous bone; and (2) death of the surviving blood vessels in the graft which causes further bone necrosis.

The Impaired Revascularization

Both cortical and cancellous homografts are revascularized more slowly than are autografts of bone. This is due firstly, to the immune response destroying patent vessels in the graft; and secondly, to the fibrosis which develops around homografts of fresh bone.

Cortical bone. In periosteal-covered transplants, there is no detectable difference between homografts and autografts until the 8th day after transplantation. Then, the inflammatory response in the periosteum of homografts obliterates the vascular bed, resulting in necrosis of the newly-forming bone (Hammack and Enneking 1960).

A different and more complex pattern has been observed in periosteal-free cortical graft inserted supra-pannicularly into rats (Zeiss *et al.* 1960). The homografts are revascularized more slowly than autografts from the very beginning (Fig. 18). Some anastomoses do occur between graft and host vessels, but the surviving graft vessels are destroyed by the inflammatory response, resulting in diminished vascularity of the bone. Ultimately, with fibrosis developing around the homograft, the blood supply is still further impaired.

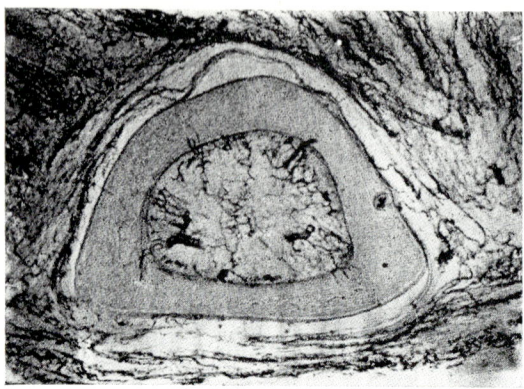

Fig. 18. A cortical tibial homograft removed 5 weeks after its insertion suprapannicularly into a rat. Note the medullary vessels (filled with Berlin blue) which are less well filled than the medullary vessels of a comparable autograft (see Part I, Fig. 10(a)). The cortical bone of the homograft is poorly vascularized. (Reproduced by kind permission of Mr. N. W. Nisbet and the Editor, *Brit. J. Exp. Path.*)

Cancellous bone. Homografts of cancellous bone are revascularized more slowly and less effectively than are the corresponding autografts (Stringa 1957).

CONCLUSION

Due to the impaired revascularization of first-set bone homografts, the remodelling of both cortical and cancellous bone is consequently impaired. No studies have yet been reported of the revascularization, if any, of second-set bone homografts (see Burwell 1962).

The Impaired Osteogenesis

The influence of the inflammatory response upon new-bone formation by a bone homograft is seen most clearly when the graft is inserted into an heterotopic site.

Such studies have shown that fresh bone homografts form new bone in two phases (Axhausen 1956), an *early phase* and a *late phase*. The early phase of new bone formation occurs in the first 1–2 weeks, is derived from the graft and dies (Chalmers 1959). After about a month, a few grafts form a small amount of *late-phase* bone, which interpreted as an inductive effect of the bone upon the tissues at the site of grafting (Axhausen 1956, Chalmers 1959).

Certain osteocytes survive in bone homografts, which has been attributed to the inability of cell-bound antibodies to gain access to the osteocytes through the canaliculi (Heslop *et al.* 1960, Nishimura *et al.* 1962).

Remodelling

The rate of remodelling of bone homografts is a function of the type of bone (cortical or cancellous), the size of the graft and the site into which it is inserted.

Cortical bone. The resorption of fresh bone homografts (split ribs) applied as onlays to the radii of dogs is delayed compared with that of fresh rib autografts. Moreover, the homografts excite a foreign-body reaction, including osteoclastic cells and fibrosis (Campbell *et al.* 1953).

In a heterotopic site (subcutaneous tissue) cortical homografts even after nine months are scarcely remodelled at all; while similar autografts show considerable replacement and new bone formation (Heslop *et al.* 1960).

Cancellous bone. Very small iliac homografts (3 × 1 mm.) inserted as inlays into the upper femora of rats, remodel about the same rate as do similar autografts (Anderson *et al.* 1965).

Large homografts inserted into cancellous bone (Bush and Garber 1948, Maatz *et al.* 1954, Ecke *et al.* 1964*a,b*) or a defect of the ulnar shaft (Heiple *et al.* 1963), heal more slowly during the first six months than do autografts; but at one year the homografts and the autografts are closely similar (Fig. 9).

In an heterotopic site, iliac homografts remodel much less than that of autografts (Chalmers 1959, Burwell 1964*a*). This difference seems to be linked to the impaired osteogenesis in homografts.

Segments of long bones. An old observation of Brooks and Hudson (1920) showed how segments of long bones inserted as fresh homografts into skeletal defects of the ulna in dogs, can bridge the gap in a high proportion of cases, though not quite as well as autografts. Thus, while the failure rate was 15·2 per cent with autografts, it was only 23·2 per cent with homografts (cf. Herndon 1960). The figures are very similar to the clinical comparisons made between fresh autografts of bone and bank bone already discussed.

CONCLUSIONS

The experimental findings are consistent and show that a fresh bone homograft excites an immune response in the host. As a consequence a cellular infiltration ('inflammatory response') occurs around the graft which halts osteogenesis derived from the graft. Vascularization also is delayed, and unless the host bed is highly osteogenic (e.g. a cancellous site), replacement of the foreign bone is slow, and, in a heterotopic site scarcely occurs at all. However, after a year a considerable proportion of homografts of cortical and cancellous bone inserted into skeletal defects are fully incorporated, though the effectiveness of a homograft to bridge a skeletal gap is less than that of an autograft.

The Fate of Preserved Homografts of Bone

In the patient it is difficult to assess the relative worth of one type of bank bone against that of another, for the good results of surgery are not necessarily due to good surgery (Roaf 1966). To achieve a critical analysis of bank bone, recourse must therefore be made to animal studies in which many of the variable factors are controlled, and after excision of the graft at selected time intervals it may be studied microscopically (see Young 1967).

The General Problems

The questions which need answering for each type of bank bone are:
- (1) Is it foreign?
- (2) Is it revascularized?
- (3) Does it influence osteogenesis?
- (4) How well does it remodel?
- (5) What is the best method of sterilization?

(1) **Is it foreign?** There are at least two ways in which a bank bone may be foreign to the tissues of the host. Firstly, it may contain residual antigenicity; and secondly, without being antigenic, it may excite a foreign-body reaction.

The antigenicity of a bone implant may be assessed by several methods which include: (1) serological studies; (2) transplantation immunity; (3) immune responses of lymph nodes; (4) inflammatory infiltrations; and (5) impairment of new bone formation (see Burwell 1964b).

A foreign-body reaction can be assessed only by microscopical examination of the cells and tissues which surround the implant. Perhaps the best guide to such a reaction is the presence of foreign-body giant cells.

(2) **Is it revascularized?** The term 'revascularization' is generally used to describe the invasion of blood vessels into dead bone. But such an invasion of capillary loops is accompanied by a cellular complex including fibroblasts, macrophages, polymorphonuclear leucocytes and lymphocytes; and, in an osseous bed, migrating and dividing osteogenic cells (Chalmers 1967).

Such 'revascularization' (or osteoconduction) will clearly be facilitated if the spaces of the bone (Haversian and intertrabecular) are large and more so if all the soft tissues are carefully cleansed from the bony spaces before its implantation (see Burwell 1964a,b).

(3) **Does it influence osteogenesis?** A bank bone might influence osteogenesis *directly* by providing living cells, or *indirectly* by stimulating osteogenesis at the site of implantation.

For practical purposes, however, bank bone is dead and cannot of itself contribute directly to osteogenesis. The exception to this rule was reported by Ray et al. (1954) who found that embryonic rat femora frozen to $-18°C$ and then freeze-dried, formed new bone when transplanted to a heterotopic site.

Osteogenesis may be stimulated indirectly, either: (1) by inducing local primitive connective tissue cells to differentiate into osteogenic cells (osteogenic induction); or (2) by stimulating mitosis in osteogenic cells at the site of implantation. There is considerable evidence that certain varieties of bank bone can initiate (1) but no evidence, as yet, that they can initiate (2) (see Burwell 1964a, 1966, 1968).

(4) **How well does it remodel?** The remodelling of a cortical bone graft is *biphasic*: resorption followed by accretion.

In a cortical bone graft accretion usually follows resorption, but this is not invariable. The reason why this does not always happen could shed considerable light upon the repair of bone and of certain pathologies in bone, e.g. essential osteolysis (see Part I: Remodelling; the mechanism of the 'switch-over' from resorption to accretion).

In appraising the remodelling of bank bone, sites of moderate osteogenesis such as the shaft of a long bone are preferable to sites of extreme osteogenesis such as cancellous bone; for a cancellous site will tend to cloud any difference in remodelling between one type of bone and that of another (Heiple et al. 1963, 1967).

(5) **What is the best method of sterilization?** The methods available for sterilizing bone include: boiling and autoclaving; chemicals such as merthiolate solution, ethylene dioxide and β-propiolactone; and high-energy irradiation.

Boiling is known now to be an inefficient method of sterilization (Bowie 1955). But autoclaving (like boiling) causes denaturation of bone proteins leading to markedly delayed resorption after implantation.

Merthiolate solution (aqueous 1/1000) is an efficient method of sterilizing bone. The bone is washed before use and no case of sensitivity to merthiolate has yet been encountered (Reynolds et al. 1951).

β-propiolactone as a 1 per cent solution (Lo Grippo et al. 1957) is more efficient than ethylene dioxide for sterilizing tissues (Sutherland et al. 1958). Its efficiency is greater in tissue procured surgically than from the postmortem room. Contaminated specimens are discarded. At the time they are used in the operating theatre the grafts are used either in the dry state (Berkin et al. 1957) or after reconstitution in a solution containing penicillin and streptomycin (see Dexter 1965, 1966).

Ionizing radiation has been employed to sterilize bone either: a beam of high-energy electrons from a Van de Graaf accelerator (Cohen 1955, Turner et al. 1956); or γ-rays from a cobalt-60 source (DeVries et al. 1955, 1958, Chalmers et al. 1960, see Dexter 1965, 1966). It has been found that a dose of about 2×10^6 *rad* is a minimal bacteriocidal level; and that some 4×10^6 *rad* are required to inactivate certain viruses (DeVries et al. 1958). After such intense irradiation the bone is discoloured.

It should be added that bone subjected to such ionizing radiation has been found to emit electron spin resonance signals indicating the presence of free radicals in the bone (Slager and Zucker 1964). The long term effect of such radicals upon the healthy surrounding tissues after transplantation is unknown (Ostrowski 1969).

Frozen Bone

Freezing provides the simplest method of preserving bone. The bone may be stored in a refrigerator at $+2°$ to $5°C$; in a 'deep-freeze' at $-79°C$; or in a liquid nitrogen at $-196°C$. At the higher temperatures a slow denaturation of proteins is believed to occur.

(1) **Residual antigenicity.** Freezing markedly impairs the antigenicity of cortical and cancellous bone grafts (Burwell and Gowland 1962, Burwell 1963, Brooks et al. 1963). In grafts frozen for only one week, however, certain antigens may persist (Burwell et al. 1963). In support of this conclusion Hancox et al. (1961) have reported that frozen $(-37°C)$ cancellous homografts inserted into drill holes at ends of limb bones in

sheep occasionally evoke large gatherings of plasma cells and lymphocytes, suggesting a lingering antibody response to antigens persisting in the bone.

(2) **Revascularization.** The revascularization of frozen cortical (Kingma and Hampe 1964) and cancellous (Deleu and Trueta 1965) bone homografts is slower and less extensive than that of similar autografts (Kiehn and Glover 1953).

(3) **Osteogenesis.** Frozen bone is dead and does not usually form new bone when transplanted into a heterotopic site (DeBruyn and Kabisch 1955, Burwell 1966, but see Wilson 1951).

Frozen bone still, however, carries the capacity to induce osteogenesis in the reticulo-endothelial cells of red marrow (Burwell 1966). This property is clearly worth retaining in a bank bone.

(4) **Remodelling.** Cortical homografts inserted into skeletal defects show delayed resorption and replacement compared with that of fresh cortical autografts (Reynolds and Oliver 1950, Kreuz et al. 1951, Marrangoni 1951, Kingma and Hampe 1964, but see Wilson 1951). Ultimately however, after 3–12 months, there is little difference between the frozen homografts and the fresh autografts.

Cancellous homografts are incorporated almost, but not quite as rapidly as autografts (Bush and Garber 1948, Marrangoni 1951, Wilson 1951, Maatz et al. 1954, Heiple et al. 1963, Freiberg and Ray 1964). Chips of rib bone inserted into the lower end of the femur of dogs are removed at about the same rate as autograft bone, though appositional new bone formation is a little more slow (Chalmers et al. 1960).

In a heterotopic site, frozen bone homografts scarcely remodel at all (Wilson 1951, Burwell 1966).

(5) **The influence of temperature and duration of storage upon remodelling.** Speed and Smith (1951) have found that bone stored at $+2°$ to $+5°C$ in doubly-sealed jars for three months becomes discoloured, dry and loses elasticity. The incorporation and remodelling of frozen bone autografts is said to be delayed after storage for only two weeks at $-24°C$ (Bush and Garber 1948); and this effect may be even more marked after 28 days storage (Maatz et al. 1954).

The use of radioactive isotope (^{32}P) has shown that homografts of bone frozen at $-26°C$ for 143 days are less well vascularized than are similar grafts frozen for 51 days (Kiehn and Glover 1953).

Herbert (1951) felt that bone could be stored at $-30°C$ for five months without impairment; but Wilson (1951) has found that frozen bone homografts stored for one year in a single jar at $+2°$ to $+5°C$ do not seem to give as satisfactory a clinical result as bone preserved for shorter periods of time.

These findings are consistent and suggest strongly that frozen bone should be stored at temperatures below $-20°C$. Indeed, in Russia temperatures of $-70°C$ are being used for storing bone (Timashkevich 1966, see Roaf 1966). Clearly more experimental work is needed.

(6) **The influence of irradiation upon remodelling.** The influence of high doses of irradiation ($2 \times 6 \times 10^6$ *rad*) on the rate of remodelling of frozen bone grafts is still uncertain.

This is because three groups of workers have produced conflicting results. Thus: one group found such doses to accelerate the rate of healing (Turner et al. 1956); a second group found it to retard the early incorporation (Heiple et al. 1963); while Cohen (1955) found irradiation to have no effect on the rate of disappearance of the grafted bone.

However there is evidence that freeze-dried (non-irradiated) bone may be rapidly resorbed than is frozen (non-irradiated) bone (Turner et al. 1956, Chalmers et al. 1960, Heiple et al. 1963) (Fig. 19), though this conclusion has recently been challenged (*vide infra*).

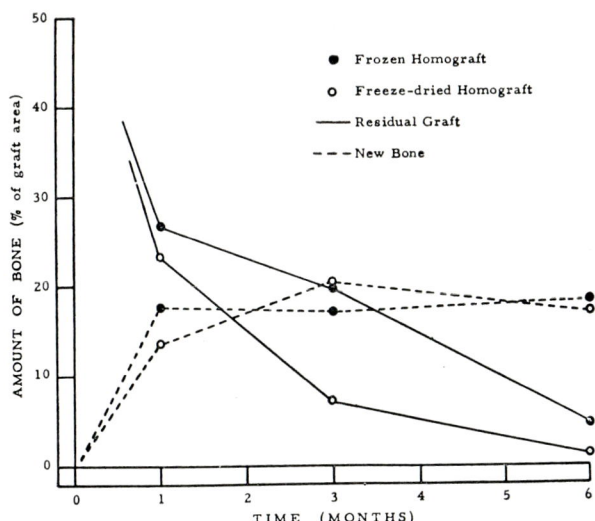

FIG. 19. A graph showing the resorption and new bone formation in frozen and freeze-dried homografts of rib bone chips inserted into the lower femora of dogs and removed for study at intervals up to 6 months. Note the more rapid removal of the freeze-dried bone. (Reproduced by kind permission of Mr. J. Chalmers and Blackwell Scientific Publications.)

(7) **Clinical results.** *Frozen bone.* Some of the clinical results using frozen bone are summarized in Tables II and III. It can be seen in Table II that the failure rate varied between 6·0 to 30·0 per cent. Some of these figures are indeed comparable to the results which have been reported with autograft bone (Table IV).

Is then frozen bone as good as autograft bone in clinical use? As already discussed (*vide supra*: a comparison of bank bone with autograft bone), the clinical evidence suggests that frozen bone is, in general, less effective than autograft bone as the grafting material; and this conclusion is substantiated by the weight of current authoritative opinion.

Frozen-irradiated bone. Despite the conflicting experimental findings concerning whether irradiation influences the rate of incorporation of frozen bone, Bassett and Packard (1959) and Swanson et al. (1963) have each reported encouraging results using frozen-irradiated bone in Man (Table II).

CONCLUSIONS

Experimentally, frozen bone is hardly antigenic and it seems to carry the capacity to induce new bone formation in susceptible tissues (e.g. red marrow). In a skeletal site it is generally resorbed more slowly than autograft bone; but this difference is slight when frozen cancellous bone is inserted into a cancellous site. However, in general it does not seem to be incorporated as well as freeze-dried bone.

Clinically, it has been used with apparently good results, though one clinical experiment showed that autograft bone for spinal fusions was three times as effective as frozen bone.

The clinical and experimental findings suggest strongly that frozen bone should be stored at temperatures below $-20°C$, preferably at $-79°C$ if prolonged preservation is required.

Freeze-dried Bone

The general principle involved in freeze-drying of tissues is the sublimation of water vapour from the frozen state, which is greatly accelerated by reducing the total pressure of the atmosphere in which the graft lies (Hyatt 1960, Dexter 1965, 1966).

The freeze-drying of bone requires special equipment and technical skill. Its advocates claim that for it several advantages lacking in frozen bone: (1) minimal protein denaturation; (2) constancy of its physical state with time; (3) a faster rate of incorporation into the tissues of the host; and (4) ease of handling, being stored at room temperature.

(1) **Antigenicity.** In freeze-dried bone certain tissue antigens may persist (Chalmers 1959, Burwell 1963, Burwell *et al.* 1963).

(2) **Revascularization.** No vascular perfusion studies of freeze-dried bone grafts have now been reported.

(3) **Osteogenesis.** Freeze-dried bone is dead, but a proportion of implants inserted intramuscularly do form a small amount of *late phase* new bone 5 to 10 months after grafting (21 per cent: Chalmers 1959).

Like frozen bone, freeze-dried bone carries the capacity to induce osteogenesis in the reticulo-endothelial cells of red marrow (Burwell 1966).

(4) **Remodelling.** In a skeletal site, cortical homografts in dogs are incorporated in the same manner as autografts, but at a slightly slower rate (Kreuz *et al.* 1951). Cancellous bone and chips of rib bone (like frozen chips) are removed almost at the same speed as autograft bone (Chalmers *et al.* 1960, Heiple *et al.* 1963).

In a heterotopic site, the remodelling of freeze-dried bone is extremely slow (Burwell 1966).

(5) **A comparison of the remodelling of freeze-dried bone with frozen bone.** Three groups of workers have each found that freeze-dried bone homografts are slightly superior to frozen-homografts in their speed of incorporation into the tissues of the dog (cortical grafts—Turner *et al.* 1955; cancellous grafts—Heiple *et al.* 1963; chips of rib bone—Chalmers *et al.* 1960) (see Figs. 19 and 20). It should be recorded however that Timashkevich (1966) using rabbits found freeze-dried

bone to be replaced more slowly than bone frozen at −70°C for 24 hours and stored at −25°C; and that Pappas and Beisaw (1968) who inserted tubular homografts into tibial defects in rats did not find any significant variation in the incorporation of bone grafts stored by freezing at −20°C, −85°C and by freeze-drying. More work in this field is needed.

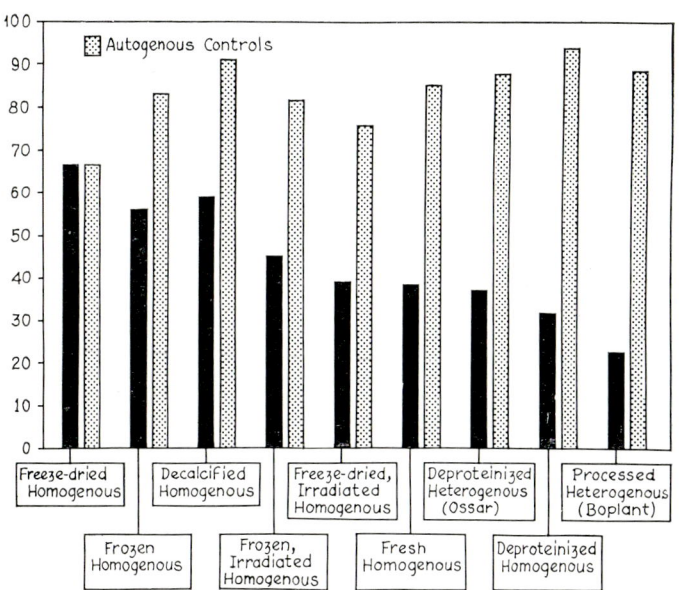

FIG. 20. Graphic representation of the numerical rating of a variety of homografts and heterografts of cancellous bone inserted into complete defects of the ulnae in dogs. The numerical rating of the foreign grafts is shown in black; and each type of graft is paired with the numerical rating of its control, namely autografts of cancellous bone inserted into the contralateral ulnae of the same dogs. Note that the best results are obtained with freeze-dried homografts and the poorest with processed heterogenous bone ('Boplant'). (Reproduced by kind permission of Dr. K. G. Heiple and the Editor, *J. Bone Jt. Surg.*)

(6) **The influence of irradiation on the remodelling of freeze-dried bone is** uncertain; for while one group of workers has found it to marginally accelerate resorption (Chalmers *et al.* 1960), another group has found it to delay incorporation (Heiple *et al.* 1963). DeVries (1955, 1958) reported that freeze-dried irradiated bone implanted into dogs and rats produced no immediate harmful effects and functioned well in stimulating new bone formation in fracture sites.

(7) **Clinical results.** *Freeze-dried bone.* Carr and Hyatt (1955) reported excellent results using freeze-dried bone (Table II). Indeed their results are quite comparable with those obtained by using the patient's

own bone as grafting material. In a subsequent paper, however, Hyatt (1960) reported a failure rate (technical and graft failure) of 31·2 per cent in 954 procedures using freeze-dried bone. He concluded "... if osteogenesis is a prime concern—it is evident that the fresh autogenous bone is the graft of choice; ..."

No comparison of freeze-dried bank bone against autograft bone as grafting material has yet been reported.

Freeze-dried irradiated bone. DeVries et al. (1958) reported encouraging clinical results in 104 operative procedures using irradiated freeze-dried bone.

Freeze-dried βPL-treated bone. In a short term clinical study, Berkin et al. (1957) published excellent results in 46 patients who had received freeze-dried βPL-treated bone grafts. Pain (1959) however, reviewing the same and additional patients at a later date found successful results in only 65·9 per cent of patients (Table II).

CONCLUSIONS

Experimentally, freeze-dried (like frozen) bone is hardly antigenic and seems to carry the capacity to induce new bone formation in red marrow. Resorption in a skeletal site is slightly delayed for cortical bone, but not for cancellous freeze-dried bone. The effects of irradiation of freeze-dried bone upon such remodelling is probably minimal.

Freeze-dried bone may be more rapidly remodelled than is frozen bone, but more work in this field is needed.

Clinically, encouraging results have been reported for freeze-dried, freeze-dried-irradiated and freeze-dried βPL-treated bone; but long term results from the latter type of bank bone have not been substantiated.

Merthiolate-preserved Bone

The merthiolate preservation of bone is claimed to be a simple inexpensive and aseptic method (Reynolds et al. 1951).

After an encouraging experimental evaluation of cortical bone in dogs (Reynolds and Oliver 1950), Reynolds and his colleagues (1951) reported the clinical results of 129 patients who had received merthiolate-preserved bone grafts (Table II). They recorded failure in 30·3 per cent and concluded: "Merthiolate-preserved bone does not compare favourably with autogenous bone grafts in that the process of fixation and replacement is definitely retarded ..." However, while they advocated its use for obliterating cavities, arthrodeses and fresh fractures, they advised against its use in the treatment of non-union.

In 1953, a Committee of the American Academy of Orthopaedic Surgeons reported a failure of 12·9 per cent in 630 patients who had received this type of bone. Moreover, it was concluded that there was less chance of success than if frozen bone grafts were used.

Most recently, failure rates of 39·5 per cent (Arden 1956) and 23·1 per cent (Carnesale and Spankus 1959) have been recorded using merthiolate-preserved bone; and when using a block graft the figure rose to 31 per cent (Carnesale and Spankus 1959).

A comparison of the clinical results using merthiolate-preserved bone with those obtained using frozen bone (Table III) shows frozen bone to be the superior grafting material.

CONCLUSION

The clinical evidence suggests that merthiolate-preserved bone is not as effective as frozen and freeze-dried. However, it may be used to fill cavities and to supplement autograft bone in certain orthopaedic conditions (Carnesale and Spankus 1959).

Boiled and Autoclaved Bone

The boiling and autoclaving of bone causes: (1) coagulation of the soft tissues in the Haversian canals and intertrabecular spaces; and (2) denaturation of the collagen in bone. With prolonged boiling the collagen passes into solution as gelatin (Eastoe 1956), and by high temperature autoclaving most of the collagen can be removed leaving behind only the bone mineral.

The coagulation mentioned above impairs the process of revascularization of a bone graft; while the denaturation of the bone proteins markedly retards its resorption by the tissues of the host.

Experimental observations. Boiled bone is not antigenic (Burwell *et al.* 1963). It probably carries little or no capacity to induce new bone formation in red marrow (Burwell 1966). The revascularization of boiled bone (assessed by the uptake of the isotope ^{32}P) is delayed and is comparable to that of frozen bone (Kiehn and Glover 1953, Ruf 1954). The remodelling of both boiled and autoclaved bone implanted into skeletal sites is severely retarded (Hey Groves 1917, Gallie 1918, Gallie and Robertson 1918, Key 1934, Orell 1937, Blaimont 1960, Chalmers *et al.* 1960).

Clinical observations. Gallie advocated that boiled bone be used for spinal fusions (tuberculosis) and recent fractures, but not for the treatment of non-union or for bridging gaps in long bones.

Lloyd-Roberts (1952), reporting his experience (Table II) with boiled cadaveric bone, wrote: "We believe that boiled bone may be used with confidence when a bone graft is required for non-union of a fracture, to supplement an intra-articular arthrodesis, or to obliterate a bone cavity or surgically produced effect. Its capacity to bridge a gap cannot as yet be assessed." Rocher (1953) supported Lloyd-Roberts from an experience of over 200 cases: he felt, however, that boiled bone should not be used to fuse a hip or spine, nor should it be used to bridge a gap in a long bone. Later, Lloyd-Roberts (1960) admitted that in the treatment of pseudarthrosis, boiled bone was less useful than fresh autogenous or deep-frozen homologous bone. Williams (1964) however, has reported a method by which boiled bone can be used effectively for the treatment of delayed union of fractures. A slot is cut across the fracture in the long axis of the bone. The slot penetrates the full thickness of the cortex exposing the medullary cavity, but without disturbing the rest of the soft tissue joining the bone ends. Boiled cadaveric iliac cancellous bone which has been minced is then used to pack both the medullary cavity and the prepared slot in the cortex. In a small series of patients, over

90 per cent of the fractures so-treated proceeded to bony union (Table II). But it has yet to be shown that established non-union can be treated successfully by this method.

There are occasions when autoclaved bone may be used with success to bridge a gap in a long bone. Kirkup (1965) described such a patient in whom the lower 10 inches of the shaft of the femur had been avulsed in a motorcycle accident. The bone, lost at the scene of the accident was found by a police dog! After autoclaving, the bone was reinserted using a Küntscher nail for internal fixation and packing chips from the fragmented patella around the dead bone. Three months later there was a strong involucrum around the implanted bone and the patient returned to work a year after the accident.

In such a case in which the replacement of the autoclaved bone must have taken a year or more the success of the adroit surgeon may be attributed to: (1) the subperiosteal avulsion of the bone; (2) the use of internal fixation; (3) the exuberant periosteal new bone; and (4) the comparative youth (20 years) of the patient.

In these rarities if the lost bone is not returned, a massive frozen homograft, if available, might be successful.

CONCLUSION

Boiled bone is probably relatively inert, but its revascularization is delayed and it takes a long time to be replaced by host bone. Clinicians with experience of its use are agreed that it is effective for obliterating cavities. Its worth for arthrodesis and the treatment of non-union is still being debated; but it can probably be safely used to bridge an acute skeletal defect in the limb bone of a young patient provided that the periosteal tube is relatively intact.

Decalcified Bone

Since the introduction of decalcified bone by Senn (1889) conflicting reports of its clinical use have been recorded (see van de Putte and Urist 1966). At the present time there is still considerable controversy about the merits of decalcified bone as a substitute for the bone autograft.

Most of the recent work in this field is experimental, and much of which is again conflicting. But some of this confusion may be resolved by the recent finding that different acids used to decalcify bone affect its biological properties in different ways (Urist 1965, van de Putte and Urist 1966, Urist *et al.* 1968a).

Antigenicity. Whether decalcified bone is antigenic, is at present uncertain (Brooks *et al.* 1963).

Revascularization of decalcified bone is said to be rapid (Freiberg and Ray 1964, Urist 1965).

Osteogenic induction. Decalcified bone is of course dead; but it can induce new bone formation in susceptible tissues of the host by the process known as osteogenic induction.

Urist has reported an extensive study of the capacity of decalcified bone grafts to induce osteogenesis in heterotopic sites (principally muscle) in a variety of mammals (Urist 1965, van de Putte and Urist 1966, Urist et al. 1967, 1968a).

In his work it was found that the incidence of osteogenic induction depended upon the acid which had been used to decalcify the bone. Thus: using 0·6 N. hydrochloric acid (HCl) induction occurred in 50–98 per cent of experiments; using diamino-ethane-tetra-acetate (EDTA at pH 7·4) there were only 28 per cent positive results; and with nitric acid (HNO_3), the bone elicited an intense inflammatory reaction and no new bone formation occurred. In his most recent papers (Urist et al. 1967, 1968a) Urist reports that the inductive capacity of HCl-decalcified bone is *enhanced* by freezing at $-70°C$ and by freeze-drying; is *unaffected* by lipid solvents, common detergents and hyaluronidase; and is *impaired* (or annulled) by heat, thrice freezing and thawing, high-energy radiation ($> 2 \times 10^6$ r.e.p.), 10 per cent β-propriolactone, formaldehyde and proteolytic enzymes. Fragmentation of freeze-dried HCl-decalcified bone into particles ($< 420\mu$) also destroys the inductive capacity, but not apparently if the particles are implanted as pellets (Urist et al. 1968b).

EDTA is known to extract some of the mucopolysaccharide from bone (Auty 1965); and this may account for the poorer results using bone decalcified with this acid. In the light of these recent findings it is unfortunate that in much of the experimental work on decalcified bone, EDTA has been used as the reagent. Nevertheless, the addition of chondroitin-sulphate to EDTA-decalcified bone has been found to accelerate the rate of bone repair (Burger et al. 1962).

Remodelling. Implanted into muscle the resorption of HCl-decalcified bone is found to be more rapid than that of undecalcified bone (Urist 1965).

In a skeletal site, conflicting results concerning the remodelling of decalcified bone have been reported. Thus: two groups of writers have found decalcified bone to be invaded and replaced more rapidly than frozen homologous bone (Ray and Holloway 1957, Hejna and Ray 1963, Freiberg and Ray 1964, van de Putte and Urist 1966); two other groups have reported that the rate of remodelling of decalcified and frozen homologous bone is about the same (Burger et al. 1962, Heiple et al. 1963) (Fig. 6); while Young (1964) and Chalmers (1966) recorded that decalcified bone was invaded less readily and remodels less well than frozen implants.

Each of these groups used EDTA-extracted bone with the exception of Urist who used HCl-decalcified bone. Clearly the experiments should be repeated using HCl as the decalcifying agent for bone.

Clinical results. Sharrard and Collins (1961) reported that decalcified (autologous) bone implanted into three children (aged 10–12 years) for spinal fusion, was perfectly acceptable to the tissues and formed a good scaffold for the appositional growth of new reparative bony callus.

CONCLUSION

The clinical results using decalcified bone grafts have been variable, though in a recent small series favourable results were reported (Sharrard and Collins 1961). The experimental findings are no less conflicting. Some of this controversy may be resolved with the recent knowledge that EDTA (which has been commonly used to decalcify bone) is much less satisfactory than HCl because it extracts some of the mucopolysaccharides from bone. HCl-decalcified bone is not only resorbed more rapidly, but in it the property of osteogenic induction is enhanced.

Further experimental work on HCl-decalcified bone is needed combined with a study of the influence of 1 per cent β-propiolactone and ethylene dioxide upon such bone.

Deproteinized Bone

Before the immunological studies of recent years showed that the transplantation antigens in bone homografts could be largely inactivated by such simple procedures as freezing and freeze-drying, empirical attempts were made to overcome the protein-bound incompatibility between host and graft by removing the proteins from bone. Thus work relates mainly to heterografts (Orell 1937, Losee and Hurley 1956, Maatz and Bauermeister 1957), but some studies have also been made on deproteinized homografts.

The removal of proteins from bone (mostly collagen) to produce macerated or 'deproteinized' bone is usually performed by drastic biochemical methods (e.g. dry heat at 500–600°C; high-temperature autoclaving; and by boiling in a potassium hydroxide-glycol solution, each of which alters the gross structure and crystal patterns of the bone) (Williams and Irvine 1954).

Less drastic ways include digestion with trypsin (Ritter 1954d), extraction with ethylenediamine (ED) (Williams and Irvine 1954), 20 per cent hydrogen peroxide solution (Maatz and Bauermeister 1957), or formamide (Fuchs et al. 1963, Fuchs 1966). After extraction by each of these latter methods, some residual protein nitrogen remains in the bone (Wheeler and Hyatt 1960, Stegeman 1966, Fuchs et al. 1963, Fuchs 1966).

Antigenicity. Brooks et al. (1963) reported the surprising finding that homografts of deproteinized bone evoked transplantation immunity in rats.

Revascularization. The revascularization of deproteinized bone is slight (Anderson et al. 1959).

Osteogenic induction. Key (1934), who inserted deproteinized bone powder into prepared ulnar defects of dogs, concluded that it did not appear to stimulate osteogenesis of the host bone. Moreover, that it was surrounded by a fibroblastic wall and was slowly resorbed.

More recent work has shown that deproteinized bone does not carry the capacity to induce osteogenesis in susceptible tissues, e.g. red marrow. Moreover, calcined bone (previously dry-heated to 660°C) is frankly inhibitory to osteogenesis in marrow (Burwell 1966).

Remodelling. Implanted into heterotopic sites, deproteinized bone homografts excite a marked foreign-body reaction (Burwell 1966).

In a prepared skeletal defect, both cortical and cancellous deproteinized bone has been found to delay healing and to be resorbed very slowly

(Ray and Holloway 1957, Rosomoff *et al.* 1959, Bassett *et al.* 1962, Heiple *et al.* 1963). Indeed Heiple and his colleagues (1963) in their careful quantitative analysis of a variety of bank bones found it to be one of the least effective of all the types which they tested (Fig. 20). It should be added, however, that Young (1964) reported that in his hands deproteinized bone rated higher than EDTA-decalcified bone, but less than frozen bone.

CONCLUSIONS

No clinical results using deproteinized bone homografts have been published. In view of the fact that the replacement of deproteinized bone by host bone is exceedingly slow, the clinical use of deproteinized bone does not seem indicated (Bassett *et al.* 1962).

OVERALL CONCLUSIONS CONCERNING HOMOGRAFTS OF BANK BONE

During the last 25 years, since Inclán (1942) introduced the bone bank, many different types of preserved homografts of bone have been tried clinically and evaluated experimentally.

Clinically, excellent results have been claimed for frozen, freeze-dried bone and boiled bone; while less certain results have been reported for merthiolate-preserved bone. There is, however, considerable difficulty in assessing clinically the worth of any bank bone material (Roaf 1966); and particularly is this so after implantation into the spine in which the incidence of pseudarthrosis can be assessed accurately only by exploration (James 1967).

A more critical analysis of bank bone can be made experimentally, though of course the applicability of such work to Man is always in question. Nevertheless, from animal studies it has been shown that there are four biological mechanisms which require careful consideration in selecting a preserved-bone homograft to serve as a substitute for the patient's own bone as grafting material. These biological mechanisms are: (1) immunological; (2) vascular and cellular invasions (osteoconduction); (3) osteogenic induction; and (4) remodelling (Burwell 1964*b*, 1967, 1968).

The types of bank bone which satisfy these criteria most certainly are frozen bone, freeze-dried bone and perhaps HCl-decalcified bone. Frozen and freeze-dried bone are each antigenically weak; each carries inductive capacity; but freeze-dried may be remodelled more quickly than bone preserved at $-15°$ to $-20°C$. However freeze-dried bone may not be remodelled more quickly than bone frozen at $-70°C$ (Timashkevich 1966).

The effectiveness of bank bone may be improved markedly by two further procedures, namely: (*a*) the cleansing of the soft tissues from the bony spaces in the graft to facilitate revascularization; and (*b*) by placing the bone graft in close apposition with host tissue of either high osteogenic capacity (such as cancellous bone) or of high osteogenic potential (such as red marrow).

More experimental work is needed:

(1) To decide the optimal temperature for preserving bone by freezing.
(2) To compare the best frozen bone against freeze-dried bone.
(3) To establish the worth of HCl-decalcified bone as a graft material.
(4) To ascertain whether osteogenic induction by bank bone can be enhanced by chemicals such as chondroitin sulphate and β-aminoproprionitrile.
(5) To appraise the best method for sterilizing bone: by high-energy irradiation?; by β-propiolactone?; or by ethylene dioxide?

The Fate of Heterografts of Bone

A heterograft (or xenograft) is the term used to indicate a graft transferred between individuals of different species.

Principles of Heterotransplantation

Skin heterografts are poorly, if at all, vascularized. Hence their survival time is much less than that of homografts of skin. In skin heterografts which are vascularized (rabbit to cat), cytological evidence of an immune response occurs in the regional lymph nodes (Egdahl et al. 1958).

The mechanism of heterograft rejection. The mechanisms leading to the death of fresh heterologous tissues are less well understood than that of homografts.

Although it is possible that natural cytotoxins in the body fluids of the host may play a role in graft rejection (see Burwell 1963), it is likely that *heterograft* transplantation immunity is mediated largely by humoral antibodies (Millonig et al. 1962); and such immunity may involve a different antibody-forming cell system (? plasma cells) than that involved in the rejection of homografts (lymphoid cell system) (Tyan and Cole 1963a,b, 1964).

The precise biochemical way in which an antigen-antibody reaction may impair osteogenesis in bone has recently been investigated by Dame Honor Fell and her colleagues at the Strangeways Laboratory, Cambridge, England (Fell et al. 1966).

In these tissue culture experiments, the effect of antisera (prepared in rabbits against chick tissues) upon chick limb rudiments, has been examined at the morphological and biochemical levels. Fell and her colleagues found that the antiserum (in the presence of complement) caused: (1) death of the most superficial cells of the explant; (2) disintegration of the intercellular material; and (3) the release of lysosomal acid protease into the tissue-culture medium.

Fell suggests that the antiserum may act directly on the cell membranes to cause release of proteolytic enzymes from lysosomes. The experiment is of fundamental importance, because it suggests the mechanism whereby an antigen-antibody reaction may cause the death of foreign tissue after transplantation. *Fresh* bone heterografts have no place in orthopaedic surgery (see Peer 1955).

Preserved Heterografts of Bone

Owing to the ready availability of animal tissues, the worth of preserved heterogenous skeletal tissues has been extensively explored in surgery; these include ivory, cow-horn and beef bone (Bircher 1887, see Peer 1955). Ivory and cow-horn are very resistant to incorporation into host bone, though beef bone remodels more rapidly (Hughes 1943).

During the last 70 years, several attempts have been made to use various types of preserved ox bone as a substitute for autograft bone.

Frozen Bone

French surgeons have used stored heterologous (calf) bone for clinical purposes for several years with apparently satisfactory results (Symposium 1958). Kingma (1960, 1967), however, who organizes the Bone Transplantation Service of the Netherlands Red Cross, has now had extensive experience with the clinical use of calf bone procured under aseptic conditions and stored at $-40°C$. He has concluded that the ultimate results with this type of bone were a serious disappointment and were far inferior to autograft bone (Table V).

Kingma has discontinued using frozen calf bone.

TABLE V

A Comparison of Frozen Calf Bone with Autograft Bone

Writer	No. of procedures		Percentage of failures	
	Heterograft	Autograft	Heterograft	Autograft
Kingma (1967)	49 operations	599 operations	34·7%	13·9%

Freeze-dried Bone ('Boplant')

In this section it is proposed to restrict discussion to the commercial preparation 'processed heterogenous' bone ('Boplant'—Squibb).

Preparation. Boplant is bone removed aseptically from young calves and which is then subjected to extraction by a detergent, a fat solvent and water, sterilization by β-propiolactone, followed by freeze-drying and packaging under a vacuum for storage at room temperature (Bassett and Creighton 1962).

Antigenicity. The protein content of the bone tissue is probably little altered. Its antigenicity has been carefully assessed and, it is claimed, is negligible (Anderson *et al.* 1962, 1964, Council on Drugs 1966); but Kramer *et al.* (1968a) have reported that some residual antigenicity may persist in 'Boplant'.

Osteogenic induction. No work has yet been published concerning the capacity of Boplant to induce osteogenesis in susceptible tissues. However, it has been found that Gelfoam soaked in an extract of calf bone paste (Squibb) produced cartilage, osteoid-like tissue, and, at times, bone when implanted into the anterior chambers of the eyes or intracranially into rats (Moss 1958, 1960, Anderson et al. 1960).

Remodelling. Cortical bone. The remodelling of Boplant cortical bone implanted as inlays into the radii of dogs is more rapid than that of fresh cortical autografts (Bassett and Creighton 1962, Karges et al. 1963). This unexpected finding has been attributed to: (*a*) the removal of fatty débris from the prepared bone; and (*b*) the large Haversian spaces of calf bone compared with those of dog bone. More recently it has been claimed that if the soft tissues are not removed during the preparation of such grafts, there is a more vigorous response of the host's tissues leading to resorption or sequestration of the implant (Gresham and Thomas 1966).

Cancellous bone. The findings for cancellous bone are conflicting. Karges et al. (1963) reported that cancellous 'Boplant' inserted as inlays into the radii of dogs compared favourably with autograft cancellous bone.

Heiple et al. (1967), however, observed: (*a*) a marked inflammatory response about the processed heterograft during the first month; (*b*) rapid removal of the processed bone; and (*c*) little evidence of new bone formation in it. These observations have been confirmed by Kramer et al. (1968a, b) who implanted Boplant into a prepared defect in the rabbit skull. In the work of Heiple and his colleages (1963) only one of eleven implants (inserted for three months or longer) achieved bony union across the defect. They concluded that Boplant was the least effective of all the types of bank bone which they tested; and "... we do not see any clear indication for the use of this material in orthopaedic surgery" (Figs. 20 and 21).

Bassett (1967) in discussing these conflicting results was of the opinion that the difference is due to Karges et al. using Boplant specially-prepared in the laboratory; while Heiple et al. used the production-line material. Accordingly, the manufacturers have withdrawn Boplant from the market, and are correcting the manufacturing process. Boplant will not be available again in this country until, at the earliest, late 1971 (Cromie, 1967).

Clinical results. The initial clinical results using Boplant were encouraging—86 per cent success in 265 operations (Anderson et al. 1963). Harmon (1964) has found Boplant to be satisfactory for bone grafting of the spine; and Scopp et al. (1966a,b) using Boplant in dental operative surgery have reported the results to compare favourably with the use of the patient's own bone as grafting material.

At the New York Orthopaedic Hospital, cancellous slabs of Boplant implanted at the first stage of scoliosis fusions and excised *in toto* after two weeks (at the time of the second stage), revealed two different histological patterns. In one group, from certain lots of Boplant, there was massive appositional osteogenesis and in the other, from different lots, a low grade inflammatory response, without evidence of new bone formation (Bassett 1967).

In a further series of 33 operations using Boplant the results have been disappointing (Pieron et al. 1968).

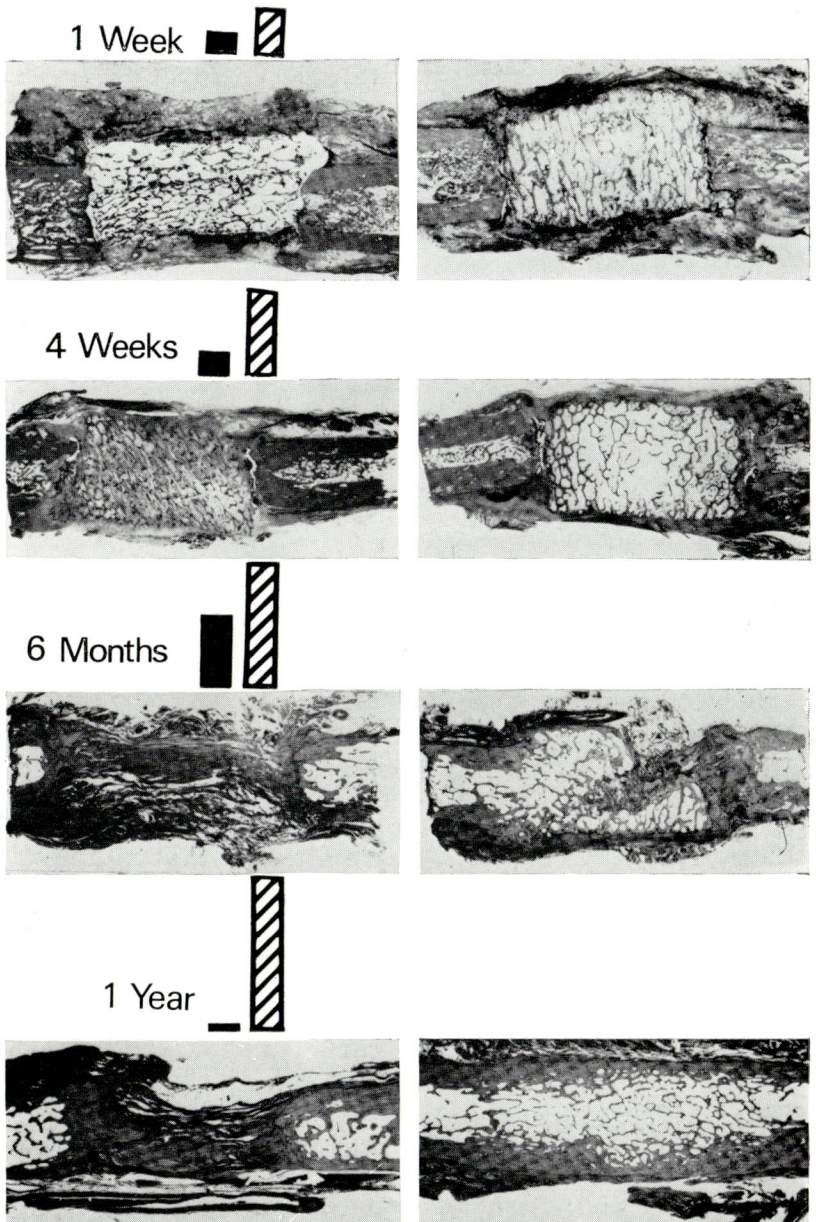

FIG. 21. Representative sections of processed heterogenous bone ('Boplant') on the left with the autogenous control on the right inserted into complete defects of the ulnae of dogs and removed for study at intervals from 1 week to 1 year. Note the resorption of the 'Boplant' and its failure to restore the continuity of the shaft of the ulna. (Reproduced by kind permission of Dr. K. G. Heiple and the Editor, *J. Bone Jt. Surg.*)

CONCLUSIONS

Boplant has been carefully evaluated experimentally and clinically. The first reports were a striking success story. More recently, however, Boplant has been found experimentally to be the least satisfactory of many types of bank bone (Heiple *et al.* 1967).

These conflicting findings may be attributable to the initial studies using processed bone prepared specially in the laboratory; and to the later studies using 'production-line' material.

Decalcified Bone

At the present time, the worth of decalcified bone as a bank bone is being re-evaluated experimentally.

It was introduced by Senn (1889) who decalcified ox bone in hydrochloric acid, sterilized it in an alcoholic solution of mercuric chloride and used it successfully to treat cavities in human bone resulting from osteomyelitis.

Decalcified bone was tried by several surgeons at the close of the nineteenth century, but its use was discontinued (see van de Putte and Urist 1966).

In recent years, Ray of Chicago has been re-evaluating decalcified bone experimentally, and has reported favourably upon it (see Preserved homografts of bone—decalcified bone).

Deproteinized Bone

It has been thought for many years that the material in ox bone which is foreign to the tissues of Man is its organic material. Hence it seemed logical to remove the organic matrix in order to overcome the histoincompatibility between the donor and the host (Orell 1937) (see Preserved homografts of bone: deproteinized bone).

In this section it is proposed to restrict attention to certain types of partially or completely deproteinized bone, namely: 'os purum'; 'Kiel bone'; 'anorganic (ethylene-diamine-extracted) bone'; and 'Oswestry bone'.

'Os purum' is bone which has been mechanically freed from soft tissues, soaked in warm potassium hydroxide to remove connective tissues, acetone to remove fat, and salt solution to remove proteins. It still, however, contains some residual collagen (Orell 1937, 1938).

Orell, its orginator, knew that for clinical success this partially-deproteinized bone needed to be implanted in close contact with living bone, supplemented at times with autograft bone or specially-prepared bony callus ('os novum'); and he was aware that its resorption was slow, taking as long as 2-3 years. He described its use in 49 patients with success. Goff (1944) used os purum in 80 operative procedures; sixteen were followed by complications, but only in 6 (10 per cent) did he attribute this to foreign bone.

The use of this bank bone, manufactured in Sweden, declined during World War II, and it has not been reincarnated since the war. Orell

(1953), however, stated that he was using finely divided bone as grafting material.

'Kiel bone.' This is a commercial, partially-deproteinized bone manufactured by Braun, Melsungen, East Germany, and marketed in the United Kingdom by the Armour Pharmaceutical Co., Ltd., Eastbourne.

Preparation. Bone is procured from freshly-killed calves which is then washed in water, extracted with hydrogen peroxide (which macerates through the oxidization of the organic substances), dried with acetone and sterilized with ethylene dioxide (Maatz and Bauermeister 1957, Stegeman 1966).

Antigenicity. The protein content is lower than that of normal bone (Stegeman 1966) and it is said to be antigen-free (Kienholz and Kemkes 1956); but Kramer *et al.* (1968a) have reported that some residual antigenicity may persist in Kiel bone.

Osteogenic induction. Maatz and Bauermeister (1957) reported that osseous metaplasia occurred in 63 per cent of hydrogen peroxide-treated heterogenous bone grafts implanted intra-muscularly into dogs; but this was not confirmed by Hancox *et al.* (1961) using sheep. Fuchs and his colleagues compared Kiel bone grafts with autografts inserted experimentally into cancellous sites and removed for study 15 days after grafting (Fuchs *et al.* 1963, Fuchs 1966). They found the amount of new bone formed to be equally great in Kiel bone as in the autografts; but that if the protein was largely removed from calf bone (by previous treatment with formamide for 24 hours), then the amount of new bone formed is also diminished. They concluded that, "there are soluble and removable components important as inducers in bone formation" (Fuchs 1966).

Remodelling. Maatz and Bauermeister (1957) inserted hydrogen-peroxide-treated heterologous bone grafts into a cancellous site in dogs. They stated that the biological results were excellent or good in 84 per cent (49/58 tests). Ecke *et al.* (1964b) compared Kiel bone with both fresh autograft and homograft bone inserted into prepared defects in the diaphysis of dogs and removed for study at intervals up to six months after grafting. They rated Kiel bone lower than fresh autograft bone but higher than fresh homograft bone.

Kingma (1967) has found Kiel cortical bone to be very slowly resorbed in rabbits. Using cancellous Kiel bone implanted into skull defects, also in rabbits, Kramer *et al.* (1968a) reported that the bone was resorbed by osteoclasts within six months, but was not invaded by host new bone, suggesting that it may exert inhibitory effect upon osteogenesis.

Clinical results. Maatz (1966) stated that he had used Kiel bone in 701 patients. Koch and Dahmen (1962) in Munster claimed 84 per cent successful results in 133 procedures using Kiel bone. Hallén (1966), however, in Sweden, found only 62 per cent good results with this type of bone. He also emphasized: (*a*) the importance of obtaining good apposition between Kiel bone and the patient's own bone at the site of grafting; (*b*) the unsuitability of Kiel bone for bridging defects of long bones; and (*c*) the slow resorption of Kiel cortical and cancellous bone which is sometimes observed. Williams (1966) reported that he had used

Kiel bone to treat 14 patients with delayed union of the tibiae; all the fractures united, though one refractured and required a sliding bone graft. Bell (1966a,b) has reported unfavourably on the use of Kiel bone for the correction of nasal deformities.

CONCLUSION

Further biological testing of Kiel bone is desirable, comparing it in various animals against the different types of homologous and heterologous bank bones.

'**Anorganic bone**' is the name generally given to bone from which the organic material has been extracted by means of the chemical, ethylenediamine (ED) (Williams and Irvine 1954). The material is brittle, can be readily carved with a knife and is sterilized by autoclaving. In it the bone crystals lie as though the collagen was still present, an effect which enormously increases the surface area of the bone (Quigley and Hjørting-Hansen 1962).

It was introduced into bone-grafting by Losee and Hurley (1956a,b) as an empirical attempt to overcome the immunological problems of heterologous bone transplantation. In a series of experiments they implanted cortical and cancellous ED-extracted bovine bone into tibial and calvarial defects in dogs (Losee and Hurley 1956a,b, Rosomoff et al. 1959) and as particles into mandibular defects of monkeys (Losee and Boyne 1957). They reported that the material was well-accepted by host tissues, did not evoke a foreign-body reaction, and was revascularized and invaded by osteogenic cells from the host.

Subsequently, however, other workers, while confirming that anorganic bone is relatively inert, have found that the material is not subject to an osteoclastic attack and is very slowly resorbed (Toto and Giannini 1961, Kramer et al. 1964, Killey et al. 1966) (Fig. 22a). Moreover, anorganic bone does not possess inductive capacity (Burwell 1966), though attempts have been made to give it an osteogenic inductive effect by means of chemical additives: calcium hydroxide has no such action (Rönning and Koski 1966) but encouraging results have been reported using β-aminopropionitrile (Gardner 1964, 1966).

In orthopaedic surgery, anorganic bone is apparently well-tolerated by human tissues. It serves best as an implant or filling material in bone defects when it acts to prevent the invasion of fibrous connective tissue and to supply an absorbable trellis through which new bone from the host may develop (Hurley et al. 1960). In dental surgery encouraging clinical results with its use have been claimed (Costich et al. 1957, Boyne 1958, for review see Gardner 1964, Costoyas and Fabaran 1966).

The marketing of anorganic bone was originally undertaken by the Armour Pharmaceutical Co., Ltd., Eastbourne, Sussex, England. It is now sold as miscellaneous-sized pieces, as granules, and in powder form under the trademark of 'Ossar' (Lääke Oy, Turku, Finland). In this connection it should be added that fragmented anorganic bone becomes more intimately incorporated into new host bone than does cortical anorganic bone, but its resorption is still very slow (Kramer et al. 1964, Killey et al. 1966) (Fig. 22b).

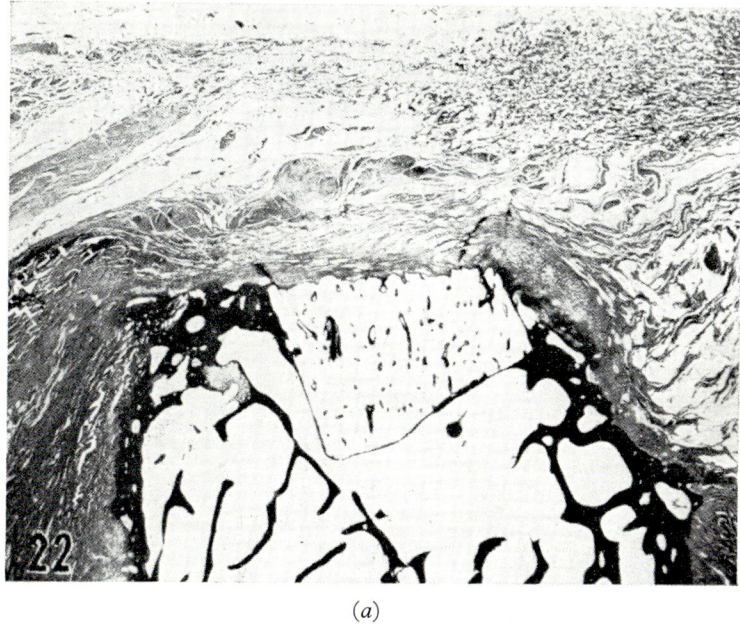

(a)

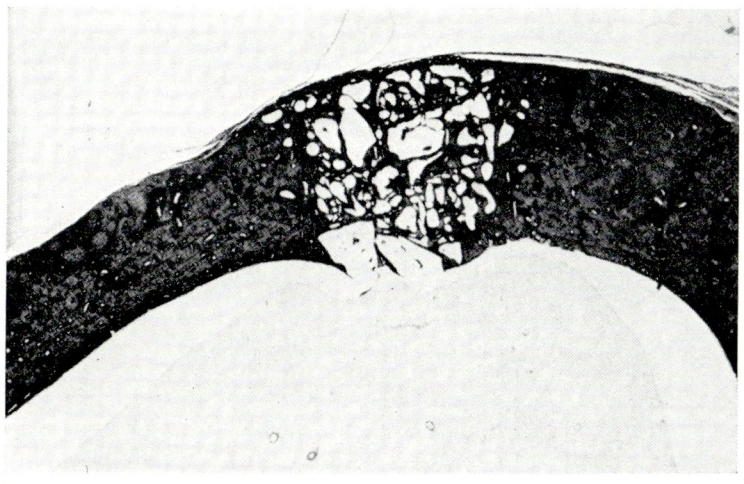

(b)

FIG. 22. (a) Heterograft of a block of anorganic bone, 372 days after implantation into the tuba coxa of the sheep. Although the block has been revascularized and new bone has formed within it, it still has a sharply-defined outline indicating that little or no resorption has occurred. (van Giesen. × 10.)

(b) Heterograft of fragmented anorganic bone, 147 days after implantation into the shaft of a long bone. Although the implant is now embedded in lamellar bone, little resorption of it has occurred. (van Giesen. × 10.) (Reproduced by kind permission of Professor I. R. H. Kramer and the Editor, *Arch. Oral Biol.*)

'Oswestry bone.' This type of deproteinized bone has been evaluated at the Robert Jones and Agnes Hunt Orthopaedic Hospital, Oswestry, Shropshire, England, by Professor Roaf and his colleagues. It is *fully* deproteinized bovine cancellous bone prepared by a double-extraction method using both hydrogen peroxide and ethylenediamine (Kershaw 1963).

Experimentally, the material has been tested in sheep and rabbits. Hancox *et al.* (1961) inserted pegs of 'Oswestry bone' into drill holes at the ends of limb bones in sheep. They reported that the material did not evoke an abnormal tissue response and, after 36 days, had been invaded by host new bone. Moreover, that on the whole, the healing of this material seemed better than that of frozen ($-37°$C) homologous bone grafts which evoked a local inflammatory response. Kramer and his colleagues (Killey *et al.* 1966, Kramer *et al.* 1968a, c), however, using rabbits, found that 'Oswestry bone' excited neither an inflammatory response nor an osteoclastic reaction. Its cancellous spaces were invaded by host new bone, but after 16 weeks little resorption had occurred, and it showed an obstruction to complete repair.

Clinically, this fully-deproteinized bone has been tried for filling defects in bone, for spinal fusions and for the treatment of ununited fractures (Roaf and Hancox 1963, Roaf 1966). Professor Roaf (personal communication) has kindly provided the following summary of Oswestry bone:

"This bone is completely non-antigenic but is of course purely a scaffolding and has bone conduction powers not bone induction powers. It is therefore only effective when placed in an excellent vascular bed in which there are plenty of potential osteogenic cells. Used in this limited way it has proved completely successful by itself in two situations, namely in filling cavities in bone and as a means of posterior spinal fusion in the thoracic region in children. It has not been consistently successful as a means of anterior lumbar fusion, and by itself I would not advise it for this purpose. It has also been successful used as an expander of the patient's own cancellous bone, where it is difficult to acquire enough of this. Naturally it is very hard to evaluate its exact potency in this situation when it is mixed with the patient's own bone."

CONCLUSIONS

The limitations imposed on the procurement of autograft bone for surgical purposes are avoided by using bone obtained from a human cadaver (as a homograft) or from another species, such as a calf (as a heterograft).

Homografts. In the last 20 years with the growth of knowledge concerning the immunity caused by skin homografts, the clinical use of *fresh* bone homografts has virtually ceased. It may be that the *prosthetic* replacement of bone and joints in Man will provide an easier method of treatment for skeletal deficiency than the use of fresh bone homografts involving, as it does, the use of tissue-typing and immunosuppressive therapy.

The storage of human bone for use as homografts has been practised widely since Inclán (1942) introduced the bone bank. Methods of storage which have been utilized include: freezing, freeze-drying and merthiolate solution. The bone has been stored either intact, or after removal of the bone protein or of the bone mineral. Sterilization of bone grafts has been attempted by heat, by chemical means and by high-energy radiation.

Many different varieties of treated bone homografts have been used empirically in clinical surgery. The clinical results using frozen and freeze-dried bone are better than those obtained with merthiolated and boiled bone (Table II and Table III). Indeed many of the results using frozen and freeze-dried bone have been as good as can be expected from the use of the patient's own bone as the grafting material. Is then such bank bone as effective in clinical use as the patient's own bone used as the graft? Unfortunately, there are very few reports in which the clinical results of bank bone have been compared with those of autograft bone (Table IV). These results are not consistent: thus while one writer has found bank bone to be as effective as autograft bone, others have shown it to be less satisfactory. In a clinical trial in which frozen bone was compared with autograft bone for spinal fusion, the autograft bone was about three times as effective as frozen bank bone (Bosworth).

In general, then, the clinical evidence suggests that autograft bone is superior to bank bone. But frozen and freeze-dried bone may be used as effectively as autograft bone if it be placed as chips of cancellous bone in intimate contact with the skeleton at the site of grafting; and perhaps especially so in sites of cancellous bone such as at the ends of long bones. It has been found clinically that bank bone should not be used as blocks; and experience has shown that it should not be used to span large defects in the shafts of long bones.

There are difficulties in assessing clinically the worth of any bank bone (Roaf) due, most probably to the numerous variables which exist in the grafting of bone into the human. The escape from this *impasse* is to appraise bank bone biologically in the animal. In the last 10 years, the biological problems of bone transplantation have been analysed more critically and have been found to relate to: (1) immunology; (2) vascular and cellular invasions; (3) osteogenesis; (4) remodelling; and (5) sterilization.

The three types of homologous bank bone which satisfy these criteria most certainly are frozen bone, freeze-dried bone and perhaps HCl-decalcified bone. Frozen and freeze-dried bone are each antigenically weak; each carries inductive capacity, but freeze-dried bone may be remodelled more quickly than frozen bone; more work in this field is needed. Boiling and autoclaving, and removing the proteins from bone, is known to have a retarding effect upon the renewal of the bone after grafting.

Recent experimental work suggests that during its preparation for the bank, the soft tissues should be cleansed from the spaces of cancellous bone in order to facilitate its revascularization after grafting. The impedance which necrotic medullary tissues can exert upon the revascularization of dead cancellous bone is seen commonly in the femoral head after sub-capital fracture (Catto 1965a,b), leading to the well-known sequela of avascular necrosis.

The main weakness of bank bone may be that it is *dead* and cannot, of itself, contribute *directly* to osteogenesis. However, certain types of bank bone (e.g. frozen, freeze-dried and HCl-decalcified) can stimulate osteogenesis *indirectly* by inducing bone formation in the tissues of the host at the site of grafting. It may be that future research will find a chemical which, as an additive, will increase the inductive capacity, and perhaps the mitogenic capacity, of bank bone (see Part I, the natural stimulation of osteogenesis). In the meantime osteogenesis in bank bone may be enhanced by placing it in the closest contact with the skeleton, particularly cancellous bone; especially at a cancellous site containing red marrow which is itself intensely osteogenic; and most markedly in children. A similar osteogenic effect may be achieved by using bank bone to supplement autograft bone for grafting purposes.

Although clinical experience has shown that bank bone should not be used for bridging large skeletal defects in the shafts of long bones, massive frozen homografts are being re-evaluated for the replacement of bone resected for tuberculosis, tumour, osteoarthritis or osteomyelitis. This trial of massive frozen homografts is a clinical experiment. The results will have to be compared against the use of custom-made prosthetic replacements.

Heterografts. *Fresh* heterografts of bone have no place in orthopaedic surgery. During the last 70 years, several attempts have been made to use various types of preserved ox bone as a substitute for autograft bone.

Frozen calf bone has been found to be far inferior to autograft bone as a grafting material.

Freeze-dried calf bone (as 'Boplant', Squibb) has been evaluated carefully both clinically and experimentally. The first reports were most encouraging, but a recent experimental analysis has found 'Boplant' to be the least satisfactory of many types of bank bone. These conflicting findings may be attributable to the initial studies using processed bone prepared specially in the laboratory; and to the later studies using 'production-line' material.

Decalcified calf bone as a grafting material is worthy of further study.

Deproteinized calf bone has been used clinically either as partially-deproteinized bone (e.g. os purum, Kiel bone and anorganic bone); and as fully-deproteinized bone (Oswestry bone). Each of these varieties of bone implants are probably resorbed more slowly than is bone from which the proteins have not been removed. **Os purum** is probably little used at the present time. **Kiel bone** is still being assessed both clinically and experimentally. **Anorganic bone** may serve best as a filling material in bone defects when it acts to prevent the invasion of fibrous connective tissue and supplies an absorbable trellis through which new bone from the host may develop. **Oswestry bone** has been successfully used for filling cavities in bone and as a means of posterior spinal fusion in the thoracic region in children.

The final word on bank bone cannot yet be stated. More *experimental* work on homologous bone is needed:

(1) To decide the optimal temperature for preserving bone by freezing ($-20°C$, $-79°C$ or $-196°C$).

(2) To compare the best frozen bone against freeze-dried bone.

(3) To establish the worth of HCl-decalcified bone as a graft material.

(4) To ascertain whether osteogenic induction by bank bone can be enhanced by chemicals such as chondroitin sulphate and β-aminopropionitrile.

(5) To appraise the best method for sterilizing bone: by high-energy radiation?; by β-propiolactone?; or by ethylene dioxide?

(6) Finally, to inquire whether any type of preserved heterologous bone will match the best homologous bank bone. If it does, then a commercially-prepared calf bone would clearly be more convenient in clinical use than a 'home-made' homologous bank bone.

Then, and only then, will it be the task of clinicians to define more clearly not only the indications for but also the limitations of the use of bank bone. In the meantime, the best bank bone available for clinical use to-day seems to be freeze-dried homologous cancellous bone sterilized by irradiation.

References

ABBOTT, LeR. C. (1944). The use of iliac bone in the treatment of ununited fractures. I. Lectures on Reconstr. Surg., Amer. Acad. Orthop. Surgeons. Michigan: Ann. arbor.

ABBOTT, L. C., SCHOTTSTAEDT, E. R., SAUNDERS, J. B. DeC. and BOST, F. C. (1947). The evaluation of cortical and cancellous bone as grafting material. A clinical and experimental study. *J. Bone Jt. Surg.*, **29**, 381.

AFANASSIEFF, A. (1967). Les reconstructions articulaires partielles ou totales par homogreffes. *La Presse Medicale.*, **75**, 669.

ALBEE, F. H. (1912). Quoted by Peer (1955).

ALBEE, F. H. (1915). Bone graft surgery. Philadelphia: W. B. Saunders & Co.

ALBEE, F. H. (1923). Fundamentals in bone transplantation. Experiences in three thousand bone graft operations. *J. Amer. Med. Assoc.*, **81**, 1429.

ALBEE, F. H. (1944). Evolution of bone graft surgery. *Amer. J. Surg.*, **63**, 421.

ALLDREDGE, R. H. (1948). In discussion after the paper of Henry (1948).

ANDERSON, K. J. (1961). The behaviour of autogenous and homogenous bone transplants in the anterior chamber of the rat's eye. A histological study of the effect of the size of the implant. *J. Bone Jt. Surg.*, **43A**, 980.

ANDERSON, C. E. and PARKER, J. (1966). Invasion and resorption in endochondral ossification. An electron microscopic study. *J. Bone Jt. Surg.*, **48A**, 899.

ANDERSON, K. J., SCHMIDT, J. and CLAWSON, D. K. (1959). The vascularization and cellular response induced by homogenous deproteinized bone transplants in the anterior chamber of the rat eye. *Plast. Reconstr. Surg.*, **24**, 97.

ANDERSON, K. J., DINGWALL, J. A., LECOCQ, J. F. and CLAWSON, D. K. (1960). Induced connective tissue metaplasia. I. Heterogenous bone extract implants in the rat anterior chamber. A preliminary report. *Plast. Reconstr. Surg.*, **25**, 399.

ANDERSON, K. J., LECOCQ, J. F. and CLAWSON, D. K. (1962). Processed heterogenous bone. A basic scientific study and preliminary clinical trial in humans. A Scientific exhibit at the 29th Annual Meeting of the American Academy of Orthopaedic Surgeons, Chicago, Illinois, January 1962.

ANDERSON, K. J., LECOCQ, J. F. and MOONEY, J. G. (1963). Clinical evaluation of processed heterogenous bone transplants. *Clin. Orthop. rel. Res.*, **29**, 248.

ANDERSON, K. J., LECOCQ, J. F., DINGWALL, J. A. and KARGES, D. E. (1964). Processed heterogenous bone. A basic scientific study with preliminary clinical trial in humans. *J. Amer. Med. Assoc.*, **193**, 127.

ANDERSON, K. J., FRY, L. R., CLAWSON, D. K. and SAKURAI, O. (1965). Experimental comparison of autogenous, homogenous and heterogenous bone grafts: a planimetric measurement study. *Ann. Surg.*, **161**, 263.

Ansari, P. (1966). Klinische Erfahrungen über 383 homioplastische Knochentransplantationen. *Zeit. für Chir.*, **91**, 875.
Arden, G. P. (1956). Experiences with a merthiolate bone bank. *Brit. J. Clin. Pract.*, **10**, 522.
Auty, J. R. (1965). Mucopolysaccharides and bone. Ph.D. Thesis. University of Leeds.
Axhausen, G. (1908). Die histologischen und klinischen Gesetze der freien Osteoplastik auf Grund von Thierversuchen. *Arch. klin. Chir.*, **88**, 23.
Axhausen, W. (1956). The osteogenetic phases of regeneration of bone. A historical and experimental study. *J. Bone Jt. Surg.*, **38A**, 593.
Baadsgaard, K. and Medgyesi, S. (1965). Muscle-pedicle bone grafts. An experimental study. *Acta. Orthop. Scandinav.*, **35**, 279.
Bain, B. and Lowenstein, L. (1964). Genetic studies on the mixed leucocyte reaction. *Science.*, **145**, 1315.
Barnes, B. A. (1965). Survival data on renal transplantation in patients. Report issued by Transplantation Unit, Dept. Surgery, Mass. Gen. Hosp., Boston. May 14, 1965. Quoted by Ceppelini et al. (1965).
Bassett, C. A. L. (1962a). Current concepts of bone formation. *J. Bone Jt. Surg.*, **44A**, 1217.
Bassett, C. A. L. (1962b). Bibliography of bone transplantation. Addendum No. V. *Plast. Reconstr. Surg.*, **29**, 476/104.
Bassett, C. A. L. (1966). Electro-mechanical factors regulating bone architecture. Proceedings of the Third European Symposium on Calcified Tissues. Edited by H. Fleisch, H. J. J. Blackwood and M. Owen. Berlin: Springer-Verlag.
Bassett, C. A. L. (1967). Discussion after the paper of Heiple et al. (1967).
Bassett, C. A. L. and Creighton, D. K. J. (1962). A comparison of host response to cortical autografts and processed calf heterografts. *J. Bone Jt. Surg.*, **44A**, 842.
Bassett, C. A. L. and Hermann, I. (1961). Influence of oxygen concentration and mechanical factors on differentiation of connective tissues *in vitro*. *Nature*, **190**, 460.
Bassett, C. A. L. and Packard, A. G., Jnr. (1959). A clinical assay of cathode ray sterilized cadavar bone grafts. *Acta. Orthop. Scand.*, **28**, 198.
Bassett, C. A. L. and Rued, T. P. (1966). Transformation of fibrous tissue to bone *in vivo*. *Nature*, **209**, 988.
Bassett, C. A. L., Creighton, D. K., and Stinchfield, F. E. (1961). Contributions of endosteum, cortex, and soft tissues to osteogenesis. *Surg. Gyn. Obstet.*, **112**, 145.
Bassett, C. A. L., Hurley, L. A. and Stinchfield, F. E. (1962). The fate of long term anorganic bone implants. *Trans. Bull.*, **29**, 423/51.
Barth, A. (1893). Ueber histologische Befunde nach Knochenimplantationen. *Arch. f. Klin. Chir.*, **46**, 409.
Bauermeister, A. (1958). Experimentelle Grundlagen für den Aufbeau einer neuen Knockenbank. Heft 58. Berlin: Springer-Verlag.
Baumgart, R. (1958). Erfahrungen mit dem ausgekochten homologen Knochenspan. *Zentr. Chir.* **31**, 1552.
Bélanger, L. F. (1959). Observations on the manifestation of osteolathyrism in the chick. *J. Bone Jt. Surg.*, **41B**, 581.
Bélanger, L. F., Semba, T., Tolnai, S., Copp, D. H., Krook, L. and Gries, C. (1966). The two faces of resorption. Proceedings of the Third European Symposium on Calcified Tissues. Edited by H. Fleisch, H. J. J. Blackwood and M. Owen. Berlin: Springer-Verlag.
Bell, R. (1966a). An interim report on the use of Kiel bone in the correction of nasal deformities. In "Symposium on Bone Grafting Materials". Eastbourne: Armour Pharmaceutical Co., Ltd., p. 117.
Bell, R. C. (1966b). Unsuccessful use of 'Kiel bone' in nasal reconstruction. *Brit. J. plast. Surg.*, **19**, 271.
Berg, E. M. and Trevaskis, A. E. (1967). Metacarpal transplant and joint reconstruction following a power mower injury. *Plast reconstr. Surg.*, **39**, 287.
Berkin, C. R. (1957). Freeze-dried bone grafts. *Lancet*, **i**, 730.

Billingham, R. E., Brent, L. and Medawar, P. B. (1954). Quantitative studies on tissue transplantation immunity. I. The survival times of skin homografts exchanged between members of different inbred strains of mice. *Proc. R. Soc.*, **143B**, 43.

Billingham, R. E. and Silvers, W. S. (1967). Studies on the conservation of epidermal specificities of skin and certain mucosas in adult mammals. *J. exp. Med.*, **125**, 429.

Bircher, H. (1887). A new method of immediate retention in fractures of the tubular bones. *Ann. Surg.*, **6**, 268.

Bisgaard, J. D. (1936). Ossification. The influence of the mineral constituents of bone. *Arch. Surg., Lond.*, **33**, 926.

Blaimont, P. (1960). Contribution expérimentale à l'etude des greffes osseuses bouilles. *Acta chir. belg.*, **59**, 871.

Blockey, N. J. (1967). Observations on the fate of fibular transplants for congenital absence of the radius. *J. Bone Jt. Surg.*, **49B**, 762.

Bloom, W. (1960). A note on osteogenesis by myeloid reticular cells. *J. infect. Dis.*, **107**, 11.

Bloom, M. A., Domm, L. V., Nalbandov, A. V. and Bloom, W. (1958). Medullary bone of laying chickens. *Amer. J. Anat.* **102**, 411.

Bohr, H., Ravn, H. O. and Werner, H. (1967). Investigations on the osteogenesis in autotransplants of bone. *Acta orthopaed. scand.*, **38**, 381.

Bohr, H., Ravn, H. O. and Werner, H. (1968). The osteogenic effect of bone transplants in rabbits. *J. Bone Jt. Surg.*, **50B**, 866.

Bonfiglio, M. and Jeter, W. S. (1962). Further experimental studies on bone transplantation. *J. Bone. Jt. Surg.*, **44A**, 1029.

Bonfiglio, M., Jeter, W. S. and Smith, C. L. (1955). The immune concept: its relation to bone transplantation. *Ann. N.Y. Acad. Sci.*, **59**, 417.

Bosworth, D. M., Wright, H. A., Fielding, J. W. and Goodrich, E. R. (1953). A study in the use of bank bone for spine fusion in tuberculosis. *J. Bone Jt. Surg.*, **35A**, 329.

Bottcher, E. J. (1962). Lathyrism in rabbits. *J. Bone Jt. Surg.*, **44A**, 717.

Bowie, J. H. (1955). Modern apparatus for sterilization. *Pharm. J.*, **174**, 473, 489.

Boyd, H. B. (1939). Congenital pseudarthrosis. Treatment by dual bone grafts. *J. Bone Jt. Surg.*, **23**, 497.

Boyd, H. B., Lipinski, S. W. and Wiley, J. H. (1960). Non-union of the shafts of the long bones: treatment and observations. *Huitième Congrès de la Société Internationale de Chirurgie Orthopedique et de Traumatologie, New York, 4–9 Septembre,* 291.

Boyd, H. B., Anderson, L. D. and Johnson, D. S. (1966). Changing concepts in the treatment of non-union. *Clin. Orthop.*, **43**, 37.

Boyne, P. J. (1958). Treatment of oral bony defects in Man with anorganic heterogenous bone. *Oral Surg.*, **11**, 322.

Brånemark, P. I. (1959). Vital microscopy of bone marrow in rabbit. *Scand. J. cli. Lab. Med.*, **2** Suppl. **38**, 1.

Brav, E. A. (1954). A comparative clinical study of autogenous and frozen homogenous bone in grafting procedures. *Cli. Orthop.*, **3**, 163.

Brav, E. A., McFaddin, J. G. and Miller, J. A. (1958). The replacement of shaft defects of long bones by metallic prostheses. *Amer. J. Surg.*, **95**, 752.

Brent, L. and Medawar, P. B. (1963). Tissue transplantation: a new approach to the 'typing' problem. *Brit. med. J.*, **ii**, 269.

Bridges, J. B. (1959). Experimental heterotopic ossification. *Intn. Rev. Cytol.*, **8**, 253.

Brookes, M. (1964). The blood supply of bone. In "Modern Trends in Orthopaedics, 4, Science of Fractures". Ed. J. M. P. Clark. London: Butterworths.

Brooks, B. (1919). Studies in bone transplantation; a study of the method of increasing the osteogenetic power of a free bone transplant. *Ann. Surg.*, **49**, 113.

Brooks, B. and Hudson, W. A. (1920). Studies in bone transplantations. An experimental study of the comparative success of autogenous and homogenous transplants of bone in dogs. *Arch. Surg.*, **1**, 282.

BROOKS, D. B., HEIPLE, K. G., HERNON, C. H. and POWELL, A. E. (1963). Immunological factors in homogenous bone transplantation. IV. The effect of various methods of preparation and irradiation on antigenicity. *J. Bone Jt. Surg.*, **45A**, 1617.

BULLOUGH, W. S. (1962). The control of mitotic activity in adult mammalian tissues. *Biol. Rev.*, **37**, 307.

BUNCKE, H. J., BUNCKE, C. M. and SCHULZ, W. P. (1966). Immediate Nicoladoni procedure in the Rhesus monkey, or hallux-to-hand transplantation, utilising microminiature vascular anastomoses. *Brit. J. plast. Surg.*, **19**, 332.

BUNCKE, H. J., JR., DANILLER, A. I., SCHULZ, W. P. and CHASE, R. A. (1967). The fate of autogenous whole joints transplanted by microvascular anastomoses. *Plast. reconstr. Surg.*, **39**, 333.

BURGER, M., SHERMAN, B. S. and SOBEL, A. E. (1962). Observations on the influence of chondroitin sulphate on the rate of bone repair. *J. Bone Jt. Surg.*, **44B**, 675.

BÜRING, K. and URIST, M. R. (1967). Transfilter bone induction. *Clin. Orthop.*, **54**, 235.

BÜRKLE DE LA CAMP, H. (1954). Knochenkonservierung und Verwendung konservierten Knochens. *Arch. klin. Chir.*, **279**, 26.

BURROWS, H. J. (1940). Treatment of ununited fractures by bone grafting without resection of the bone ends. *Proc. roy. Soc. Med.*, **33**, 157.

BURROWS, H. J. (1968). Major prosthetic replacement of bone: lessons learnt in 17 years. *J. Bone Jt. Surg.*, **50B**, 225.

BURROWS, H. J. and LETTIN, A. W. F. (1964). Fibular replacement of the upper humerus after segmental resection for chondrosarcoma. *Proc. roy. Soc. Med.*, **57**, 90.

BURWELL, R. G. (1962). Studies in the transplantation of bone. IV. The immune responses of lymph nodes draining second-set homografts of fresh cancellous bone. *J. Bone Jt. Surg.*, **44B**, 688.

BURWELL, R. G. (1963). Studies in the transplantation of bone. V. The capacity of fresh and treated homografts of bone to evoke transplantation immunity. *J. Bone Jt. Surg.*, **45B**, 386.

BURWELL, R. G. (1964*a*). Studies in the transplantation of bone. VII. The fresh composite homograft-autograft of cancellous bone. An analysis of factors leading to osteogenesis in marrow transplants and in marrow-containing bone grafts. *J. Bone Jt. Surg.*, **46B**, 110.

BURWELL, R. G. (1964*b*). Biological mechanisms in foreign bone transplantation. In "Modern Trends in Orthopaedics, 4, Science of Fractures". Ed. J. M. P. Clark. London: Butterworths.

BURWELL, R. G. (1965). Osteogenesis in cancellous bone grafts considered in terms of cellular changes, basic mechanisms and the perspective of growth-control and its possible aberrations. *Clin. Orthopaed. and Rel. Res.*, **40**, 35.

BURWELL, R. G. (1966). Studies in the transplantation of bone. VIII. Treated composite homograft-autografts of cancellous bone: an analysis of inductive mechanisms in bone transplantation. *J. Bone Jt. Surg.*, **48B**, 532.

BURWELL, R. G. (1968). The scientific basis of bone homotransplantation. In "The Scientific Basis of Medicine, Annual Reviews". University of London: Athlone Press.

BURWELL, R. G. and GOWLAND, G. (1961). Studies in the transplantation of bone. II. The changes occurring in the lymphoid tissue after homografts and autografts of fresh cancellous bone. *J. Bone Jt. Surg.*, **43B**, 820.

BURWELL, R. G. and GOWLAND, G. (1962). Studies in the transplantation of bone. III. The immune responses of lymph nodes draining components of fresh homologous cancellous bone and homologous bone treated by different methods. *J. Bone Jt. Surg.*, **44B**, 131.

BURWELL, R. G., GOWLAND, G. and DEXTER, F. (1963). Studies in the transplantation of bone. VI. Further observations concerning the antigenicity of homologous cortical and cancellous bone. *J. Bone Jt. Surg.*, **45B**, 597.

BUSER, P. (1959). Erfahrungen mit Kältekonservierten Knochenspänen. *Arch. klin. Chir.*, **290**, 289.

Bush, L. F. and Garber, C. Z. (1948). The bone bank. *J. Amer. med. Assoc.*, **137**, 588.
Bush, L. F. (1947). The use of homogenous bone grafts. A preliminary report on the bone bank. *J. Bone Jt. Surg.*, **29**, 620.
Byars, L. T. (1952). Toe to finger transplant. *Plast. reconstr. Surg.*, **9**, 274.
Calne, R. Y. (1967). Renal transplantation. 2nd Ed. London: Edward Arnold.
Cameron, D. A. (1961). Erosion of the epiphysis of the rat tibia by capillaries. *J. Bone Jt. Surg.*, **43B**, 590.
Campbell, C. J., Brower, T., Macfadden, D. G., Payne, E. B. and Doherty, J. (1953). Experimental study of the fate of bone grafts. *J. Bone Jt., Surg.*, **35A**, 332.
Carnesale, P. L. and Spankus, J. D. (1959). A clinical comparative study of autogenous and homogenous bone grafts. *J. Bone Jt. Surg.*, **41A**, 887.
Carr, C. R. and Hyatt, G. W. (1955). Clinical evaluation of freeze-dried bone grafts. *J. Bone Jt. Surg.*, **37A**, 549.
Carroll, R. E. (1966). Use of the fibula for reconstruction in congenital absence of the radius. *J. Bone Jt. Surg.*, **48A**, 1012.
Catto, M. (1965a). A histological study of avascular necrosis of the femoral head after transcervical fracture. *J. Bone Jt. Surg.*, **47B**, 749.
Catto, M. (1965b). The histological appearances of late segmental collapse of the femoral head after transcervical fracture. *J. Bone Jt. Surg.*, **47B**, 777.
Ceppelini, R., Curtoni, E. S., Leigheb, G., Mattiuz, P. L., Miggiano, V. C. and Visetti, M. (1965). An experimental approach to genetic analysis of histocompatibility in Man. In "Series Haematologica, **11**, Histocompatibility Testing". Copenhagen: Munksgaard.
Chalmers, D. G., Coulson, A. S., Evans, C. and Yealland, S. (1966). Immunologically stimulated human peripheral blood lymphocytes in vitro. II. Mixed lymphocyte cultures with related and unrelated donors. *Int. Arch. Allergy*, **30**, 177.
Chalmers, J. (1959). Transplantation immunity in bone homografting. *J. Bone Jt. Surg.*, **41B**, 160.
Chalmers, J. (1966). In "Symposium on Bone Grafting Materials". p. 141. Eastbourne: Armour Pharmaceutical Co. Ltd.
Chalmers, J. (1967). Bone transplantation. In "Symposium Tissue Organs Transplant". (Suppl. *J. clin. Path.* **20**, 540.)
Chalmers, J., Lea, L., Stewart, L. and Sissons, H. A. (1960). Freeze-dried bone as grafting material. In "Recent Research in Freezing and Drying". Ed. A. S. Parkes and Audrey U. Smith. Oxford: Blackwell Scientific Publications.
Chalmers, J. and Ray, R. D. (1962). The growth of transplanted foetal bones in different immunological environments. *J. Bone Jt. Surg.*, **44B**, 149.
Chandler, R. and Clarkson, P. (1958). A toe-to-thumb transplant with nerve graft. *Amer. J. Surg.*, **95**, 315.
Chase, S. W. and Herndon, C. H. (1955). The fate of autogenous and homogenous bone grafts. A historical review. *J. Bone Jt. Surg.*, **37A**, 809.
Chesterman, P. (1965). Cartilage for joint repair. *New Scientist*, July 22, p. 210.
Clark, K. (1959). A case of replacement of the upper end of the humerus by a fibular graft reviewed after 28 years. *J. Bone Jt. Surg.*, **41B**, 365.
Clarkson, P. (1955). Reconstruction of hand digits by toe transfers. *J. Bone Jt. Surg.*, **37A**, 270.
Clarkson, P. (1962). On making thumbs. *Plast. reconstr. Surg.*, **29**, 325.
Cleveland, M. and Winant, E. M. (1952). Treatment of non-union in compound fractures with infection. *J. Bone Jt. Surg.*, **34A**, 554.
Cohen, J. (1955). Cathode ray sterilization of bone grafts. *Arch. Surg.*, **71**, 784.
Coley, B. L. and Higinbotham, N. L. (1949). Use of bank bone in the treatment of central lesions of bone. *Amer. J. Surg.*, **78**, 587.
Committee of the American Academy of Orthopaedic Surgeons (1953). Report to the Committee to study the preservation of bone. *J. Bone Jt. Surg.*, **35A**, 774.

CONWAY, H. (1962). Digital lengthening by insertion of a composite graft of bones, joints and tendons into pedicled tissue. *Amer. J. Surg.*, **104,** 111.

CORKERY, P. H. (1965). The 'bolt' bone grafting technique. *Brit. J. cli. Pract.*, **19,** 289.

COSTICH, E. M., AVERY, J. K. and HAYWARD, J. R. (1957). Heterogenous 'anorganic' bone grafts in humans. *Trans. Bull.*, **4,** 130.

COSTOYAS, N. R. and FABARAN, J. B. (1966). The filling of bone cavities with anorganic bone. *Rev. Assoc. odont. Argent.*, **54,** 91.

COUNCIL ON DRUGS (1966). A new implant material for use in reconstructive surgical procedures. Surgibone (Boplant). *J. Amer. med. Ass.*, **195,** 167.

CRAWFORD ADAMS, J. (1966). Ischio-femoral arthrodesis. London: E. & S. Livingstone Ltd.

CROMIE, B. W. (1967). Personal communication and a subsequent communication from E. R. Squibb and Sons Ltd., 14th February, 1969.

CURRAN, J. P. and MCGAW, W. H. (1968). Postero-lateral spinal fusion with pedicle grafts. *Clin. Orthop.*, **59,** 125.

CURTISS, P. H., JR. and WILSON, P. D. (1953). A comparison of the healing of homogenous and autogenous fresh bone grafts with and without the administration of cortisone. *Surg. Gynec. Obstet.*, **96,** 155.

DAUSSET, J., IVANYI, P. and IVANYI, D. (1965). Tissue alloantigens in humans: identification of a complex system (Hu-1). Series Haematologica II, Histocompatibility Testing 1965. Copenhagen: Munksgaard.

DAVIS, J. B. and TAYLOR, A. N. (1952). Muscle pedicle bone grafts. Experimental study. *Arch. Surg.*, **65,** 330.

DAVIS, J. E. (1964). Toe-to-hand transfers (pedochirodactyloplasty). *Plast. reconstr. Surg.*, **33,** 422.

DE BRUYN, P. P. H. and KABISCH, W. T. (1955). Bone formation by fresh and frozen autogenous and homogenous transplants of bone, bone marrow and periosteum. *Amer. J. Anat.*, **96,** 375.

DELEU, J. and TRUETA, J. (1965). Vascularisation of bone grafts in the anterior chamber of the eye. *J. Bone Jt. Surg.*, **47B,** 319.

DEVRIES, P. H., BRINKER, W. O. and KEMPE, L. (1955). Utilisation of radioactive cobalt in the sterilization of homogenous bone transplants. *Surg. Forum.*, **6,** 546.

DEVRIES, P. H., BADGLEY, C. E. and HARTMAN, J. T. (1958). Radiation sterilization of homogenous-bone transplants utilizing radio-active cobalt. *J. Bone Jt. Surg.*, **40A,** 187.

DEWAR, F. P. and YABSLEY, R. H. (1967). Fracture-dislocation of the shoulder. Report of a case. *J. Bone Jt. Surg.*, **49B,** 540.

DEXTER, F. (1965). The preservation of tissue for surgical transplantation and subsequent formation of a tissue bank. *J. sci. Technol.*, **11,** 149.

DEXTER, F. (1966). The preservation of tissue for surgical transplantation and subsequent formation of a tissue bank. *J. sci. Technol.*, **12,** 1.

DINEEN, J. R. and GRESHAM, R. B. (1962). Rib osteoperiosteal grafts. A preliminary report of their use in the treatment of fresh and ununited fractures of the long bones. *J. Bone Jt. Surg.*, **44A,** 1653.

DOBROWOLSKAJA, N. A. (1916). On the regeneration of bone in its relation to the cultivation of bone tissue. *Brit. J. Surg.*, **4,** 332.

EASTOE, J. E. (1956). The organic matrix of bone. Ch. IV. In "The Biochemistry and Physiology of Bone". Ed. G. H. Bourne. New York: Academic Press Inc.

ECKE, H., ROMFEL, K. and GRABOW, L. (1964a). Tierexperimentelle Untersuchungen zur Bestimmung der Qualität von Knochenspänen verschiedener biologischer Herkunft für Transplantationzwecke Teil I. Austestung Herkömmlichen Spanmaterials. *Arch. klin. Chir.*, **307,** 169.

ECKE, H., ROMPEL, K. and GRABOW, L. (1964b). Tierexperimentelle Untersuchungen zur Bestimmung der Qualität von Knochenspänen verschiedener biologischer Herkunft fur Transplantationzwecke. Teil II. Austestung nicht Herkommlichen Spanmaterials. *Arch. klin. Chir.*, **307,** 179.

EGDAHL, R. H., VARCO, R. L. and GOOD, R. A. (1958). Local reaction and lymph node response to skin heterografts exchanged between rabbits and rats. *Int. Arch. Allergy. Basel*, **13,** 129.

Eger, W. and Kämmerer, H. (1967). On the regeneration of bone tissue examined with tetracycline in transparent bone sections. *Symp. biol. Hung.*, **7,** 179.
Ehalt, W. (1954). Ergebnisse bei der Verwendung konservierter Knochen. *Arch. klin. Chir.*, **279,** 44.
Eichwald, E. J. and Silmser, C. R. (1955). No title. *Transpl. Bull.* **2,** 148.
Ellmer and Schminke (1925). A $15\frac{1}{2}$ year old homeoplastic bone graft. *J. Amer. med. Assoc.*, **84,** 1463 (Abstract).
Eloesser, L. (1920). Rib grafting operations for the repair of bone defects and their end-results. *Arch. Surg.*, **1,** 428.
Elves, M. W. and Israëls, M. C. G. (1965). Lymphocyte transformations in cultures of mixed leucocytes. A possible test of histocompatibility. *Lancet* **i,** 1184.
Elves, M. W. and Nisbet, N. W. (1969). Symposium on Transplantation antigens and tissue typing. Oswestry: The Robert Jones and Agnes Hunt Orthop. Hosp. Management Committee.
Enlow, D. H. (1963). Principles of bone remodelling. Springfield: C. C. Thomas.
Enneking, W. F. (1957). Histological investigation of bone transplants in immunologically prepared animals. *J. Bone Jt. Surg.*, **39A,** 597.
Entin, M. A., Alger, J. R. and Baird, R. M. (1962). Experimental and clinical transplantation of autogenous whole joints. *J. Bone Jt. Surg.*, **44A,** 1518.
Erdélyi, R. (1963). Reconstruction of ankylosed finger joints by means of transplantation of joints from the foot. *Plast. reconstr. Surg.*, **31,** 140.
Evans, F. G. (1957). Stress and strain in bones. Their relation to fractures and osteogenesis. Springfield: Chas. C. Thomas.
Fang, H. C. and Miltner, L. J. (1934). Comparison of osteogenic power of periosteal transplants from rib and tibia. *Proc. Soc. exp. Biol., N.Y.*, **31,** 386.
Farmer, A. W. (1952). The use of a composite pedicle graft for pseudarthrosis of the tibia. *J. Bone Jt. Surg.*, **34A,** 591.
Fell, H. B. (1956). Skeletal development in tissue culture. Ch. XIV. In "The Biochemistry and Physiology of Bone". Ed. G. H. Bourne. New York: Academic Press. Inc.
Fell, H. B., Dingle, J. T. and Coombs, R. R. A. (1966). Recent experiments on the degradation and synthesis of bone and cartilage matrix in organ culture. In "Fourth European Symposium on Calcified Tissues". Abridged proceedings. Ed. P. J. Gaillard, A. van den Hoof, and R. S. Steedijk. Amsterdam: Exc. Med. Foundation.
Felts, W. J. L. (1961). *In vivo* implantation as a technique in skeletal biology. *Int. Rev. Cytol.*, **12,** 243.
Ferguson, A. B., Laing, P. G., Grebner, M. and Madancy, L. (1959). Study of revascularization of autogenous cortical bone grafts in rabbit using radiophosphorus. *Arch. Surg.*, **78,** 57/551.
Freeman, B. S. (1956). Reconstruction of thumb by toe transfer. *Plast. reconstr. Surg.*, **17,** 393.
Freeman, B. S. (1965). The results of epiphyseal transplants by flap and by free graft: a brief survey. *Plast. reconstr. Surg.*, **36,** 227.
Freiberg, R. A. and Ray, R. D. (1964). Studies of devitalized bone implants. *Arch. Surg.*, **89,** 417.
Fuchs, G. (1966). The inter-relation of bone graft chemistry and its fate. In "Symposium on Bone Grafting Materials". Eastbourne: Armour Pharmaceutical Co. Ltd., p. 5.
Fuchs, G., Stegemann, H. and Eber, W. (1963). Der transplantierte Knochenspan und seine Qualität nach partieller und vollstandiger Enteiweissung bei erhaltener anorganischer Substanz. *Arch. klin. Chir.*, **303,** 240.
Gabrielson, A. E. and Good, R. A. (1967). Chemical suppression of adaptive immunity. *Adv. Immun.*, **6,** 91.
Gage, A. A., Greene, G. W., Jr., Neiders, M. E. and Emmings, F. G. (1966). Freezing bone without excision. An experimental study of bone cell destruction and manner of regrowth in dogs. *J. Amer. med. Ass.*, **196,** 770.
Gallie, W. E. (1918). The use of boiled bone in operative surgery. *Amer. J. Orthop. Surg.*, **16,** 373.

GALLIE, W. E. and ROBERTSON, D. E. (1918). The transplantation of bone. *J. Amer. med. Ass.*, **70**, 1134.
GALLINARO, P., MASSÉ, G., CACAI, F. and COSCIA, P. L. (1966). Studi sull' immunità da trapianto. VII. Effeto dell' omogenato osseo omologo sulla reattività del ricevente. *Minerva Ortop.*, **17**, 305.
GARDNER, A. F. (1966). Beta-aminopropionitrile anorganic bone in the repair of oral and maxillofacial wounds. *J. dent. Res.*, **46**, 181.
GHORMLEY, R. K. (1939). Choice of bone graft methods in bone and joint surgery. *Ann. Surg.*, **115**, 1942.
GHORMLEY, R. K. and STUCK, W. G. (1954). Experimental bone transplantation with special reference to the effect of 'decalcification'. *Arch. Surg.*, **28**, 742.
GOFF, C. W. (1944). The os purum implant. A substitute for the autogenous implant. *J. Bone Jt. Surg.*, **26**, 758.
GOLDHABER, P. (1961). Osteogenic induction across millipore filters *in vivo*. *Science*, **133**, 2065.
GÖTHMAN, L. (1960). The arterial pattern of the rabbit's tibia after the application of an intramedullary nail. A microangiographic study. *Acta Chir. Scand.*, **120**, 211.
GÖTHMAN, L. (1961). Arterial changes in experimental fractures of the monkey's tibia treated with intramedullary nailing. A microangiographic study. *Acta Chir. Scand.*, **121**, 56.
GÖTHMAN, L. (1962). Local arterial changes associated with diastasis in experimental fractures of the rabbit's tibia treated with intramedullary nailing. A microangiographic study. *Acta Chir. Scand.*, **123**, 1.
GRAHAM, W. C. (1954). Transplantation of joints to replace diseased or damaged articulations in the hands. *Amer. J. Surg.*, **88**, 136.
GRAHAM, W. C., BROWN, J. B., CANNON, B. and RIORDAN, D. C. (1947). Transposition of fingers in severe injuries of the hand. *J. Bone Jt. Surg.* **29**, 998.
GRAHAM, W. C. and RIORDAN, D. C. (1948). Reconstruction of a metacarpophalangeal joint with a metatarsal transplant. *J. Bone Jt. Surg.*, **30A**, 848.
GRESHAM, R. B. and THOMAS, E. D. (1966). Histological study of processed bovine-bone heterografts implanted into guinea pigs. *J. Bone Jt. Surg.*, **48A**, 1227.
HAAS, S. L. (1921). Function in relation to transplantation of bone. *Arch. Surg.* **3**, 425.
HAAS, S. L. (1957). The viability of preserved bone. *Surg. Gynec. Obstet.*, **105**, 449.
HALDEMAN, K. O. (1933). The influence of periosteum on the survival of bone grafts. *J. Bone Jt. Surg.*, **15**, 302.
HALLÉN, L. (1966). Heterologous transplantation with Kiel bone. An experimental and clinical study. *Acta orthopaed. scand.*, **37**, 1.
HAM, A. W. (1930). A histological study of the early phases of bone repair. *J. Bone Jt. Surg.*, **12**, 827.
HAM, A. W. (1952). Some histiophysiological problems peculiar to calcified tissues. *J. Bone Jt. Surg.*, **34A**, 701.
HAM, A. and GORDON, S. (1952). The origin of bone that forms in association with cancellous bone transplanted into muscle. *Brit. J. plast. Surg.*, **5**, 154.
HAM, S. W. and HARRIS, W. R. (1956). Repair and transplantation of bone. In "The Biochemistry and Physiology of Bone". Ed. G. H. Bourne. New York: Academic Press Inc.
HAMMACK, B. L. and ENNEKING, W. F. (1960). Comparative vascularization of autogenous and homogenous bone transplants. *J. Bone Jt. Surg.*, **42A**, 811.
HANCOX, N. (1956). The osteoclast. Ch. VIII. In "The Biochemistry and Physiology of Bone". Ed. G. H. Bourne. New York: Academic Press Inc.
HANCOX, N. M. and BOOTHROYD, B. (1964). Ultrastructure of bone formation and resorption. Ch. III. In "Modern Trends in Orthopaedics Science of Fractures." Ed. J. M. P. Clark. London: Butterworths.
HANCOX, N. M., OWEN, R. and SINGLETON, A. (1961). Cross-species grafts of deproteinized bone. *J. Bone Jt. Surg.*, **43B**, 152.
HARMON, P. H. (1945). A simplified surgical approach to the posterior tibia for bone-grafting and fibular transference. *J. Bone Jt. Surg.*, **27**, 496.

HARMON, P. H. (1964). Processed heterogenous bone implants. (Boplant, Squibb) as grafts in spinal surgery. *Acta orthop. scand.*, **35,** 98.
HARRIS, W. H., TRAVIS, D. F., FRIBERG, U. and RADIN, E. (1964). The *in vivo* inhibition of bone formation by alizarin red S. *J. Bone Jt. Surg.*, **46A,** 493.
HARRIS, W. H., LAVORGNA, J., HAMBLEN, D. L. and HAYWOOD, E. A. (1968). The inhibition of ossification *in vivo. Clin. Orthop.*, **61,** 52.
HARTMAN, T. and RAPP, R. (1965). The effects of Roentgen therapy on the host acceptance of autogenous bone grafts in dogs. *Radiology*, **85,** 532.
HATTNER, R., EPKER, B. N. and FROST, H. M. (1965). Suggested sequential mode of control of changes in cell behaviour in adult bone remodelling. *Nature*, **206,** 489.
HAY, B. M. (1954). A review of the results of bone grafting. *J. Bone Jt. Surg.*, **36B,** 681.
HEIPLE, K. G., CHASE, S. W. and HERNDON, C. H. (1963). A comparative study of the healing process following different types of bone transplantation. *J. Bone Surg.*, **45A,** 1593.
HEIPLE, K. G., KENDRICK, R. E., HERNDON, C. H. and CHASE, S. W. (1967). A critical evaluation of processed calf bone. *J. Bone Jt. Surg.*, **49A,** 1119.
HEIPLE, K. G., HERNDON, C. H., CHASE, S. W. and WATTLEWORTH, A. (1968). Osteogenic induction by osteosarcoma and normal bone in mice. *J. Bone Jt. Surg.*, **50A,** 311.
HEJNA, W. F. and RAY, R. D. (1963). Comparative study of bone implants. *Surg. Forum*, **14,** 448.
HELLER, M., MCLEAN, F. C. and BLOOM, W. (1950). Cellular transformations in mammalian bones induced by parathyroid extract. *Amer. J. Anat.*, **87,** 315.
HELLSTADIUS, A. (1955). Studies on osteogenesis around autoplastic bony transplants in bony defects. *Acta orthop. scand.*, **24,** 278.
HENRY, M. O. (1948). Homografts in orthopaedic surgery. *J. Bone Jt. Surg.*, **30A,** 70.
HERBERT, J. J. (1951). Homografts and the bone bank. *J. Bone Jt. Surg.*, **33B,** 316.
HERNDON, C. H. (1960). Principles of bone graft surgery—different methods of operative procedure and indications for each. *American Academy of Orthopaedic Surgeons, Instructional Course Lecture*, **17,** 149.
HESLOP, B. F., ZEISS, I. M. and NISBET, N. W. (1960). Studies on transference of bone. I. A comparison of autologous and homologous bone implants with reference to osteocyte survival, osteogenesis and host reaction. *Brit. J. exp. Path.*, **41,** 269.
HEY GROVES, E. (1917). Methods and results of transplantation of bone in the repair of defects caused by injury or disease. *Brit. J. Surg.*, **5,** 185.
HOLMSTRAND, K. (1957). Biophysical investigations of bone transplants and bone implants. An experimental study. *Acta orthop. scand.*, Suppl. **26,** 1.
HOLUB, K. (1958). The importance of bony constituents in production of blood elements. *Blood*, **13,** 300.
HUGHES, C. W. (1943). Rate of absorption and callus stimulating properties of cown horn, ivory, beef bone and autogenous bone. *Surg. Gynec. Obstet.*, **76,** 665.
HURLEY, L. A., ZEIER, F. G. and STINCHFIELD, F. E. (1960). Anorganic bone grafting. Clinical experiences with heterografts processed by ethylenediamine extraction. *Amer. J. Surg.*, **100,** 12.
HUTCHINSON, J. (1952). The fate of experimental bone autografts and homografts. *Brit. J. Surg.*, **39,** 552.
HYATT, G. W. (1960). The bone homograft—experimental and clinical applications. *American Academy of Orthopaedic Surgeons, Instructional Course Lecture*, **17,** 133.
INCLÁN, A. (1942). The use of preserved bone graft in orthopaedic surgery. *J. Bone Jt. Surg.*, **24,** 81.
IRVING, J. T. and MIGLIORE, S. A. (1965). Connective tissue response to altered collagen and bone implants. *Amer. J. Anat.*, **117,** 151.
JAMES, J. I. P. (1967). Scoliosis. Edinburgh: E. & S. Livingstone Ltd.

Jansen, M. (1920). On bone formation. Its relation to tension and pressure. Manchester: University Press.
Joyce, J. L. (1918). A new operation for the substitution of a thumb. *Brit. J. Surg.*, **5,** 499.
Judet, J. and Judet, R. (1960). L'ostéogénèse et les retards de consolidation et les pseudarthroses des os longs. Huitième Congrès de la Société Internationale de Chirurgie Orthopedigue et de Traumatologie, New York.
Kaplan, I. (1967). Pollicization. Ch. VI. In "Modern Trends in Orthopaedics". Fifth Ed. W. D. Graham. London: Butterworths.
Karges, D. E., Anderson, K. J., Dingwall, J. A. and Jowsey, J. (1963). Experimental evaluation of processed heterogenous bone transplants. *Clin. Orthop. & Rel. Resl*, **29,** 230.
Keith, W. S. (1934). Small bone grafts. *J. Bone Jt. Surg.*, **16,** 314.
Kershaw, R. (1963). Preparation of anorganic bone grafting material. *Pharm. J.*, **190,** 537.
Key, J. A. (1934). The effect of a local calcium depot on osteogenesis and healing of fractures. *J. Bone Jt. Surg.*, **16,** 176.
Kiehn, C. L., Friedell, H. L. and McIntyre, W. J. (1948). Study of the vitality of tissue transplants by means of radioactive phosphorus: preliminary report. *Plast. reconstr. Surg.*, **3,** 335.
Kiehn, C. L., Friedell, H., Benson, J., Berg, M. and Glover, D. M. (1950). A study of the viability of autogenous frozen bone grafts by means of radioactive phosphorus. *Ann. Surg.*, **132,** 427.
Kiehn, C. L., Cebul, F., Berg, M., Gutentag, J. and Glover, D. M. (1952). A study of the vascularization of experimental bone grafts by means of radioactive phosphorus and the transparent chamber. *Arch. Surg.*, **136,** 404.
Kiehn, C. L. and Glover, D. M. (1953). A study of the revascularization of experimental bone grafts by means of radioactive phosphorus. *Plast. reconstr. Surg.*, **12,** 233.
Kienholz, M. and Kemkes, B. (1956). Untersuchungen über den immunobiologischen Wert heteroplastischer konservierter Knochenspäne. *Arch. orthop. Unfallchir.*, **48,** 632.
Killey, H. C., Kramer, I. R. H. and Wright, H. C. (1966). The effects of implanting heterogenous compact and cancellous anorganic bone into the long bones of rabbits. *Arch. Oral Biol.*, **11,** 1117.
Kingma, M. J. (1960). Results of transplantations with preserved calf bone. *Arch. chir. Neerl.*, **12,** 221.
Kingma, M. J. (1967). Deep frozen calf bone. In "Dixième Congrès de la Société internationale de Chirurgie Orthopedique et de Traumatologie". Paris.
Kingma, M. J. and Hampe, J. F. (1964). The behaviour of blood vessels after experimental transplantation of bone. *J. Bone Jt. Surg.*, **46B,** 141.
Kirkup, J. R. (1965). Traumatic femoral bone loss. *J. Bone Jt. Surg.*, **47B,** 106.
Klinkerfuss, G. H. (1924). A study of the growing power of periosteal callus when transplanted to costal cartilages. *Surg. Gynec. Obstet.*, **38,** 625.
Koch, W. and Dahmen, G. (1962). Experimental and clinical experience with the heterogenous bone bank graft. *Z. Orthopäd.*, **96,** 348.
Kovalenko, D. G. and Vereshchagin, A. P. (1966). Homografts in reconstructive surgery for tuberculosis of joints. *Vestn. Khir.* (Grekov), **9,** 93 (Exc. Med., Section **9B, 12,** No. 1059).
Kramer, I. R. H., Killey, H. C. and Wright, H. C. (1964). The pattern of healing following implantation of heterogenous anorganic compact bone in sheep. *Arch. Oral Biol.*, **9,** 671.
Kramer, I. R. H., Killey, H. C. and Wright, H. C. (1968a). The replacement of bone. *Austr. Dental J.*, **13,** 17.
Kramer, I. R. H., Killey, H. C. and Wright, H. C. (1968b). The response of the rabbit to implants of processed calf bone (Boplant). *Arch. Oral Biol.*, **13,** 1262.
Kramer, I. R. H., Killey, H. C. and Wright, H. C. (1968c). A histological and radiological comparison of the healing of defects in the rabbit calvarium with and without implanted heterogenous anorganic bone. *Arch. Oral Biol.*, **13,** 1095.

Kreuz, F. P., Hyatt, G. W., Turner, T. C. and Bassett, C. A. L. (1951). The preservation and clinical use of freeze-dried bone. *J. Bone Jt. Surg.* **33A**, 863.
Krupko, I. L., Tkachenko, S. S. and Malevski, A. M. (1966). *Vestn. Khir* (Grekov), 9/97, 87. (Abstract in Exc. Med., Section **9B, 12** No. 1205.)
Küpperman, W. and Schwier, von H. (1964). Quoted by Petrokov *et al.* (1967). *Sym. biol. Hung.*, **7,** 87.
Lacroix, P. (1951). The Organization of Bones. Translated by S. Gilder. London: J. & A. Churchill, Ltd.
Lagier, R. and Rutihauser, E. (1965). Osteoarticular changes in a case of essential osteolysis. An anatomical and radiological study. *J. Bone Jt. Surg.*, **47B,** 339.
Lagrot, F., Costagliola, N. Py. M. and Micheau, Ph. (1966). L'utilité et la valeur du greffon costal osseux. *Ann. chir.* **20,** 1453.
Lawson Dick, I. (1946). Iliac-bone transplantation. *J. Bone Jt. Surg.*, **28,** 1.
Levander, G. (1938). A study of bone regeneration. *Surg. Gynec. Obstet.* **67,** 705.
Lexer, E. (1925). Joint transplantation and arthroplasty. *Surg. Gynec. and Obstet.* **40,** 782.
Littler, J. W. (1953). The neurovascular pedicle method of digital transposition for reconstruction of the thumb. *Plast. reconstr. Surg.*, **22,** 303.
Lloyd-Roberts, G. C. (1952). Experiences with boiled cadaveric bone. *J. Bone Jt. Surg.*, **34B,** 428.
Lloyd-Roberts, G. (1960). Personal communication to Blaimont (1960).
Lo Grippo, G. A., Burgess, B., Teodoro, R. and Fleming, J. L. (1957). Procedure for bone sterilization with beta-propiolactone. *J. Bone Jt. Surg.*, **39A,** 1356.
Losee, F. L. and Boyne, P. J. (1957). Response of oral tissues to grafts of ethylene-diamine-treated heterogenous bone. *Nature*, **179,** 818.
Losee, F. L. and Hurley, L. A. (1956a). Bone treated with ethylenediamine as a successful foundation material in cross-species bone grafts. *Nature*, **177,** 1032.
Losee, F. L. and Hurley, L. A. (1956b). Successful cross-species bone grafting accomplished by removal of the donor organic matrix. *Res. Rep. naval Med. Res. Inst.* **14,** 911.
Maatz, R. (1966). The Kiel bone graft. Development, chemistry and clinical results. In "Symposium on Bone Grafting Materials". Eastbourne: Armour Pharmaceutical Co., Ltd., p. 21.
Maatz, R. and Bauermeister, A. (1957). A method of bone maceration. *J. Bone. Jt. Surg.*, **39A,** 153.
Maatz, R., Lentz, W. and Graf, R. (1954). Spongiosa test of bone grafts for transplantation. *J. Bone Jt. Surg.*, **36A,** 721.
McElroy, D. K. (1963). Failure of bank bone. *J. Bone Jt. Surg.*, **45A,** 1555.
Macewen, W. (1887). The osteogenetic factors in the development and repair of bone. *Ann. Surg.*, **6,** 289.
Macewen, W. (1912). The Growth of Bone. Observations on osteogenesis. An experimental inquiry into the development and reproduction of diaphyseal bone. Glasgow: J. Maclehose & Sons.
McFarland, B. (1951). Bone grafts. *Medical Press*, **225,** 284.
Maggregor, I. A. and Simonetta, C. (1964). Reconstruction of the thumb by composite bone-skin flap. *Brit. J. Plast. Surg.*, **17,** 37.
McLean, F. C. (1965). Internal remodelling of compact bone. Proceedings of the Second European Symposium on Calcified Tissues. Ed. L. J. Richelle and M. J. Dallemagne. Collection des Colloques de l'Université de Liège.
Marmor, L. (1964). The treatment of infected nonunion of the tibia. *J. Trauma*, **4,** 301.
Marrangoni, A. G. (1951). The fate of frozen homogenous bone transplants. *Amer. J. Surg.*, **82,** 378.
Massé, G., Gallinaro, P., Garelli, R. and Siliquini, P. L. (1965a). Studi sull' immunità da trapianto. IV. Induzione di risposte accelerate e iperimmuni dopo 'primo trapianto' omologo allogenico di corticale ossea. *Minerva Ortopedica,* **16,** 530.
Massé, G., Gallinaro, P., Coscia, P. L. and Garelli, R. (1965b). Studi sull' immunità de trapianto. III. Osservazioni sul 'primo' e 'secondo' trapianto osseo omologo allogenico. *Minerva Ortopedica,* **16,** 527.

MEDAWAR, P. B. (1944). The behaviour and fate of skin autografts and skin homografts in rabbits. *J. Anat., Lond.*, **78,** 176.
MEDAWAR, P. B. (1945). A second study of the behaviour and fate of skin homografts in rabbits. *J. Anat., Lond.*, **79,** 157.
MEDAWAR, P. B. (1959). In "Cellular and Humoral Aspects of Hypersensitive States". Ed. H. S. Lawrence. London: Cassell.
MEDGYESI, S. (1965). Healing of muscle-pedicle bone grafts. An experimental study. *Acta orthop. Scand.*, **35,** 294.
MERLE D'AUBIGNÉ, R., MËARY, R. and THOMINE, J. M. (1966). La resection dans le traitement des tumeurs des os. *Rev. Chir. Orthop.*, **52,** 305.
MILLER, R. C. and PHALEN, G. S. (1947). The repair of defects of the radius with fibular bone grafts. *J. Bone Jt. Surg.*, **29,** 629.
MILLONIG, R. C., AMREIN, B. J. and BORMAN, A. (1962). Antigenicity of bovine cortical bone. *Proc. Soc. exp. Biol., N.Y.* **109,** 562.
MITCHELL, D. F. and SHANKWALKER, G. B. (1958). Osteogenic potential of calcium hydroxide and other materials in soft tissue and bone wounds. *J. dent. Res.*, **37,** 1157.
MOORE, J. R. (1948). Cartilaginous cup arthroplasty in ununited fractures of the neck of the femur. *J. Bone Jt. Surg.*, **30A,** 313.
MORRISON, G. M., JOHNSON, H. L. and HAZARD, J. B. (1937). Promotion of fracture repair. *J. Bone Jt. Surg.*, **19,** 425.
MOSIMAN, R. S. (1950). Quoted by Kiehn, C. L., Cebul, F., Berg, M., Gutentag, J. and Glover, D. M. (1952). *Arch. Surg.*, **136,** 404.
MOSS, M. L. (1958). Extraction of an osteogenic inductor factor from bone. *Science*, **127,** 755.
MOSS, M. L. (1960). Experimental induction of osteogenesis. In "Calcification in Biological Systems". Ed. F. Sognnaes. Washington D.C. Publication No. 64 of the American Association for the Advancement of Science.
MOSS, M., KRUGER, G. O. and REYNOLDS, D. C. (1965). The effect on chondroitin sulphate on bone healing. *Oral Surg.*, **20,** 795.
MOVIN, R. (1963). On the use of muscle-pedicle bone grafts in fresh sub-capital fractures of the femur. *Acta orthop. Scand.*, **33,** 382.
MOWLEM, R. (1941). Bone and cartilage transplants. *Brit. J. Surg.*, **29,** 182.
MOWLEM, R. (1944). Cancellous chip bone-grafts. Report on 75 cases. *Lancet* **ii,** 746.
MOWLEM, R. (1952). Editorial. *Brit. J. plast. Surg.*, **4,** 231.
MÜLLER, M. (1963). Internal fixation for fresh fractures and non-union. *Proc. roy. Soc. Med.*, **56,** 455.
MÜLLER, M. E. (1966). Treatment of non-unions by compression. *Clin. Orthop.*, **43,** 83.
NICOLL, E. A. (1956). The treatment of gaps in long bones by cancellous insert grafts. *J. Bone Jt. Surg.*, **38B,** 70.
NISBET, N. W. (1966). Immunology of bone transplantation. *Clin. Orthopaed. & Rel. Res.*, **47,** 199.
NISHIMURA, K. K., YAEGER, J. A. and SABET, T. K. (1962). Fate of osteocytes in adult mouse whole bone isografts and homografts. *Anat. Rec.*, **144,** 85.
ORELL, S. (1937). Surgical bone grafting with 'os purum', 'os novum' and 'boiled bone'. *J. Bone Jt. Surg.*, **19,** 873.
ORELL, S. (1938). The use of os purum in bone implantations with special reference to its use in tuberculous bone and joint lesions. *Surg. Gynec. Obstet.*, **66,** 23.
ORELL, S. (1953). Implantation of autoplastic, homoplastic and heteroplastic bone. *J. intern. Surg.*, **23,** 238.
OSTROWSKI, K. (1969). Current problems of tissue banking. *Trans. Proc.*, **1,** 126.
OWEN, O. E., JACOB, S. W., MOLONEY, W. C. and DUNPHY, J. E. (1958). Studies in autologous bone marrow transplantation. *Trans. Bull.*, **5,** 129.
OTTOLENGHI, C. E. (1966). Massive osteoarticular bone grafts. *J. Bone Jt. Surg.*, **48B,** 646.
PAIN, A. B. (1959). Unpublished observations. Personal communication.

Pappas, A. M. and Beisaw, N. E. (1968). Bone transplantation: correlation of physiological and histological aspects of graft incorporation. *Clin. Orthop.*, **61**, 179.

Parrish, F. F. (1966). Treatment of bone tumours by total excision and replacement with massive autologous and homologous grafts. *J. Bone Jt. Surg.*, **48A**, 968.

Peacock, E. E. (1962). Metacarpal transfer following amputation of a central digit. *Plast. reconstr. Surg.*, **29**, 345.

Peer, L. A. (1951). The fate of autogenous human bone grafts. *Brit. J. plast. Surg.*, **3**, 233.

Peer, L. A. (1955). Transplantation of Tissues. Vol. I. Cartilage, Bone, Fascia, Tendon and Muscle. Baltimore: Williams & Wilkins.

Peltier, L. F. (1961). The use of plaster of paris to fill defects in bone. *Clin. Orthop. and Rel. Res.*, **21**, 1.

Petrokov, V., Vukelic, F. and Schenk, R. (1967). Bridging over of large diaphyseal defects (clinical and experimental results). *Sym. biol. Hung.*, **7**, 87.

Pfeiffer, C. A. (1948). Development of bone from transplanted marrow in mice. *Anat. Rec.*, **102**, 225.

Phemister, D. B. (1914). The fate of transplanted bone and regenerative power of its various constituents. *Surg. Gynec. Obstet.*, **19**, 303.

Phemister, D. B. (1931). Splint grafts in the treatment of delayed and non-union of fractures. *Surg. Gynec. Obstet.*, **52**, 376.

Phemister, D. B. (1947). Treatment of ununited fractures by onlay bone grafts without screw or tie fixation and without breaking down of the fibrous union. *J. Bone Jt. Surg.*, **29**, 946.

Pieron, A. P., Bigelow, D. and Hamonic, M. (1968). Grafting with Boplant. Results in Thirty-three cases. *J. Bone Jt. Surg.*, **50B**, 364.

Ponseti, I. V. (1957). Skeletal lesions produced by aminonitriles. *Clin. Orthop. and Rel. Res.*, **9**, 131.

Ponseti, I. V. and Shepard, R. S. (1954). Lesions of the skeleton and of other mesodermal tissues in rats fed sweet-pea (Lathyrus odoratus) seeds. *J. Bone Jt. Surg.*, **36A**, 1031.

Post, R. H., Heiple, K. G., Chase, S. W. and Herndon, C. H. (1966). Bone grafts in diffusion chambers. *Clin. Orthop and Rel. Res.*, **44**, 265.

Pritchard, J. J. (1961). Ossification. *Scot. med. Surg. J.*, **6**, 177.

Puranen, J. (1966). Reorganization of fresh and preserved bone transplants. An experimental study in rabbits using tetracycline labelling. *Acta orthopaed. Scand.*, Suppl. **92.**

Quigley, M. B. and Hjørting-Hansen, E. (1962). Crystal arrangement in anorganic bone. *Acta odont. scand.*, **20**, 359.

Ray, R. D. (1956). Bone grafting: transplants and implants. *American Academy of Orthopaedic Surgeons Instruction Course Lecture*, **13**, 177.

Ray, R. D. and Holloway, J. A. (1957). Bone implants. Preliminary report of an experimental study. *J. Bone Jt. Surg.*, **39A**, 1119.

Ray, R. D., Mosiman, R. and Schmidt, J. (1954). Tissue culture studies of bone. *J. Bone Jt. Surg.*, **36A**, 1147.

Ray, R. D. and Sabet, T. Y. (1963). Bone grafts: cellular survival versus induction. An experimental study in mice. *J. Bone Jt. Surg.*, **45A**, 337.

Reeves, B. (1968). Studies of vascularised homotransplants of the knee joint. *J. Bone Jt. Surg.*, **50B**, 226.

Reid, D. A. (1960). Reconstruction of the thumb. *J. Bone Jt. Surg.*, **42B**, 444.

Reynolds, F. C. and Oliver, D. R. (1950). Experimental evaluation of homogenous bone grafts. *J. Bone Jt. Surg.*, **32A**, 283.

Reynolds, F. C., Oliver, D. R. and Ramsey, R. (1951). Clinical evaluation of the merthiolate bone bank and homogenous bone grafts. *J. Bone Jt. Surg.*, **33A**, 873.

Richany, S. F., Sprinz, H., Kraner, K., Ashby, J. and Merrill, T. G. (1965). The role of the diaphyseal medulla in the repair and regeneration of the femoral shaft in the adult cat. *J. Bone Jt. Surg.*, **47A**, 1565.

RITTER, U. (1956a). Klinischer Verlauf und Ergebnisse nach Implantation ungeeignet konservierter Knochenspane am Menschen. *Zbl. Chir.*, **81**, 111.
RITTER, U. (1956b). B. Konservierungsversuche von Knochengewebe durch Trockensterilisation des Implantationsmaterials. *Zbl. Chir.*, **81**, 163.
RITTER, U. (1956c). C. Konservierungsversuche von Knochengewebe durch Alkohollagerung des Implantationsmaterials. *Zbl. Chir.*, **81**, 196.
RITTER, U. (1956d). D. Konservierungsversuche von Knochen gewebe durch Trypsin-Enteiweissung des Implantationsmaterials. *Zbl. Chir.*, **81**, 259.
RITTER, U. (1956e). E. Konservierungsversuche mit zu Mehl vermahlenem Knochen gewebe. *Zbl. Chir.*, **81**, 290.
RITTER, U. (1956f). F. Implantationsversuche mit einem 'kunstlichen Knochenspan'. *Zbl. Chir.*, **81**, 323.
RIORDAN, D. C. (1955). Congenital absence of the radius. *J. Bone Jt. Surg.*, **37A**, 1129.
RIORDAN, D. C. (1962). In the discussion after the paper by Entin *et al.* (1962).
RIZZO, P-C. and LEHMANN, O. (1947). The 'latch' graft. A combination of inlay and intramedullary graft which is self-retaining. *J. Bone Jt. Surg.*, **29**, 354.
ROAF, R. (1966). Experience of using deproteinised bone, especially the assessment of its value heterologically and radiologically. In "Symposium on Bone Grafting Materials". Eastbourne: Armour Pharmaceutical Co. Ltd., p. 93.
ROAF, R. and HANCOX, N. (1961). Fate of heterogenous deproteinised bone implants. *J. Bone Jt. Surg.*, **45B**, 617.
ROCHER, H. L. (1953). Dead bone grafts in orthopaedic surgery. *J. Bone Jt. Surg.*, **35B**, 328.
RÖNNING, O. and KOSKI, K. (1966). The fate of anorganic implants in the subcutaneous tissue of the rat. *Plast. reconstr. Surg.*, **37**, 121.
ROSENBERG, N. J., REICH, R. S. and BRAHMS, M. (1955). Experimental and clinical use of bone milled in the kitchen blender. *J. Bone Jt. Surg.*, **37A**, 640.
ROSOMOFF, H. L., HURLEY, L. A. and LOSEE, F. L. (1959). Cranial reconstruction with ethylenediamine-treated bone. *Amer. J. Surg.*, **97**, 721.
ROSS, G. E. (1966). Effect of diethylstilboestrol, prednisolone, and isoniazid on the healing rate of bone defects filled with certain bone grafting materials. *Amer. J. vet. Res.*, **27**, 1745.
RUF, F. (1954). Zur Vitalität von Knochenspänen. Untersuchungen mit Radiophosphor und Radiocalcium. *Arch. klin. Chir.*, **279**, 829.
SAKO, K. and MARCHETTA, F. C. (1966). Delayed autogenous bone and callus transplants and prepared host beds. *Arch. Surg.*, **92**, 771.
SANDISON, J. C. (1928). A method for the microscopic study of the growth of transplanted bone in the transparent chamber of the rabbit's ear. *Anat. Rec.*, **40**, 41.
SCALES, J. T., DUFF-BARCLAY, I. and BURROWS, H. J. (1965). Some engineering and medical problems associated with massive bone replacement. In "Biomechanics and Related Bio-Engineering Topics". Ed. R. M. Kenedi. London: Pergamon Press.
SCHWIER, V. (1960). Zu den Problemen der Osteosynthese, der Knochenneubildung und der Knochenverpflanzung. *Chirurg.*, **31**, 220.
SCOPP, I. W., KASSOUNY, D. Y. and MORGAN, F. H. (1966a). Bovine bone (Boplant). *J. Peridont.*, **37**, 48/400.
SCOPP, I. W., MORGAN, F. H., DOONER, J. J., FREDERICS, H. J. and HEYMAN, R. A. (1966b). Bovine bone (Boplant) implants for infrabony oral lesions (clinical trial in humans). *Periodontics* **4**, 169.
SCOTT, B. L. (1967). ³H-Thymidine electron microscope radioautography of osteogenic cells in the fetal rat. *J. cell. Biol.*, **35**, 115.
SENN, N. (1889). On the healing of aseptic bone cavities by implantation of antiseptic decalcified bone. *Int. J. med. Sci.*, **98**, 1889.
SEVASTIKOGLOU, J. A. (1965). Operative treatment of non-united fractures of long bones. *Acta orthopaed. scand.*, **36**, 192.
SHARRARD, W. J. W. and COLLINS, D. H. (1961). The fate of human decalcified bone grafts. *Proc. roy. Soc. Med.*, **54**, 1101.

SICARD, A. and BINET, J.-P. (1950). La conservation des transplants osseux et leur emploi en chirurgie. *Pr. méd.*, **58,** 433.
SIFFERT, R. S. (1955). Experimental bone transplants. *J. Bone Jt. Surg.*, **37A,** 742.
SIFFERT, R. S. and BARASH, E. S. (1961). Delayed bone transplantation. An experimental study of early host-transplant relationships. *J. Bone Jt. Surg.*, **43A,** 407.
SISSONS, H. A. (1956). The growth of bone. Ch. XV. In "The Biochemistry and Physiology of Bone". Ed. G. H. Bourne. New York: Academic Press Inc.
SIEBER, E. (1954). XI. Ergebnisse mit kältekonservierten homoioplastischen Knochenspänen, speziell bei der Pseudarthrosenoperation nach Phemister. *Arch. klin. Chir.*, **279,** 69.
SLAGER, U. T. and ZUCKER, M. J. (1962). The occurrence of electron spin resonance signals in bone grafts sterilized with high voltage electron beams. *Plast. reconstr. Surg.*, **30,** 536/146.
SMITH, A. D. (1937). Use of homologous bone grafts in cases of osteogenesis imperfecta. *Arch. Surg., Lond.*, **34,** 687.
SPEED, J. S. and SMITH, H. (1951). Quoted by Kreuz *et al.* (1951).
SPIRA, E. E. (1963). Bridging of bone defects in the forearm. *J. Bone Jt. Surg.*, **45A,** 215.
SPIRA, E. and FARIN, I. (1964). Epiphyseal transplantation. A case report. *J. Bone Jt. Surg.*, **46A,** 1278.
STEGEMAN, H. (1966). In the discussion after the paper by Roaf (1966).
STRINGA, G. (1957). Studies of the vascularisation of bone grafts. *J. Bone Jt. Surg.*, **39B,** 395.
SUTHERLAND, T. W., WILLIAMSON, G. M., ZINNEMANN, K. and SHUCKSMITH, H. S. (1958). Graft sterilization. A bacteriological and histological study of the relative merits of ethylene oxide and β-propiolactone as tissue sterilizing agents, with special reference to arterial grafts. *Brit. med. J.* **i,** 734.
SUZUKI, H. K. (1959). Estradiol valerate-induced endosteal ossification in autogenous transplants in mice tibiae. *Trans. Bull.*, **6,** 414.
SWANKER, W. A. and WINFIELD, J. M. (1952). Use of gelatinized bone in skeletal trauma. *Amer. J. Surg.*, **83,** 332.
SWANSON, A. B., GLESSNER, J. R., BURDICK, H. W. and MAHANEY, R. C. (1963). Seven years experience with irradiated bone graft material. *Surg. Gynec. Obstet.*, **117,** 573.
SYMPOSIUM (1958). Symposium sur l'os heteroplastique. *Rev. Chir. Orthop.*, **45,** 1.
TARSOLY, E. and TOMORY, I. (1966). Osteogenic action of the Kiel type of bone and that of pulverized egg-shell. *Acta chir. Acad. Sci., Hung.*, **7,** 263 (Abstract in *Excerpta med.*, Section **9B, 12,** (6) No. 902).
TARSOLY, E. and TOMORY, I. (1967). The healing process in bone cavities filled up with a mixture of egg-shell and plaster. (Animal experiments.) *Symp. biol., Hung.*, **7,** 415.
TIMASHKEVICH, K. D. (1966). A comparative study of bone homografts by various methods. *Byull. eksp. Biol. Med.*, **62,** 93. (In Exc. Med. Section **9B,** 12 No. 903).
TONNA, E. A. and CRONKITE, E. P. (1961). Autoradiographic studies of cell in the proliferation of intact and fractured femora of mice utilizing DNA labeling with H^3-thymidine. *Proc. Soc. exp. Biol., N.Y.*, **107,** 719.
TONNA, E. A. and CRONKITE, E. P. (1962). An autoradiographic study of periosteal cell proliferation with tritiated thymidine. *Lab. Invest.*, **11,** 455.
TONNA, E. A. and CRONKITE, E. P. (1963). The periosteum: autoradiographic studies on cellular proliferation and transformation utilizing tritiated thymidine. *Clin. Orthopaed. & Rel. Res.*, **30,** 218.
TOTO, P. D. and GIANNINI, J. (1961). Fate of subcutaneous anorganic bone implants. *J. dent. Res.*, **40,** 1127.
TSESARSKAYA, T. P. (1960). Bone marrow osteoblasts. *Abstr. Soviet Med.* **4B,** 1210.
TURNER, T. C., BASSETT, C. A. L., PATE, J. W. and SAWYER, P. N. (1955). An experimental comparison of freeze-dried and frozen cortical bone-graft healing. *J. Bone Jt. Surg.*, **37A,** 1197.

TURNER, T. C., BASSETT, C. A. L., PATE, J. W., TRUMP, J. G. and WRIGHT, K. (1956). Sterilization of preserved bone grafts by high voltage cathode irradiation. *J. Bone Jt. Surg.*, **38A**, 862.
TYAN, M. L. and COLE, L. J. (1963a). Differential radiosensitivity of first and second-set responses to allogeneic and xenogeneic skin grafts in lethally irradiated mice. *Transplantation*, **1**, 365.
TYAN, M. L. and COLE, L. J. (1963b). Differential radiosensitivity of first and second-set response to allogeneic and xenogeneic skin grafts in sublethally irradiated mice. *Transplantation*, **1**, 546.
TYAN, M. L. and COLE, L. J. (1964). Adoptive transfer of sensitivity to allogeneic versus xenogeneic skin grafts in mice. *Transplantation*, **2**, 515.
URIST, M. R. (1965). Bone: formation by autoinduction. *Science*, **150**, 893.
URIST, M. R. and MCLEAN, F. C. (1952). Osteogenic potency and new bone formation by induction in transplants to the anterior chamber of the eye. *J. Bone Jt. Surg.*, **34A**, 443.
URIST, M. R., WALLACE, T. H. and ADAMS, T. (1965). The function of fibro-cartilaginous fracture callus. Observations on transplants labelled with tritiated thymidine. *J. Bone Jt. Surg.*, **47B**, 304.
URIST, M. R., SILVERMAN, B. F., BÜRING, K., DUBUC, F. L. and ROSENBERG, J. M. (1967). The bone induction principle. *Clin. Orthop.*, **53**, 243.
URIST, M. R., DOWELL, T. A., HAY, P. H. and STRATES, B. S. (1968a). Inductive substrates for bone formation. *Clin. Orthop.*, **59**, 59.
URIST, M. R., DOWELL, T. A. and LEIBOVITCH, R. T. (1968b). Inductive substratum for osteogenesis in pellets of particulate bone matrix. *Clin. Orthop.*, **61**, 61.
VAINIO, S. (1950). Observations on the regeneration of an autogenous transplant of the bone. An experimental investigation. *Acta chir., scand.*, **100**, 86.
VAN DE PUTTE, K. A. and URIST, M. R. (1966). Osteogenesis in the interior of intramuscular implants of decalcified bone matrix. *Clin. Orthopaed. and Rel. Res.*, **43**, 257.
VAN NES, C. P. (1948). Transplantation of the tibia and fibula to replace the femur following resection. 'Turn-up' plasty of the leg. *J. Bone Jt. Surg.*, **30A**, 854.
VAN ROOD, J. J., LEEUWEN, A. VAN, SCHIPPERS, M. J., VOOYS, W. H., FREDERIKS, E., BALNER, H. and EERNISSE, J. G. (1965). Leucocyte groups, the normal lymphocyte transfer test and homograft sensitivity. Series Haematologica, II, Histocompatibility Testing. Copenhagen: Munksgaard.
VOLKOV, M. V. and IMAMALIEV, A. S. (1966). Problème de l'homoplastie des articulations et des parties osseuses articulaires. Dixieme Congrès de le Société Internationale de Chirurgie Orthopédique et de Traumatologie, Paris, 4–9 Septembre, 699.
VREDEVOE, D. L., TERASAKI, P. I., MICKEY, M. R., GLASSOCK, R., MERRILL, J. P. and MURRAY, J. E. (1965). Serotyping of human lymphocyte antigens. III. Long term kidney homograft survivors. In "Series Haematologica, II, Histocompatibility Testing. Histocompatibility Testing". Copenhagen: Munksgaard.
WADE, H. (1920). Report of a patient six years after the implantation of a homoplastic bone graft. *Edinb. med. J.*, N.S., **24**, 37.
WATSON-JONES, R. (1933). The repair of skull defects by a new pedicle bone-graft operation. *Brit. med. J.*, **i**, 780.
WATSON-JONES, R. (1946). Fractures and joint injuries. 3rd Ed. Edinburgh: E. & S. Livingstone Ltd.
WEAVER, J. B. (1949). Experiences in the use of homogenous (bone bank) bone. *J. Bone Jt. Surg.*, **31A**, 778.
WHEELER, T. E. and HYATT, G. W. (1960). A study of the residual nitrogen in bone following extractions with ethylenediamine. *J. Bone Jt. Surg.*, **42A**, 1435.
WILLIAMS, G. (1964). Experiences with boiled cadaveric cancellous bone for fractures of long bones. *J. Bone Jt. Surg.*, **46B**, 398.
WILLIAMS, J. B. and IRVINE, J. W. (1954). Preparation of the inorganic matrix of bone. *Science*, **119**, 771.

WILLIAMS, J. J. (1966). The use of Kiel bone in delayed union of tibial fractures. In "Symposium on Bone Grafting Materials". Eastbourne: Armour Pharmaceutical Co. Ltd., p. 57.
WILSON, J. N. (1966). Epiphyseal transplantation. A clinical study. *J. Bone Jt. Surg.*, **48A**, 245.
WILSON, P. D. (1947). Experiences with a bone bank. *Ann. Surg.*, **126**, 932.
WILSON, P. D. (1951). Follow-up study of the use of refrigerated homogenous bone transplants in orthopaedic surgery. *J. Bone Jt. Surg.*, **33A**, 307.
YOUNG, M. H. (1964). The repair of experimental defects in rabbit skulls. Observations after implantation with decalcified, deproteinized and deep frozen homogenous whole bone. *J. Bone Jt. Surg.*, **46B**, 329.
YOUNG, M. H. (1967). Bone and derivatives of bone for repair of skeletal defects. *Clin. Orthopaed. & Rel. Res.*, **50**, 257.
YOUNG, R. W. (1963). Nucleic acids, protein synthesis and bone. *Clin. Orthopaed. & Rel. Res.*, **26**, 147.
ZADEK, R. E. and ROBINSON, R. A. (1967). The healing of osteal-periosteal discontinuity of standard length, in skeletally mature and immature canine radii. In "The Healing of Osseous Tissue". A workshop sponsored by the Committee on the Skeletal System, Division of Medical Sciences, National Academy of Sciences. Ed. R. A. Robinson. Washington: National Research Council.
ZEISS, I. M. (1966). The fate of simultaneous and successive male to female skin grafts in an inbred strain of rats. *Transplantation*, **4**, 48.
ZEISS, I. M., NISBET, N. W. and HESLOP, B. F. (1960). Studies on transference of bone. II. Vascularization of autologous and homologous implants of cortical bone in rats. *Brit. J. exp. Path.*, **41**, 345.
ZUCMAN, P., MAURER, P. and BERBESSON, C. (1968*a*). The effect of autografts of bone and periosteum in recent diaphysial fractures. *J. Bone Jt. Surg.*, **50B**, 409.
ZUCMAN, J., MAURER, P., BERBESSON, C. and BARBOT, J. (1968*b*). Etude expérimentale de l'action ostéogénique des greffes de périoste, des greffes de moelle osseuse et de l'alesage centromédullaire. *Rev. Chir. Orthop.*, **54**, 221.

Chapter 7

THE PREPARATION, PRESERVATION AND TRANSPLANTATION* OF ARTICULAR BONE ENDS

A. S. IMAMALIEV

FOREWORD *by Professor M. V. Volkov*

The problem of replacing articular bone ends by transplants is, at the present time, of great importance in the field of orthopaedics and traumatology. During the last ten years much work has been done on the subject and many surgeons are now experimenting in this branch of surgery with increasing success.

A. S. Imamaliev's publication is the outcome of the researches which the author carried out at the Soviet Ministry of Health's Central Institute of Traumatology and Orthopaedics (C.I.T.O.). Here he worked on the preparation and preservation of transplants, studying the interdependence of the transplant and surrounding tissues and clarifying the reasons for success and failure in the transplantation of articular bones.

The author has the advantage of coming to the clinical work after many experiments on animals. By comparing these with his clinical cases and correlating X-ray and morphological data, he was able to obtain information about the state of articular material transplanted into another organism.

Using material which had been treated at low temperatures for varying lengths of time, he was able to determine the optimal period for preservation. The author demonstrates that the duration of the time of preservation affects the fate of the transplant.

In the clinical section there are descriptions of a large number of patients who were operated on using his methods with good results. The operations were performed by leading orthopaedic surgeons at the institute, including Imamaliev himself; the surgical technique he evolved is noteworthy because of the use of compression between the bone ends—a method which permits joint movement without impairing bony fixation and subsequent union.

A separate section is devoted to an appraisal of the isolated cases of failure at C.I.T.O. Such an analysis of complications can help to prevent them from happening in the future.

A. S. Imamaliev's publication is the first devoted to the problem of articular bone transplants and is particularly valuable in that it covers observation of patients for a period of more than ten years. It will be received with interest not only by orthopaedic and general surgeons but also by doctors in other branches of medicine.

* The literal translation from the Russian is 'homoioplastic transplant', meaning that tissues are transplanted from one animal to another of the same species. For simplicity the word 'transplant' alone has been used throughout.

EDITOR'S NOTE: The remainder of this chapter, by Professor A. S. Imamaliev, was originally submitted as a monograph; regrettably this was too long for inclusion in this book. After translation it was therefore re-arranged and abbreviated. Every effort has been made to preserve not only the fundamentals of this important work, but also to include sufficient technical information. In the process of translating and editing, errors of detail may have crept in; the surgeon wishing to undertake this work is therefore advised to contact the author direct.

Introduction

Reconstructive bone surgery is an ancient art. Even in the time of Hippocrates surgeons were attempting to use animal tissues as transplant material, but the obstacles and difficulties were enormous. More recent efforts were attacked on religious grounds and doctors' lives were

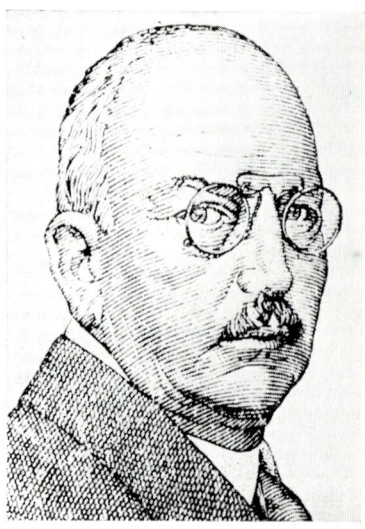

FIG. 1. Erich Lexer, originator of clinical transplantation of joints.

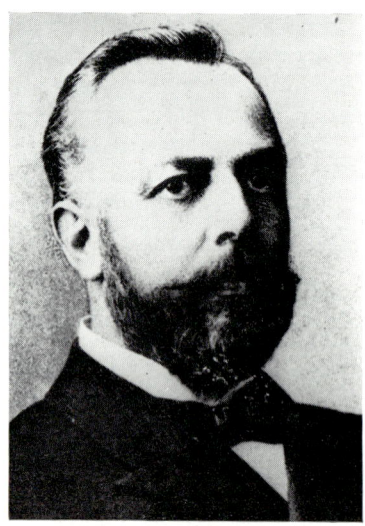

FIG. 2. Yuri Romanovich Penski, originator of experimental transplantation of joints and articular bone ends.

threatened by fanatical priests. Professor Erich Lexer (Fig. 1) cites the case of a woman who, a few years previously, had received a knee joint transplant; under the influence of the Catholic church, she demanded its removal because it might have come from someone of another denomination.

The difficulties in using tissues from the dead were just as great. Not only was there the same religious prejudice, but also legal problems, for in no country did the law provide for taking cadaveric tissue. Moreover, in the pre-aseptic and antiseptic era attempts at transplant surgery usually failed because of suppuration.

The great break-through was achieved by Pasteur; his work on microorganisms led the way to antisepsis and asepsis. A fresh impetus was given to experimental research (Yu. R. Penski 1893 (Fig. 2), Zh. Zhyude 1902, Tittse 1903, etc.) and to clinical experience in the development of transplant operations (E. Lexer, H. Küttner 1913, V. N. Pavlov-Silvanski 1914, K. Petraschews 1913 and others).

Once more failures and disappointments awaited the surgeons. Transplanted tissues either did not survive or were absorbed. The new problem, incompatibility between the donor's and the recipient's tissues, is still far from solved. At the moment work is proceeding in three main directions: (1) the influence of the donor; (2) the preparation of the recipient; and (3) the treatment of the transplanted tissue or organ. In his recent work Medawar is exploring a fourth direction—the selection of donor and recipient according to the qualitative indices of blood leucocytes; this is still only experimental.

To develop transplant surgery it was essential to have enough material, and therefore to use cadaveric tissues if possible. The problem was to preserve these for long periods in a biologically active state. An early worker in this field was P. I. Bakhmetyeva who in 1912 preserved mammalian tissue at a temperature of $-10°C$. She stated that, in lowering the temperature, "we have a new state of the organism in which it is neither dead nor alive—and this is anabiosis". Her work stimulated the use of low temperatures for preservation of tissues and organs.

In the post-war years, with the increasing clinical use of human tissue, special laboratories began to be set up for preserving transplant material. In the U.S.A. these were called 'Bone Banks' (L. F. Bush 1947), and in the Soviet Union 'laboratories for the preservation of tissues and organs' (Leningrad 1952, Moscow 1956).

Eventually, the use of cadaveric tissue became possible in all large clinics throughout the Soviet Union, so that a great fund of clinical experience accumulated (N. N. Priorov, N. P. Novachenko, V. D. Chaklin, P. P. Kovalenko, I. L. Krupko, S. S. Tkachenko, M. V. Volkov, L. I. Shulutko, I. S. Ginsburg, B. D. Golovanov, O. N. Gudushauri, G. S. Yumashev, E. A. Abalmasova, G. V. Golovin, B. V. Petrovski, N. N. Blokhin *et al.*).

At the Central Institute of Traumatology and Orthopaedics (C.I.T.O.) in the U.S.S.R. a series of experiments was carried out using tissues preserved at low temperatures ($-70°C$) (A. S. Imamaliev, G. S. Gladkova, S. I. Degtyareva, L. A. Pobelnenko). The material was available for use in various establishments in the country as well as in the C.I.T.O. clinics. Experience in orthopaedic and traumatological cases highlighted certain aspects of tissue preservation and permitted comparative evaluation of the various methods.

I should like to express my thanks to all my colleagues in the Laboratory for the Preservation of Tissues who have actively collaborated in the presentation of this work.

The Evolution of Tissue Preservation

Although examples of surgeons using human and animal tissues were described as early as the 15th and 16th centuries, these were isolated instances. Only at the end of the 19th century was tissue replacement surgery given a theoretical basis and scientific direction (N. N. Pirogov,

Z. Ollier 1867, E. I. Bogdanovski 1861, I. A. Bredikhin 1862 *et al.*). The development can be divided into three periods.

First period: This was characterized by unsuccessful experiments in transplanting organs or parts of them into humans. These operations, in the pre-aseptic period, usually ended in sepsis and destruction of the transplant.

In 1570 Jacques Mecrin carried out plastic surgery on a defective human skull with bone taken from a dog. Ambroise Paré, operating on a princess, substituted for a badly decayed tooth a healthy one from her fiancé. McEwan in 1878 replaced the damaged humerus of a three-year-old child with an amputated bone. All these transplants failed; the material was taken by primitive methods, without asepsis and without understanding incompatibility.

Second period: This was characterized by the introduction of asepsis and antisepsis. Transplant surgery took on a new lease of life; at the end of the 19th century and the beginning of the 20th, great strides were made. A series of surgeons were occupied in bone transplant surgery (N. I. Pirogov, M. Rudnev 1880, Yu. R. Penski, A. A. Abrazhanov 1900, I. I. Grekov 1901, B. I. Bashkirtsev 1911 and others), while others were transplanting tendons and nerves.

Donor material for transplants was taken from limbs amputated for trauma. Only freshly removed tissues were used, which meant that the amputation and the transplant had to be done simultaneously. This difficulty led to the search for methods of storing tissues.

Third period: This is concerned with the development of preservation techniques. One of the first methods used to preserve bone was boiling and annealing. At the beginning of the 20th century a series of operations using this method were performed (I. I. Grekov 1898, A. A. Abrazhanov 1912, G. I. Turner 1927, S. Orell 1934 and others). The results were bad and the method was soon abandoned (F. Reynolds 1913, H. Judet and others).

In 1931 S. Orell suggested a chemical method for preserving bone tissue by maceration, using 2 per cent solution of caustic alkali + 96 per cent alcohol; this found little clinical application. The researches of I. S. Ginsburg (1946) confirmed the view that macerated bone should only be employed as scaffolding and then only in dealing with small bones.

F. C. Reynolds and O. C. Oliver (1950) reported on the use of bone preserved in an aqueous solution of Merthiolate. Other workers (M. Lange, H. Bürkle, etc.) preserved bone in Cyalite, another organic mercury compound. Providing either solution is renewed every two weeks it is possible to store tissues at room temperature, but the incidence of infection where such tissues had been used was no less than 5 per cent (Stuttgart 1955). Moreover these mercurials had toxic properties which adversely affected tissue preservation.

Karrel suggested storing tissues in a nutrient medium—for example Ringer's Solution, or in blood plasma. Other workers used this idea with some success; their solutions differed from those originally suggested but were similar in principle. Nutrient solution 199 gave fully satisfactory results in preserving skin for periods of up to one month. N. G. Sushko (1963), A. F. Pavlova (1955–56) and K. D. Timashkevich (1963–66) showed that bone and cartilage preserved in physiological and hypertonic solutions at a temperature of $+4°C$ for 2–3 weeks were satisfactory for transplantation.

A suggested method of preserving tissue in a solution of honey (I. A. Akoibya 1966) gave splendid results, both experimentally and clinically, but was not widely favoured because of the expense. Many other methods were suggested but nearly all failed because antibodies were formed by the recipient in response to the foreign protein.

Meanwhile, V. N. Shamov and M. K. Kostyukov (1929) and S. S. Yudina (1930) showed that it was possible to use a man's blood after his death. In the following year a series of specialized laboratories was organized in the Soviet Union (Moscow, Leningrad) where work was done on the collection, treatment and clinical use of cadaveric blood.

In 1931 V. P. Filatov (stimulated by the work of P. I. Bakhmetyev) transplanted the cornea of an eye taken from a corpse and kept for more than 24 hours in a refrigerator at $+4°C$. Subsequently, he used other cadaveric tissues for transplants, also after storage at low temperatures. So original was Filatov's work that interest was renewed in studying tissues under these conditions, particularly their viability and biological activity.

The first reports of orthopaedic operations using bone stored at $+4°$ to $+5°C$ came from A. Smit in 1937. Then, in 1940, at the Second Congress of Traumatology and Orthopaedics in the Ukraine, I. L. Zaychenko announced the results of experimental investigations with this method. Clinical studies were presented by A. Inclan, who soon realized that, although transplanted grafts cannot compete with autografts, nevertheless they had great advantages and held the key to the future of bone graft surgery.

Low-temperature preservation was also used for other tissues—skin, tendons, etc. Thus, Baxter and Entin (1951), F. I. Pepper (1954), R. Georgiade (1956) and others recommended that skin should be stored at $+4°$ to $+5°C$. N. M. Michaelson (1938) and A. G. Fedokentov (1959) both recommended preserving cartilage in nutrient solutions at a temperature of $+2°$ to $+5°C$, a method which found support in other countries (L. Massey 1952, T. Gibson 1959 et al.). S. I. Degtyareva used temperatures of $+2°$ to $+5°C$ for tendon preservation but later used still lower temperatures $-70°$ to $-30°C$.

Tissue preservation at low temperatures won support by its results, but further research showed reduced viability and biological activity after storage for a few weeks, thereby dashing the hope of accumulating supplies. Further study showed that, in the state of anabiosis induced by temperatures of $+2°$ to $+5°C$, biological processes are not arrested, they are only slowed down; hence the deterioration which occurred 2–5 weeks after preservation. To preserve the cell structure still lower temperatures were needed.

A group of physicists (Smit and others) showed that rapid freezing to $-45°$ or $-50°C$ created conditions for the transition of liquid to an amorphous state, without undergoing crystallization. J. Herbert, 1949, with these results in mind, first suggested using temperatures in the region of −50° to −70°C for prolonged tissue-preservation. He found that quick 'deep' freezing led to the transition of the liquid in the tissues to an amorphous state, and did not cause destruction of the cells or their contents.

This view was supported by many research workers (A. Sicard, J. P. Binet 1950, Yu. I. Barkov 1955, A. S. Imamaliev 1955, G. V. Golovin 1956, E. A. Abalmasova and R. L. Ginsburg 1956 et al.). As a result the low-temperature régime was introduced into practical medicine for the preservation of all tissues of the motor system. Different temperature régimes, from −40° to −269°C, were subjected to experimental and clinical trials (P. P. Kovalenko 1953, M. I. Panova 1960, Yu. V. Beringer and A. A. Zykov 1959, A. N. Filatov 1958, I. V. Saburova 1963, N. G. Sushko 1965, M. L. Moin 1964 et al.).

Histological investigations showed that at these temperatures tissue structure was preserved for prolonged periods: bone up to six months, skin for four months (M. N. Pavlova 1962, E. Flosdorf 1949, G. Bell 1952 and others). Biochemical studies showed that tissue viability also was preserved, though the period of survival varied with different tissues (T. Ya. Balaba 1959, V. P. Torbenko 1962 et al.).

Low temperatures reduce the viability of some tissues (skin, nerves and vessels), more than others; to counteract this loss protective agents were tried, e.g. glycerine (C. Rob 1954, A. Smit 1956, L. Ray 1962, R. Klen 1962 and others), vaseline (A. G. Lapchinski 1962), and dimethyl-sulphoxide (N. G. Sushko 1965). Other workers tried rapid freezing to −60° or even −196°C (A. S. Silayeva, Yu. V. Beringer and others) and then storage at −25° to −30°C, but this seemed to reduce biological activity.

The use of very low temperatures presented many technical (and economic) problems, so that other methods continued to be sought. Preservation in lyophilic colloid was described by d'Arsonval and Borda (1906). The first attempts to preserve bone by this lyophilic method date from 1951 (F. Kreuz, G. Hyett, T. Tener, K. Basset). Next a series of papers appeared on the experimental and clinical use of tissues treated in this way (E. Flosdorf, G. Hyett 1952, G. S. Yumashev 1957, Q. Judet 1954 et al.). The advantage of the lyophilic method is that the dried tissue can be kept for years in vacuum containers. When subsequently placed in a physiological solution the colloidal state of the protein is completely restored and the morphological structure of the tissue partially re-established. However, the disadvantage of this method is that the tissues lose their viability.

The preservation of tissue in hard substances is worthy of consideration. A method of preserving bone in paraffin wax briquettes (A. P. Nadein and A. B. Savchik 1960 and others) was adopted in the Leningrad laboratories. Preserved in this way bone retains its viability for three months, and survives transplantation. Briquettes can be kept in a domestic refrigerator. However, this method too has drawbacks: the briquettes are fragile, the wax melts if exposed to warmth during transport, and the opacity of the wax makes it impossible to detect air bubbles in contact with the bone.

Paton's idea of storing bone in artificial resins was based on the preservation of perishable materials in amber, where they can survive for 1,000 years (K. Idelberger 1961). In 1959, at a symposium in Berlin, he reported on the possibility of storing bone in a quick-setting resin, and G. Garstensen reported experimental results with vascular material preserved in the same way. My colleagues and I at C.I.T.O. (M. B. Vugodskaya, G. N. Kramarenko, M. N. Palova, S. I. Merkina 1961) carried out experimental and clinical trials on bone tissue preserved in plastics for up to three years; we concluded that good results could be obtained.

The Collection of Cadaveric Tissue

The human body is the basic source of donor material and in our clinical practice we are orientated to cadaveric material or, as we call it, 'Spets-donor' (Special Donor).

Preparations of cadaveric tissue are made only from cases of sudden death due to cardio-vascular disorders, asphyxia, to hanging (suicide), arterio-sclerosis, and alcoholic poisoning. Those who die from shock, massive blood loss, extensive skin damage, poisoning, infections or drowning are unsuitable. Gout and rheumatoid disease make the subjects unsuitable donors for bone and joint material.

An ambulance or police van collects the victim of sudden death from the street or his home. Before the Spets-donor is admitted to the mortuary a medico-legal expert or the doctor on duty at the laboratory certifies death. After a thorough external examination, he gives consent for the removal of certain tissues from the dead person. The tissues are removed within six hours of death, but this may be extended to 12, 24 or even 30 hours, if the body is kept cool ($-4°C$); consequently 24-hour attendance of a medico-legal expert is not obligatory.

Blood is removed from the jugular vein during the first six hours after death; this is done by a trained nurse immediately on receipt of the body and even without an examination by the medico-legal expert.

The removal of tissues is performed by a doctor and a nurse under sterile conditions in a special theatre using full aseptic technique. If speed is important a second doctor may assist. The order of removal is as follows: skin, aponeurosis, tendons, nerves and vessels, capsule, bones, joints and costal cartilages. The removed tissues are placed for 30–40 mins. in a physiological solution with antibiotics (1 gm. Streptomycin + 1 million units Penicillin/litre).

The doctor carefully records which tissues were removed, their source and quantity. A copy of these details is attached to the medico-legal documents.

Next the body is taken to another part of the mortuary where a post-mortem is carried out, after which the body is carefully tidied up.

Further investigations include a medical history taken from the relatives and studying the medical record card. Samples of blood and tissues are subjected to bacteriological and other laboratory investigation.

DOCUMENTATION

Careful and accurate documentation is essential; it begins as soon as the body is received.

After the doctor on duty has decided which tissues are to be taken, a statutory document is prepared consisting of: the medico-legal expert's permission, details of the diagnosis and the cause of death, research subject of the laboratory concerned, X-rays of removed joints, and registration cards.

The material is labelled immediately after its removal. On to each container is stuck a label recording the serial number of the donor, the nature and condition of the transplant material, and the date.

All the material from one donor (each tissue in a separate container) is put into a sterile bag which is sealed. To the bag is attached a card recording the name of the donor, the name of the doctor and details of the initial preparation. The bag is then placed in a low-temperature chamber (below $-50°C$), and stored there until receipt of the necessary analyses and permission from the doctor responsible.

When the post-mortem findings and laboratory results have been received (histology of each tissue, Wassermann reaction, blood bilirubin, etc.) the tissues are ready for delivery on the signature, as witness, of the doctor responsible.

The Preservation of Cadaveric Tissues

Sterilization. Sterilization by ionizing irradiation has the advantage that the exact dose can be readily calculated and the process speedily carried out (a fraction of a second is sufficient). The density of the material is important in calculating the penetration required. X-rays and gamma-rays have great depths of penetration. Not all micro-organisms are equally sensitive to irradiation; the most resistant (spore-forming) are destroyed by a dose of 2 million Röntgen but some viruses require 4 million Röntgen. So the dose must exceed 4 million Röntgen.

The technique is well known; the tissues, housed in glass containers or polyethylene bags, are exposed to gamma rays or fast electrons. The sterilized tissues are not taken out of their packaging until just before they are needed for operation.

Other methods of sterilization available include Merthiolate, Cyalite, beta-propriolactone and ethylene oxide gas.

Preservation

> "The problem of the transplantation of organs and tissues cannot be successfully solved without the creation of effectual methods of preservation".
> —Academician B. V. Petrovski.

The term 'preservation' (or conservation) is familiar in connection with keeping food. The preservation of human tissues for use in transplant surgery means the creation of conditions under which their viability and biological properties are retained for long periods.

Preservation of Tissues at Low Temperatures

The use of low temperatures for preserving tissues began with the work of V. P. Filatov in 1933. Although at first this made little impression, over the years its popularity gradually increased.

At present, temperatures varying from $+4°$ to $-269°C$. are used: obviously 'low-temperature' needs more precise definition. P. P. Kovalenko proposed that temperatures from $+2°$ to $+4°C$ be termed 'cooling', of $-1°$ to $-10°C$ 'simple freezing', and anything lower 'deep freezing'. We prefer to divide the last phase into two: from $-11°$ to $-50°C$, and from $-50°$ to $-269°C$. The rapidity of freezing also is important: during the gradual freezing of tissues the liquid goes through a phase of crystallization, expands, and in so doing causes mechanical damage to tissue cells; if however the temperature is rapidly lowered to $-50°C$, the liquid quickly passes into an amorphous state—i.e. a state which does not damage the cellular structure of the tissue.

Herbert (1949), who drew attention to this, suggested a 2-stage method: quick freezing to a temperature of $-40°$ to $-70°C$, and then storage at $-15°$ to $-25°C$. Many research workers use this method, believing Herbert's auguments to be well founded (Sicart and Binet 1950, Yu. I. Barkov 1955, A. S. Imamaliev 1955, G. V. Golovin 1956, E. A. Abalmasova, R. L. Ginsburg 1956 et al.).

Experience has shown that storage at low temperatures ($-60°$ to $-70°C$) preserves tissues in a biologically active state for at least six months (P. P. Kovalenko, N. N. Priorov, S. S. Tkachenko, Yu. I. Barkov, G. V. Golovin, A. S. Imamaliev et al.). After this period, the biological activity falls and by the end of a year is very low. So that the period of storage and the actual temperature are both important.

Transplanted tissue behaves differently according to the length of time it has been preserved. This reflects profound biological processes within the tissue itself as well as the reaction of the recipient's tissues. Compared with stored frozen transplants, fresh unfrozen ones become incorporated more quickly and completely with the surrounding tissues and so stimulate a more vigorous immunological response. The absorption of a frozen transplant is slower; it proceeds *pari passu* with the process of substitution and this allows the transplant to retain its shape and structure until substitution is complete.

Low temperature preservation has disadvantages quite unconnected with the biological processes involved: a bone transplant is at first mechanically weak; and the process of maintaining constant low temperature conditions is technically difficult.

Reaching a temperature of $-70°C$ is simple enough: dry ice (solid carbon dioxide) in a Dewar flask achieves just that temperature. The evaporation of dry ice in a Dewar flask is slight, and a flask with a capacity of 2,000 ml. remains at this temperature for up to four days. Longer periods demand expensive refrigerating equipment, a constant supply of electric current and round-the-clock supervision. The technique we use is to immerse the material for 30 minutes in a physiological solution containing antibiotics; it is then transferred to a glass container or polyethylene bag which is hermetically sealed and put into a temperature of $-50°$ to $-70°C$.

Deterioration of preserved tissues. Two important factors operate—micro-organisms and enzymes. Precautions against damage by bacteria have been outlined. With regard to enzymes V. P. Torbenko showed that storage at a temperature of $-70°C$ preserved, for up to six months, the enzyme activity so important for the success of a transplant.

There are various ways of determining whether autolysis has occurred in the preserved bone tissue: biological, biochemical, histological and so on. In practice only two investigations are needed: determination of the pH, and of the alkaline phosphatase activity (V. P. Torbenko, 1963). These should be obligatory in every laboratory dealing with tissue-preservation.

Methods of Minimizing Tissue Incompatibility

The subject of incompatibility occupies at the moment a central place in the problem of transplanting tissues and organs. Different methods of preservation have been tried with the aim of lowering the immunological reactions to transplants: cooling, freezing, dehydration and preservation in different liquids. A conference devoted to the results of this research was held in the U.S.A. in 1954. At the end of 1957 a similar conference took place in Czechoslovakia with Soviet scientists participating. In Moscow some months later an All-Union conference on Tissue Incompatibility was held, and in London in April 1958, several sessions of the second International Symposium on the Preservation of Tissues were devoted to the problem.

Research aimed at lessening or eliminating tissue incompatibility has been pursued in several directions: the selection of donor and recipient from the same blood group; the selection of animals of the same colouring and even from the same litter; and reducing the host's immunological reactions in such ways as medicated sleep, treatment with adrenaline, preliminary blood transfusion from the donor, hypothermia, etc. All these methods are now being studied.

Limberg (1942) in his facio-maxillary work used an interesting 2-stage procedure. First a piece of bone was transplanted into the region of a damaged lower jaw, then moved to the actual site of the lesion 6–8 weeks later (perhaps when the host is accustomed to the graft). Out of 134 transplants of this sort 13 failed because of suppuration. Despite these results, the method has not been adopted in facio-maxillary surgery because it demands such complicated technique.

The Influence of Low Temperature Techniques on the Immunological Response

Amongst the early work on this subject, the research of I. L. Zaychenko (1938) and Tuclan (1942) is outstanding. They preserved and stored tissues at temperatures of $+4°$ to $-4°C$. Low temperature preservation of transplant material quickly found favour (Wilson 1947, Bush 1947, Hult 1950, Oliver 1950, A. N. Filatov 1958, Yu. I. Barkov 1955, G. V.

Golovin 1954, E. E. Abalmasova, R. L. Ginsburg 1956, P. P. Kovalenko 1956 and others). In 1947 Bush reported to the New York Academy of Medicine on bone transplants preserved at $-25°C$., a technique which gave good clinical results.

Despite the considerable work on bone preserved at low temperatures, transplants of whole joints and of articular bone ends from one animal to another were seldom attempted. In recent years, however, in American literature much interest has been shown in the problem. The experimental work of Chase and Herndon (1952, 1954 and 1956) dealt with auto- and homo-transplants of knee joints which had been preserved in a bone bank at low temperatures for periods varying from a few hours up to several weeks.

Some writers (A. S. Imamaliev, G. V. Golovin, A. N. Filatov and others) believe that the precise temperature used for storing bone transplants undoubtedly affects their fate; this is also influenced by the conditions and duration of conservation.

It is well-known that, following transplantation of foreign protein, specific immunizing bodies are formed in the recipient which cause conflict between the transplant and the host tissue; these antibodies usually damage or destroy the transplant. In other words the host and donor are biologically incompatible.

Tissues subjected to low temperatures and then transplanted, seem, however, to be retained longer in the recipient and to produce less reaction than fresh unfrozen transplants (A. A. Zykov—skin, N. I. Krakovski—vessels, G. V. Golovin—bone, A. S. Imamaliev—joints). A study of the literature, together with our own experimental and clinical observations, had led us to agree completely with this view: preserved transplants are more successful than fresh ones.

TRANSPLANTATION EXPERIMENTS

The creation of a laboratory for the preservation of tissues at C.I.T.O. gave us an opportunity to carry out research on the transplantation of articular bone ends treated at low temperatures. We were able to demonstrate their advantage over fresh transplants, and to formulate the most favourable temperature conditions and periods of preservation.

Materials and methods of research. The experimental study was carried out on 104 dogs, in the course of which 104 transplants of articular bone ends from one animal to another were performed. The animals were selected for age, size and weight. Experience showed that the sex, colouring and pelt were not important for the outcome of experiments: nevertheless we took them into account.

Generally we used dogs aged from 3-6 years. With younger dogs (up to two years old) whose epiphyses were still cartilaginous, the result was early absorption of the transplant at the growth disc, with deformity of the transplanted joint surface and impaired movement. Figure 3 shows this very early absorption at the growth disc; this phenomenon occurs because the vascular collaterals have not yet developed (M. G. Prives 1938).

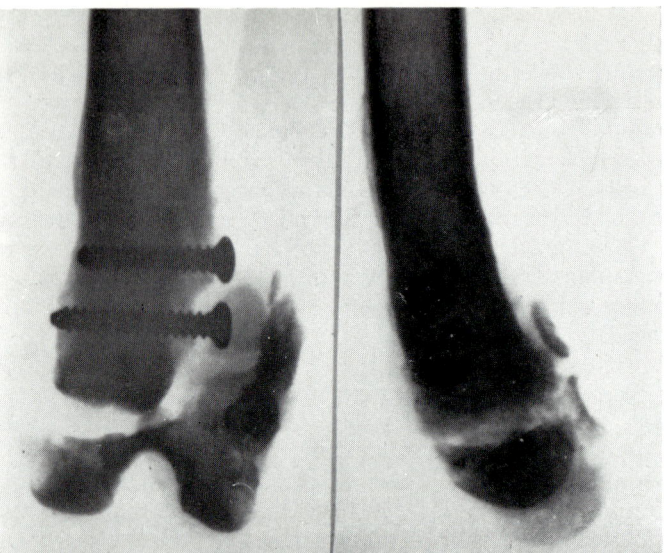

Fig. 3. Absorption along the epiphyseal line of a transplant.

We performed seven series of articular transplants. In the first series the dogs received material stored at −60° to −70°C for a period of five days; in the second series from 6–10 days; and in each subsequent series the transplants had been preserved at the same low temperatures for five days longer than the previous series. In the sixth series, material was transplanted after preservation for 26–60 days. The seventh was a control series: fresh unfrozen material was transplanted (Table I).

TABLE I
Experimental Series of Transplants

No. of series	Period of preservation (in days)	Preservation Temperature	No. of dogs
I	1–5	−60°−−70°	14
II	6–10	−60°−−70°	15
III	11–15	−60°−−70°	15
IV	16–20	−60°−−70°	15
V	21–35	−60°−−70°	15
VI	26–60	−70°−−70°	12
VII (Control)	Fresh	Room temp.	18

The conditions of freezing and preservation were the same in all the first six series. The transplants were taken from dead animals under sterile operating conditions. Each was placed in a sterile glass vessel with a ground-glass stopper and stored in a thermos with dry ice where a temperature of −60° to −70°C was produced. The temperature was measured with a thermometer fitted into the thermos. More dry ice was added every 2–3 days. Immediately before operating, the transplant was placed for 30–40 minutes in a penicillin solution.

We paid special attention to working out the transplantation technique, trying to mimic clinical conditions and paying particular attention to:

(1) The need for strong attachment of the transplant to the host bone. (2) The restoration of capsule and ligaments, to prevent the joint from dislocating. (3) The prevention of active movement for one month after operation.

The operations were carried out under general anaesthesia. After an intramuscular injection of morphia, a barbiturate solution was injected very slowly into the ulnar vein, using 1 ml. per kg. of body weight.

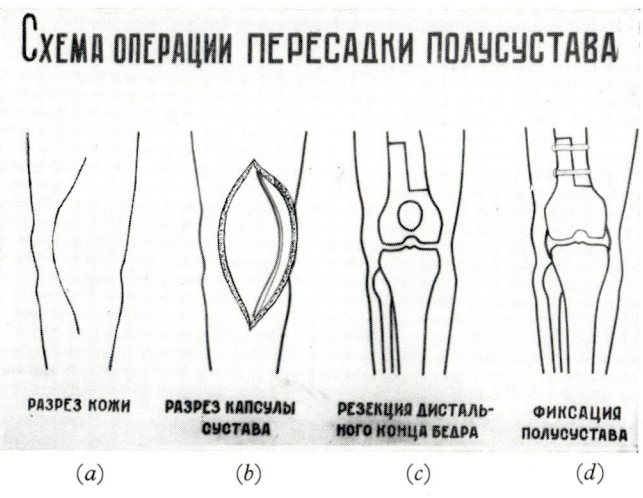

Fig. 4. Stages in the insertion of an articular bone end transplant: (a) skin incision; (b) opening the capsule; (c) line of bone section; (d) fixation of transplant.

Operative technique. A longitudinal incision is made on the lateral aspect of the recipient animal's knee.

The subcutaneous tissues are dissected to expose both sides of the joint, and the capsule opened on the medial side (so that suture lines of skin and capsule do not coincide). Protective skin towels are applied. With the help of a palette knife, the patella, with its ligament, is dislocated. The lateral ligaments are severed at their distal attachments. The cruciate ligaments are cut, leaving part attached to the femur. All these manoeuvres are performed with great care, avoiding damage to the popliteal artery and the menisci. The muscles attached to the back of the lower femur are separated by blunt dissection.

With an electric saw the distal femur is divided as shown in Fig. 4 and the lower end is removed. The transplant is then fitted into place and fixed to the host bone with two stainless steel screws.

The ends of the lateral ligaments are stitched. The patella is replaced and the deep surface of its ligament sewn to the crest of the tibia. The muscles on the back of the femur are pulled up with catgut stitches as close to the femur as possible. The capsule is repaired, the skin sutured with catgut, and penicillin introduced into the wound. Plaster is applied extending to the upper thigh, with the knee at 100°–110°. Over the next 2–3 days the dog is given injections of penicillin, 5 per cent glucose solution, and a high calorie diet.

Correct alignment and matching of transplant to host is very important, not only for the establishment of movement, but also to prevent deformity and subsequent arthrosis. In one case the transplant was offset by

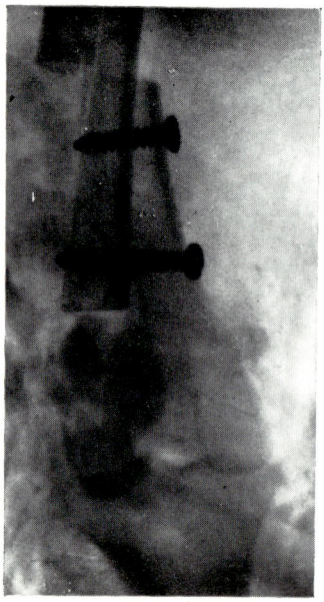

FIG. 5. The saw-cuts were mismatched and the transplant is offset.

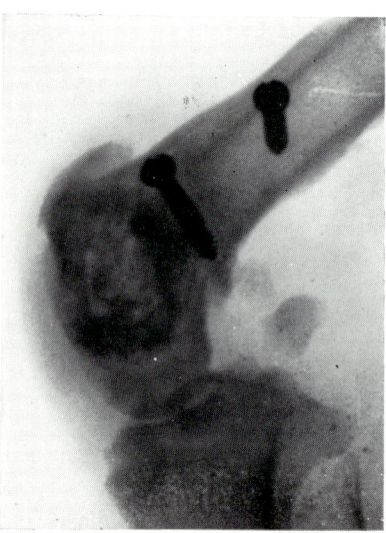

FIG. 6. The same animal 5 years later —the transplant is deformed.

mistake; we had to accept side-to-side union (Fig. 5). An X-ray 5 years after operation (Fig. 6) shows sound bony union but some deformity of the lower end of the femur.

In one case we had not sutured the lateral and cruciate ligaments: Fig. 7 shows the transplanted articular end of the femur after operation and three months later (Fig. 8) with backward dislocation.

To avoid such complications we paid special attention to the ligaments. The lateral ligaments, retained on the transplant, were stitched with silk to the recipient's ligamentous stumps; three to four months later they were indistinguishable from normal. The cruciate ligaments of the host were cut flush, those on the donor femur left long; as soon as the transplant had been fixed these long ends were placed in their correct position on the host tibia. To ensure 'rooting' of the cruciate ligament in its new

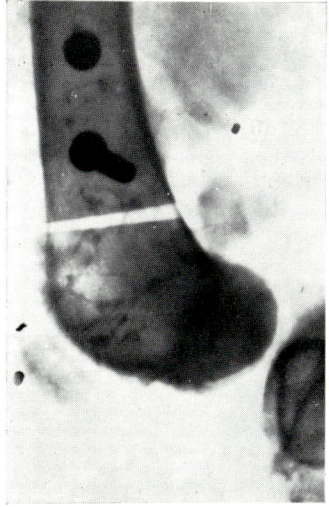
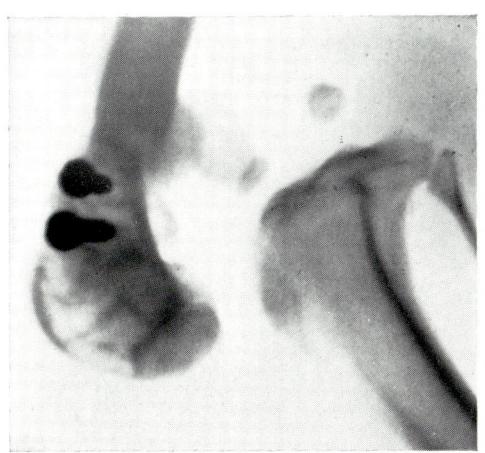

Fig. 7. In this transplant the ligaments were not sutured.

Fig. 8. The same dog, 3 months later—the knee is dislocated.

place, the knee joint must be kept immobile for 30–40 days. Figure 9 shows two examples of successful 'rooting'.

Firm and accurate fixation of the transplant to the host bone was stressed by Lexer and widely endorsed (V. N. Pavlov-Silvanski, N. N. Petrov, N. N. Priorov, N. P. Novachenko, F. R. Bogdanov and others):

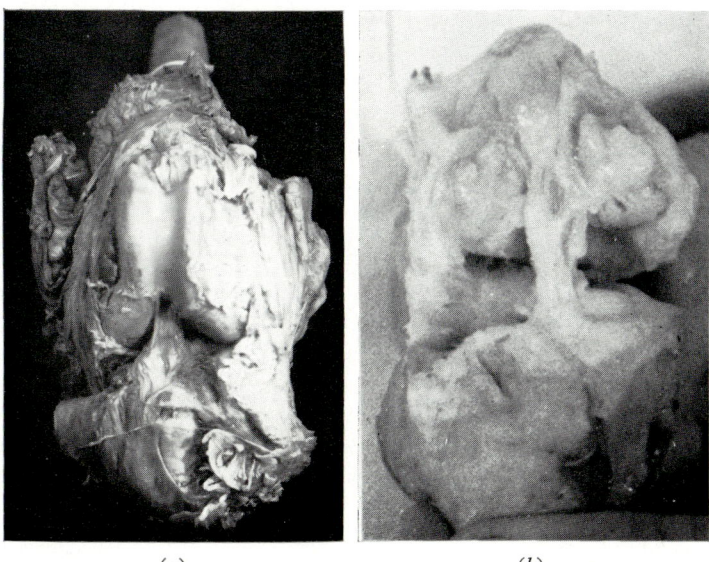

(a) (b)

Fig. 9. Newly-formed cruciate ligaments in two dogs: (a) after 120 days; (b) after 1370 days.

we also regard fixation as extremely important. It is an essential prerequisite for early joint movement. With a z-shaped bone section, two stainless steel screws, introduced transversely across the longitudinal bone cuts and passing through both cortices, are adequate.

We also tried a scythe-like bone section and an oblique cut, in each case with fixation by two screws: neither technique provided sufficient rigidity (Fig. 10). Even slight movement between the fragments led to separation of the transplant from the host bone, with consequent fibrous or cartilaginous 'union'. Unless bony union occurs the transplant is likely to fail.

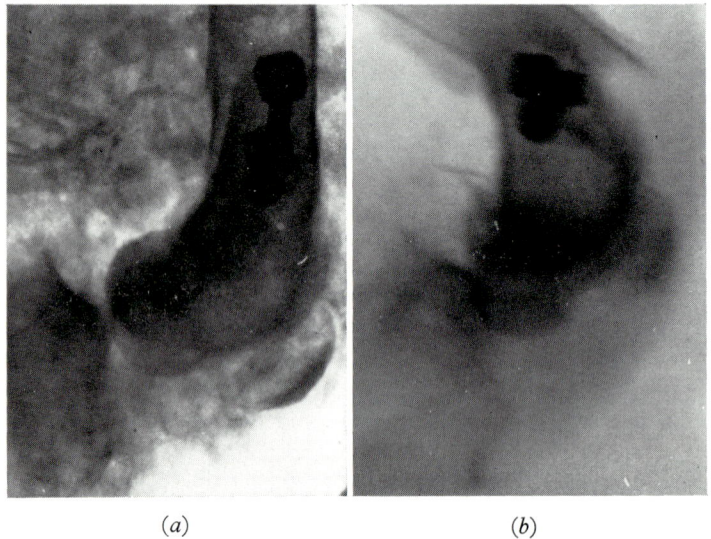

(a)   (b)

FIG. 10a and b. Fixation by an oblique cut and screws has proved inadequate.

No less important are reattachment of capsule and ligaments for joint stability; and the suturing of muscles in close contact with the transplant —otherwise the dead space invites haematoma-formation.

If the technique described is adhered to, then joint movement is, in the majority of cases, fully restored in 6–8 months.

Convalescence: During the early post-operative period the wound usually heals and any haematoma resolves. The animal usually remains inactive. The plaster is removed at one month. The most important early complication is suppuration.

After about two months, as the ligaments and muscles strengthen, the dog begins to take increasing weight on the leg. Full weight-bearing usually occurs at about four months. During this period union of the transplant and host bone takes place, and substitution of the transplant by newly-formed bone. Providing all is well, full function with a full range of joint movement should be restored by 6–8 months from operation. But if the process of substitution does not keep pace with absorption

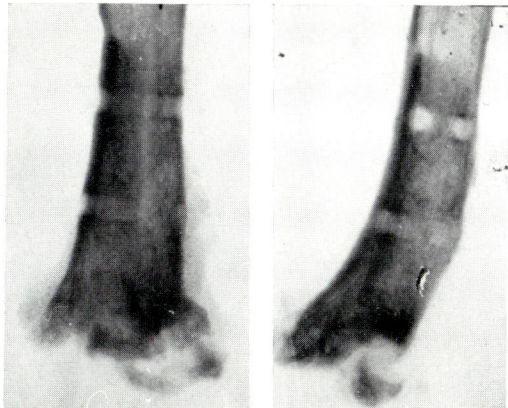

FIG. 11. This transplanted bone end has been largely absorbed and is deformed.

of the transplant, then deformity ensues (Fig. 11) with impaired joint function.

Analysis of Results:

Good results—with full restoration of function of the limb; and X-rays showing the transplant intact and firmly united to the host bone.

Fair results—with a fully weight-bearing limb but limited knee movement (20°–25°); and X-rays showing marginal damage to the transplant at the joint surfaces, and where substitution of the transplant was associated with a periosteal reaction.

Poor results—with joint deformity and grossly limited movement; and X-rays showing absence of union of transplant with the host bone, and absorption of the transplant with failure of substitution.

Table II shows the results in all the series. The fresh unfrozen transplants nearly all did badly, undergoing absorption without substitution.

TABLE II

Results of Experiments

No. of series	Period of preservation (in days)	No. of tests	Good	Result Fair	Poor
I	1–5	10	2	5	3
II	6–10	10	4	4	2
III	11–15	10	7	3	—
IV	16–20	9	6	3	—
V	21–26	10	8	2	—
VI	27–60	4	4	—	—
VII (Control)	Fresh	12	2	2	8
	Totals	65	33	19	13

With the frozen transplants the duration of storage was important. In series I and II where preservation was no more than 10 days complete absorption was noted in five cases and partial absorption in nine. In series III and IV, in 19 'clean' experiments there was no case of complete

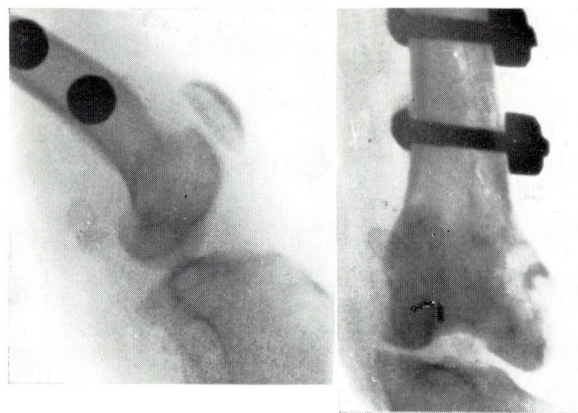

Fig. 12.

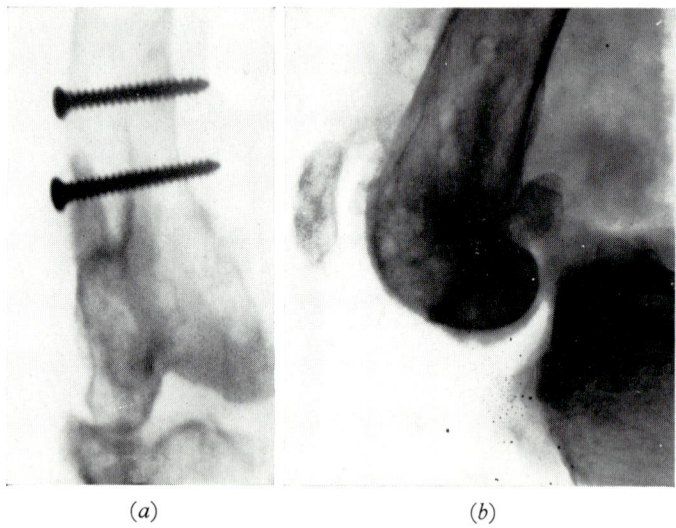

(a) (b)
Fig. 13.
Successful transplants after 220 days (Fig. 12), 1100 days (Fig. 13a) and 2000 days (Fig. 13b).

absorption and partial absorption in six. In series V and VI there was not one example of complete absorption and partial absorption in only 2 out of 14 cases.

From Table II it is obvious that after preservation for three weeks, a transplant does not undergo absorption without substitution.

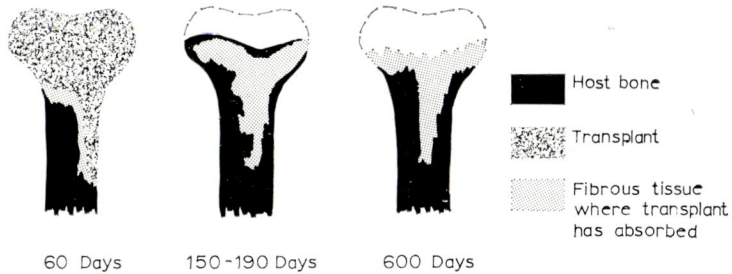

Fig. 14a. Control group (fresh unfrozen transplants).

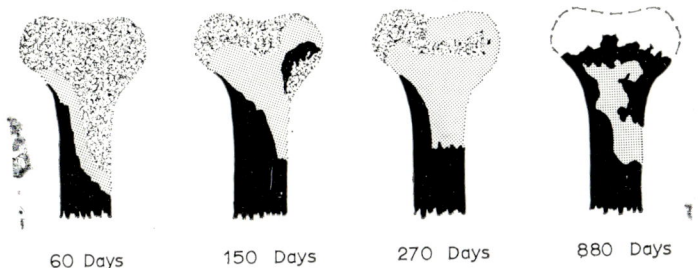

Fig. 14b. Transplant preserved for 2–10 days.

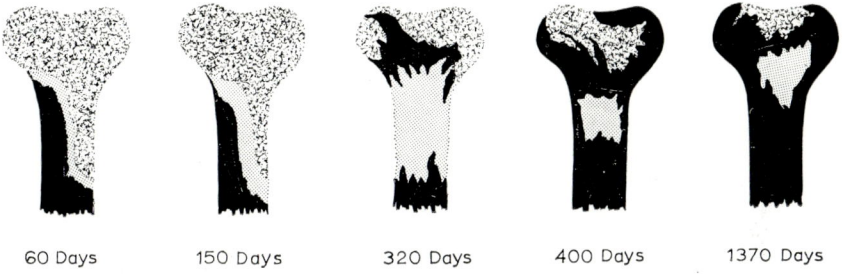

Fig. 14c. Transplant preserved for 20–25 days.

Fig. 14. Fate of transplants. Drawings prepared from histological specimens. In all groups absorption begins at the junction of host with transplant: in (a) the transplant is completely absorbed and largely replaced by fibrous tissue; in (b) absorption is less extensive; in (c) new bone from the host has grown in to replace the transplant almost completely.

Basically our experiments convinced us that freezing permits the preservation of a transplant as a whole (its shape) and, also, of its biological properties. Absorption of the transplant proceeds *pari passu* with its replacement by newly-formed tissue from the recipient. The homoio-transplant (from the same species), kept at a low temperature ($-60°$ to $-70°$) for not less than 25 days provides the best material. The ideal circumstances occur when the processes of absorption and substitution by new bone tissue occur synchronously.

Prolonged observation of the animals experimented on in the fifth series has shown that after five years the transplants still retain their shape and structure (Figs. 12, 13, 14).

Fate of the Transplant

This depends on several factors:

(1) *Infection.* This is avoided by careful aseptic techniques throughout, the use of antibiotics, and early evacuation of any haematoma.

(2) *Security of fixation.* This was achieved by shaping the bone ends to lock securely, reinforced by screw fixation and plaster splintage.

(3) *Congruity of surfaces.* The transplant selected must be of the correct size to ensure joint congruity.

(4) *Stability.* The capsule and ligaments must be reconstituted to ensure stability and good function.

(5) *Age of the donor.* Immature dogs with cartilaginous epiphyses were unsuitable, for large masses of cartilage are not satisfactorily remoulded in the process of substitution.

(6) *Treatment of the donor tissue.* Fresh donor material fared badly. Preserved frozen material was superior. Satisfactory incorporation occurred when absorption of the transplant and substitution by the host tissues kept pace with each other; this was optimum when the donor tissue was frozen at $-60°$ to $-70°C$, and stored at this temperature for 25–30 days.

THE CLINICAL TRANSPLANTATION OF ARTICULAR BONE ENDINGS

"A corpse must no longer be regarded as dead: it not only continues to live in its separate parts but can still present the living with gifts of great value—fully viable tissues and organs."—V. N. Shamov, 1949.

Our clinical data is based on 88 patients who received transplants of articular bone ends. Seventy-four patients had bone tumours which were removed by resecting the articular bone end and a transplant substituted. The remaining 14 included patients with osteomyelitis, tuberculosis, bone absorption, joint deformity after faulty healing of a fracture, and echinococcus infection.

TABLE III

Clinical Material

No.	Diagnosis	Number of patients
(1)	Tumours	74
(2)	Bone defects following trauma, tuberculosis, etc.	6
(3)	Others	8
	Total	88

Forty-six of the patients were men and 42 women. Sixty-five were aged between 12 and 30, 12 between 31 and 40 and 11 between 41 and 55. We performed no transplants on young children, because, in an unossified zone these readily undergo absorption (A. S. Imamaliev 1959) leading to joint deformity and impaired function.

Indications and Contra-indications for the Transplantation of Articular Bone Ends

(1) *Absolute indications:* These comprise cases of acquired bone defect in which it is impossible to retain one articular bone end; the opposing articular surface is intact and normal; and the state of the surrounding soft tissues is favourable.

(2) *Relative indications.* When the patient is aged over 45 the prolonged immobilization which transplants require may be unwise; autografts might be safer. Other relative indications include certain cases of tuberculosis, osteomyelitis and post-traumatic joint deformities—always providing that the transplant involves less risk than other surgical methods.

Contra-indications. Malignant tumours or deposits are a contra-indication. Nor should a transplant be done where a joint has been heavily irradiated (more than 12,000 r), or necrosis and infection follow. The surgeon must of course be certain that the transplant has been removed aseptically and preserved correctly.

METHODS OF TRANSPLANTING ARTICULAR BONE ENDS

The technique was, basically, carried over from the experimental to the clinical phase. We found it important to choose a transplant of the correct size, and to fix it rigidly so that we could start joint movement as early as possible. Strict attention to the demands enumerated in the experimental work led to the use of various types of sawcuts and combined methods of bone fixation.

After thorough clinical investigation the patient is prepared for operation. The day before, a bath is taken, the area is shaved and the skin treated with disinfectant. The night before operation, he is sedated. Most of the patients were operated on under a general anaesthetic but a few under local anaesthesia. During operations a blood transfusion was given.

The joint is opened by means of a longitudinal incision. The soft tissues and ligaments, as far as possible, are carefully preserved. After resection of the affected part of the bone, the site is ready to receive the transplant.

The transplant is brought to the theatre at the beginning of the operation, transferred to a penicillin solution, and a small piece sent for bacteriological tests. It is carefully shaped to fit the host bone. An accurate interlocking technique which we call the 'Russian lock' is illustrated in Fig. 15. Fixation can be augmented by sutures, wires, screws, intramedullary bone pegs and in other ways. More recently we have supplemented the Russian lock with compression (Fig. 16), using Gudushauri's apparatus (see below).

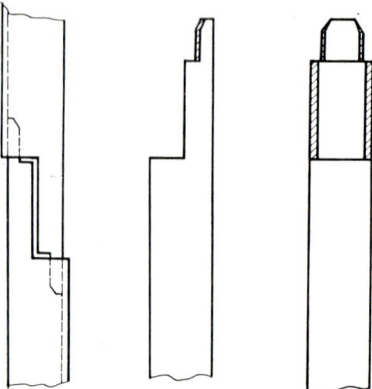

Fig. 15. The 'Russian lock' technique for fixing the fragments together (according to S. T. Zatsepin).

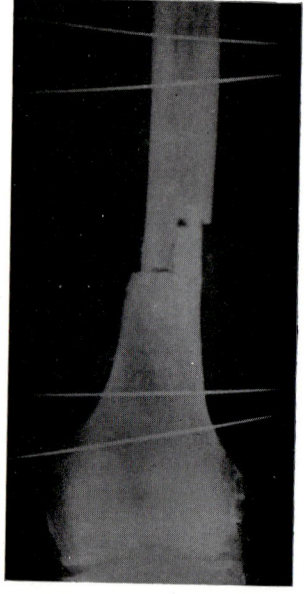

Fig. 16. The 'Russian lock' with wires for applying compression using Gudushauri's apparatus.

Once the transplant is secured the capsule and ligaments are repaired. An original method was suggested and applied by S. T. Zatsepin. The host's ligaments and joint capsule are preserved. At the proposed site of capsule and ligament attachments of the transplant fine drill holes are made. The host's capsule is attached with two nylon semi-pouched stitches; one end of each is threaded through the drill hole to meet the other, and tied tightly. In this way the capsule can be applied closely to the transplant (Fig. 17). This method provides correct alignment of the joint surfaces, facilitating restoration of function, but cannot be used where the capsule is attached at different levels. During operation penicillin solution is instilled into the wound, and at the end of the operation some is introduced into the soft tissues.

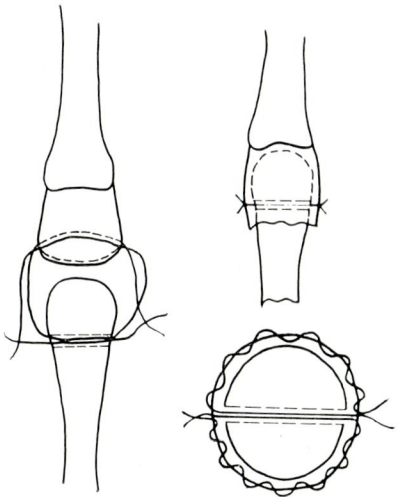

FIG. 17. Zatsepin's technique for suturing the capsule.

If Gudushauri's apparatus is being used, then, after suturing, lines are marked on the skin as shown in Fig. 18. Kirschner wires are then

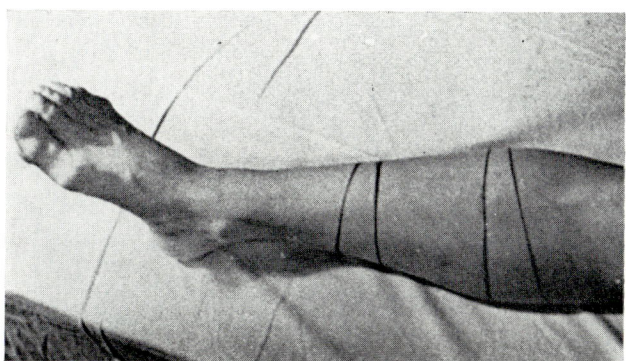

FIG. 18. Lines marked on the skin indicating where the Kirschner wires will be inserted.

inserted parallel to these lines, two through the transplant and two through the host bone. Skin tension must be avoided. Gudushauri's apparatus is attached to the wires and compression applied (Fig. 19). This technique accelerates union. The value of compression techniques in transplants had never been previously assessed; we found that the results were very good (Figs. 20, 21, 22).

Gudushauri's apparatus provides such rigid fixation that a complete

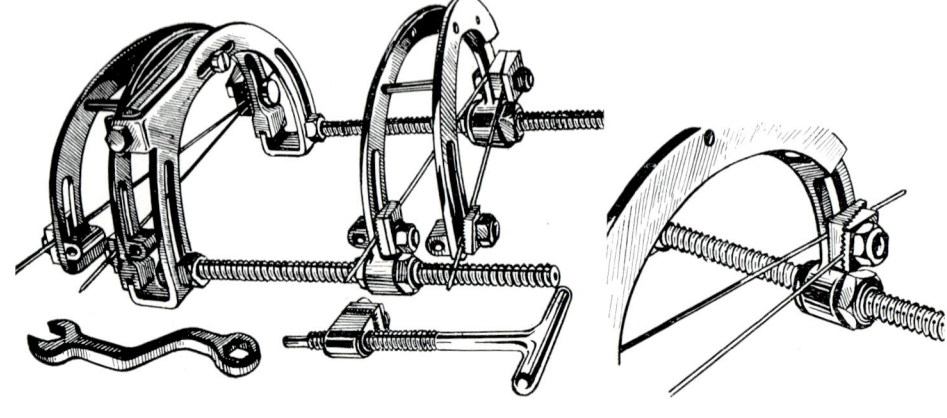

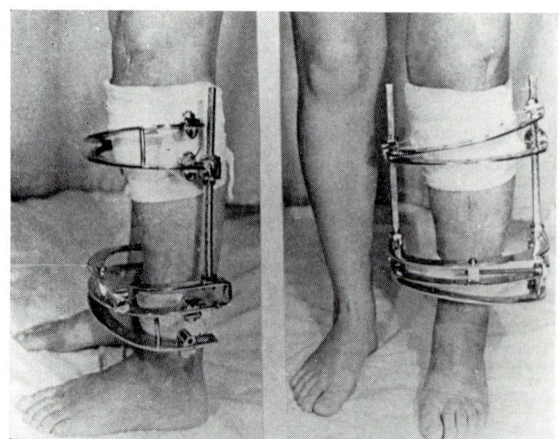

Fig. 19. Drawings of Gudushauri's apparatus, and the apparatus in position—note that the patient is able to walk.

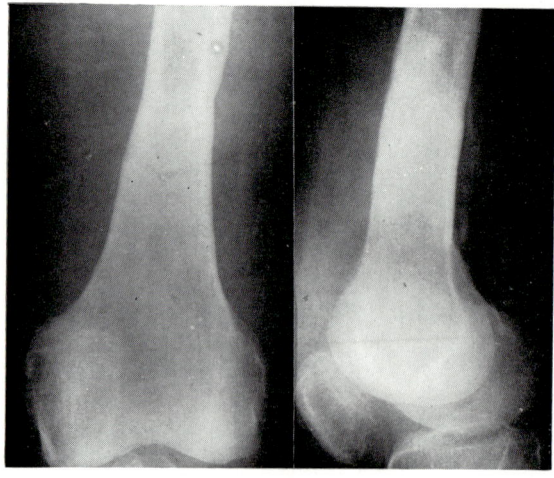

Fig. 20. Transplanted lower end of femur 6 years after operation.

plaster is not needed—a black slab is sufficient. After four weeks this is replaced by a Böhler's or Bogdanov's splint, and passive movements are started. At 6–8 weeks the patient begins walking with crutches. At 3–4 months the apparatus is removed and a hinged plaster applied which is retained until there is X-ray evidence of union between the transplant and the host bone; this takes from six months to a year. During this time the patient is given remedial exercises.

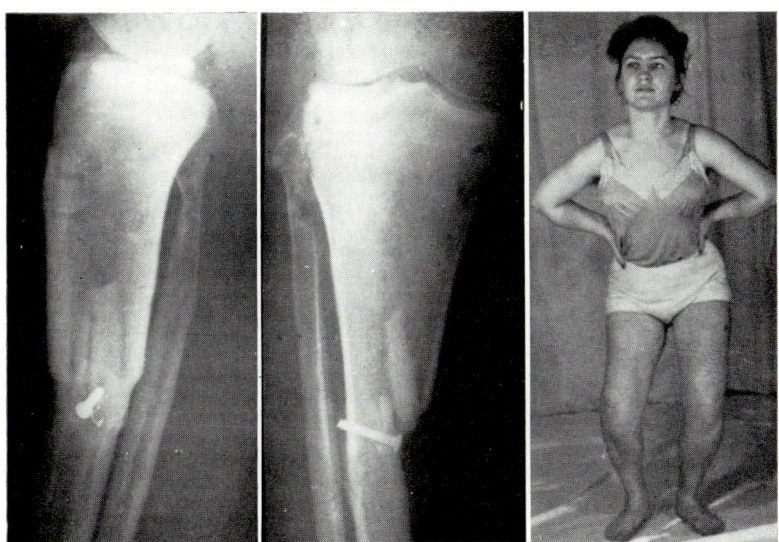

Fig. 21.   Fig. 22.

FIG. 21. Transplanted upper end of tibia 6 years after operation.
FIG. 22. The same patient bending her knee.

REACTION OF THE PATIENT TO AN ARTICULAR TRANSPLANT

Transplantations of articular bone endings, especially of large joints, are major procedures, which may take 3–4 hours. The incision is usually extensive and blood transfusion and antibiotics are needed. Nevertheless, all our patients underwent surgery without serious complications.

Pain in the first few days is relieved by analgesics and narcotics. Pain after 10 days suggests complications—suppuration, incorrect application of plaster, or inadequate fixation of the transplant.

One reaction is a raised temperature (up to $38.5°$–$39°C$) for two weeks; over the succeeding days it gradually comes down, then for up to a month in some patients it is subnormal in the evening ($37.1°$–$37.3°$).

Laboratory and blood tests showed that the organism's reaction was not severe. For the first few days there was a leucocytosis and a raised E.S.R. Then the number of leucocytes returned to normal but the E.S.R. remained high for several months, sometimes up to a year. Often there was also a post-operative eosinophilia. The appearance in the peripheral blood of an erythropoietic shift to the left, with an increase in the number of leucocytes was, in our cases, evidence either of deep-seated haematoma or of suppuration. Evacuation of a haematoma will prevent threatened suppuration.

We also analysed the blood groups of recipient and donor; when the groups were incompatible the transplants behaved no differently from when they corresponded. Thus different blood groups in donor and recipient does not prejudice the result of articular bone end transplants.

CLINICAL AND X-RAY ASSESSMENT

On analysing the clinical data of patients after transplantation of articular bone ends, we divided them into three groups:

(1) Good results. X-rays of these patients showed firm union of the transplanted bone with the host bone, with normal shape and structure of the transplant. The joint space was within normal limits and the correlation of the articular surfaces good. The limb was fully weight-bearing and often the joint had full movement, but any limitation did not interfere with normal use.

(2) Satisfactory results. These patients had incomplete restoration of limb function with limited movement due to incongruity of the articular surfaces and to adhesions.

(3) Bad results. These patients could not use the limb, which, in some cases, had to be amputated.

TABLE IV

Clinical Results of Transplantation of Articular Bone Ends

	Result	
Good	Satisfactory	Bad
57 (64%)	14 (16%)	17 (20%)

Transplantation of Articular Bone Ends in the Upper Limb: Illustrative Case Histories

Example 1. I.J. 26 years old, a lathe operator, came to C.I.T.O. on the 25th January 1958, with an enchondroma in the left hand (Fig. 23). As the tumour grew the hand became weaker, and surgical intervention became necessary.

On the 31st January, 1958, the diseased part of the metacarpal was resected and replaced by an articular transplant fixed with wire. The post-operative period was uneventful. After 10 months the patient returned to work with full movement in the fingers and full power in his hand.

Seven years later he was still doing his job as a lathe operator. X-rays (Fig. 24) show union of the transplant with the host bone. The transplant retains its shape and structure; the joint space is normal. The fingers have full movement (Fig. 25).

Example 2. A.V. 35 years old, a draughtsman, came to C.I.T.O. with a deformity which had first become apparent in 1944. The clinical and X-ray appearances are shown in Figs. 26 and 27.

On the 17th March, 1959, the affected area of the radius was removed. The defect was replaced by an articular transplant (Fig. 28). At first the

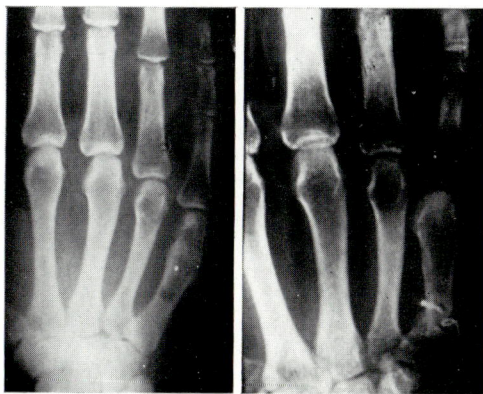

FIG. 23.   FIG. 24.

FIG. 23. Enchondroma of fifth metacarpal.
FIG. 24. X-ray some years after transplant.

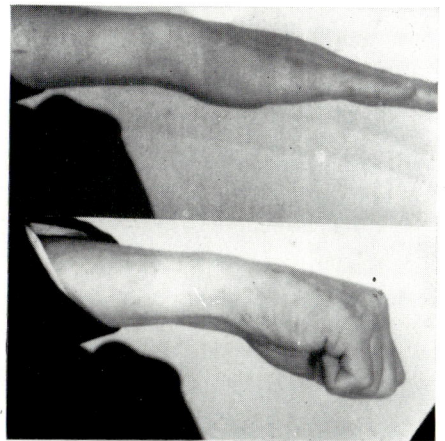

FIG. 25. Range of movement in this patient.

arm was splinted in plaster, then in a leather appliance. A year after operation the patient was able to do his own job as a draughtsman. He had good gripping power (14–16 kg.). Movements in the wrist joint were markedly improved and the deformity of the hand eliminated (Fig. 29).

Example 3. K.M. presented with an osteoclastoma of the upper humerus (Fig. 30). The affected area was resected and replaced by a

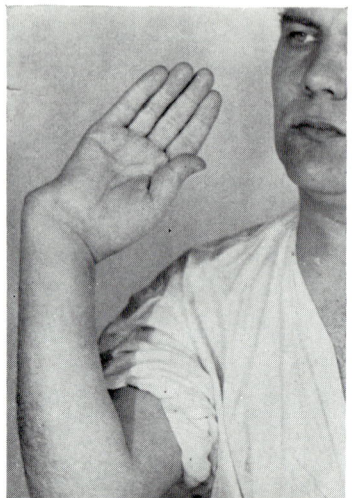

Fig. 26.   Fig. 27.
Clinical and X-ray appearance of patient A.V.

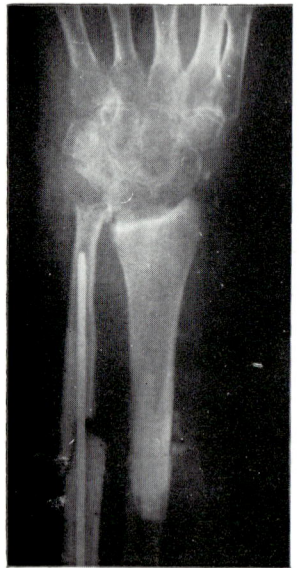

Fig. 28.
A.V. after transplant of lower end of radius.

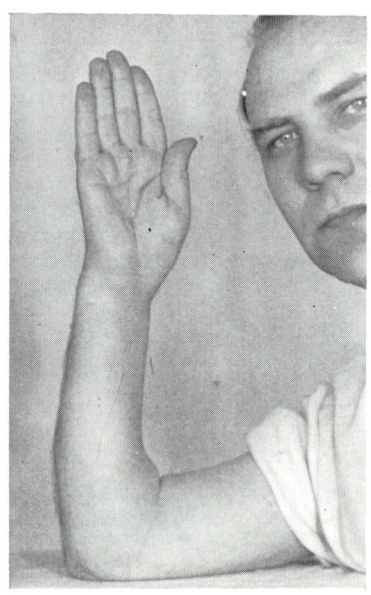

Fig. 29.
Five years after operation.

transplant. The fragments were fixed by an intramedullary bone peg. A thoraco-brachial cast was retained for two months. When this was removed, passive movements were begun with the limb only held in plaster. After 3–4 months, when there was bony union, the patient was encouraged to begin active movements. Three years after operation X-rays show good union of the transplant with the host bone; the transplant has retained its shape and structure, and the joint space is normal (Fig. 31).

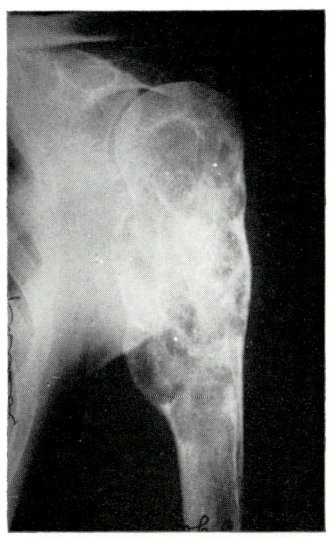

FIG. 30. Patient K.M. with large osteoclastoma.

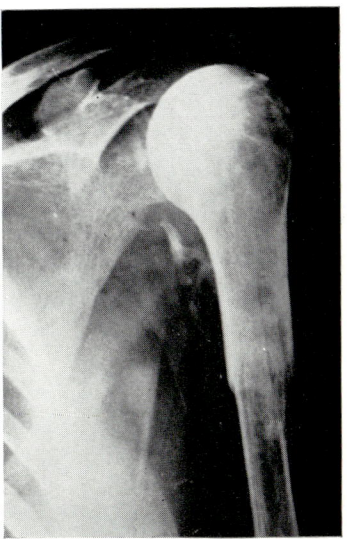

FIG. 31. Three years after transplant of the upper humerus.

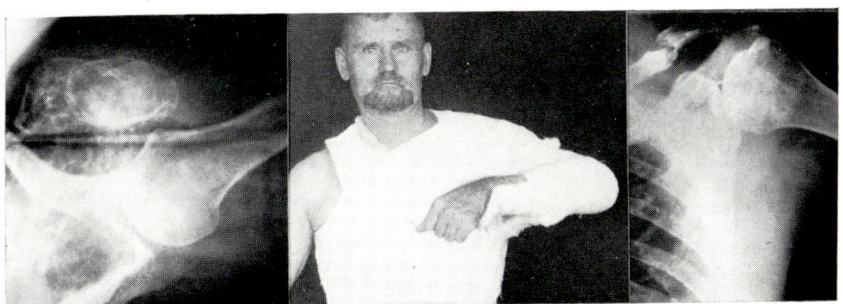

FIG. 32.   FIG. 33.   FIG. 34.

Patient A.P. with a large osteochondroma of the scapula (Fig. 32); in plaster after transplant operation (Fig. 33); and 2 years after operation (Fig. 34).

Example 4. The patient, A.P., had a large osteochondroma of the scapula (Fig. 32) which was resected and replaced by a transplant. The capsule was repaired and the biceps and triceps re-attached. He remained in plaster (Fig. 33) for one year. Subsequently he developed full shoulder movement and the X-ray after 2 years is shown in Fig. 34.

Transplantation of Articular Bone Ends in the Lower Limb: Illustrative Case Histories

The plan for replacing an upper end of femur is shown in Fig. 35.

Example 1. R.A. 25 years old, came to C.I.T.O. in August 1959, because of a destructive lesion following osteomyelitis of the upper third of the right femur (Fig. 36). The defective bone was replaced by a transplant fixed by means of a saw-cut of the 'Russian Lock' type and three screws (Fig. 37). A hip spica was applied. At six months passive movements were begun and at eight months active movements. Eight years after operation the patient has good function, taking full weight without a splint. There is 5–6 cm. of shortening, and a range of hip movement as follows: flexion—70, extension—30, abduction—30.

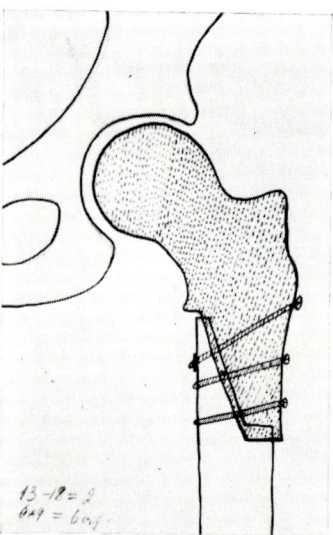

FIG. 35. Technique of upper femoral transplant.

This patient, who for four years had dragged his leg uselessly, had both weight-bearing and hip movement restored by means of a transplanted articular end of the femur. Figures 38a and 38b show the appearance five years later.

Example 2. P.V., 50 years old, came to C.I.T.O. on 16th November, 1961, with an echinococcus infection of the proximal femur, $\frac{2}{3}$ of the length of the bone being affected. He had first complained of pain and limp in 1944. Physiotherapy and spa treatment failed to help. Over a period of nine years he sustained six pathological fractures of the femur. He was treated in several medical establishments where varying diagnoses were made: fibrous dysplasia, giant-cell tumour, etc.

When seen at C.I.T.O. he limped badly and used a stick. The left femur was short, swollen and deformed; the deformity increased when he took weight, and weight-bearing was painful. Hip movements were

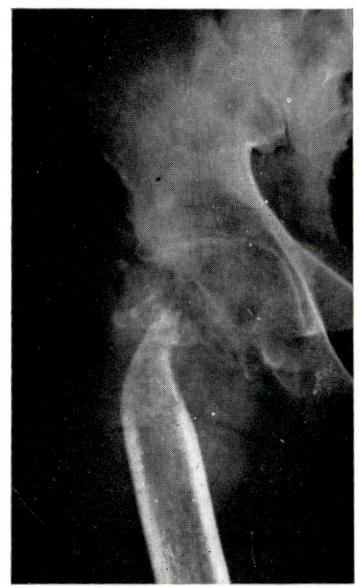
Fig. 36. Patient R.A. with a destroyed upper end of femur.

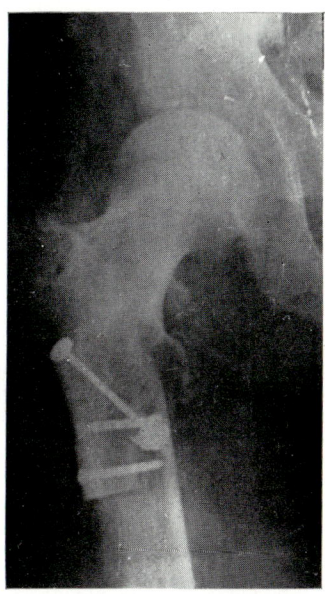
Fig. 37. Soon after transplant.

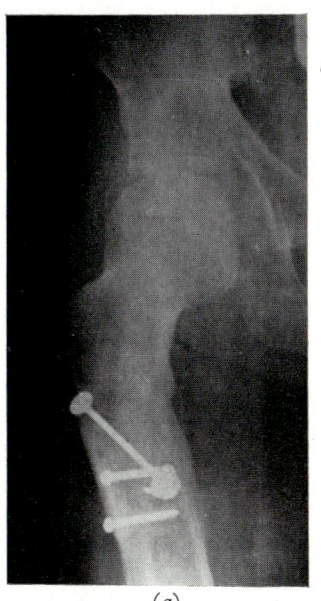
(a)

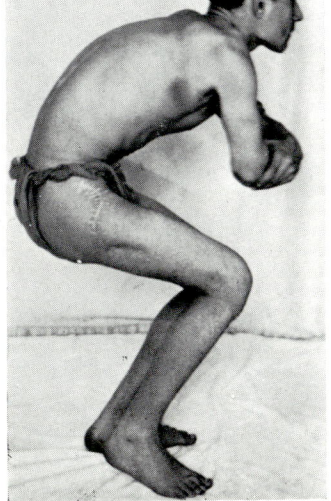
(b)

Fig. 38. (a) X-ray 5 years later, and (b) range of hip movement.

limited, but there was telescoping of up to 4 cm. When lying he could not lift the leg, and the thigh was tender.

X-ray showed a deformed upper shaft of femur with cysts; the neck was missing and the head abnormal (Fig. 39). A diagnosis of echinococcal infection was made.

Operation: Under general anaesthesia, the patient was secured to the operating table inclining ¾ to the right side. The skin and subcutaneous tissue were opened by a longitudinal incision from the crest of the ilium to the great trochanter and then along the artero-lateral aspect of the thigh. Echinococcal cysts between the muscles, and in the soft tissues, were removed. The femoral shaft which was swollen, uneven and bumpy,

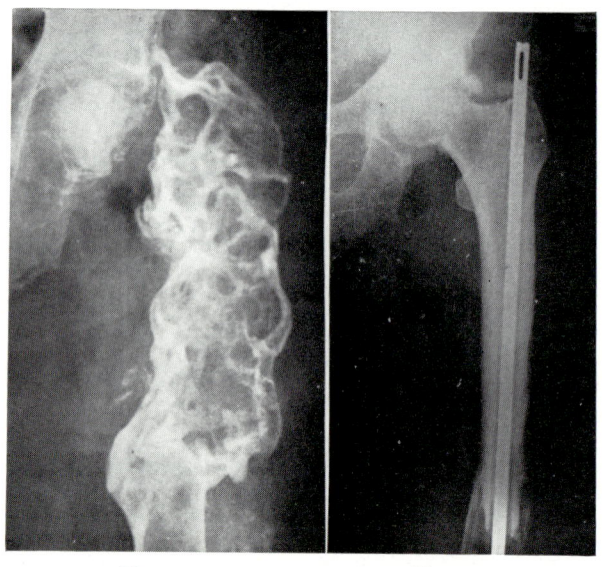

FIG. 39.   FIG. 40.

FIG. 39. Echinococcus infection of the upper femur.
FIG. 40. Appearance 1 year after transplant.

was divided in its lower third with a Gigli saw and removed. The head of the femur, also affected by echinococcal parasites and partly adherent to the acetabulum, was scraped out. The acetabular bone, also cystic and deformed, was reamed out with a milling cutter until healthy bone was reached. The wound was washed with peroxide with a solution of formalin (3 per cent), and haemostasis secured. The distal end of the articular transplant was then wedged into the remains of the host femur. The proximal end was introduced into the acetabulum and the capsule attached to it. The transplant was fixed to the host bone by an intramedullary nail of the C.I.T.O. variety. Around the junction of the transplant with the host shaft were placed two bone homografts fastened by catgut stitches. The muscles were sewn to the great trochanter. One million units of streptomycin was introduced into the wound which was sutured in layers. The wound was drained and a double hip spica applied. During operation 1,250 ml. of blood and 500 ml. of physiological solution were used.

The first post-operative week was difficult. Antibiotics and blood transfusions were given and the patient's condition gradually improved. The blood picture returned to normal, except that the E.S.R. remained high. Every day or two haematomata were aspirated from around the transplant: in all, nearly 700 ml. of blood and fluid were removed. This was sterile on culture.

Two weeks after operation the plaster was removed and the leg placed in a Böhler's splint. Movements were not permitted and oedema subsided very slowly. Three months after operation a pelvic plaster was applied and the patient sent home. Six months after operation the patient himself removed the plaster and never used it again. After a further six months he was able to walk, using one crutch. The leg was a good shape but 6–7 cm. short. Movements at the hip were present but limited. Clinically, there was fusion of the transplant with the host bone X-ray confirms the bony union and shows that the transplant has retained its shape and structure (Fig. 40).

We wish to emphasize the importance of adequate drainage to avoid haematoma formation. Delay in aspirating the blood can be disastrous and during the first week repeated aspiration is important.

Distal end of femur. In six cases of transplantation of the distal end of the femur we obtained a good result in one and satisfactory results in four.

Example. N.A. 30 years old, came to C.I.T.O. some time after an

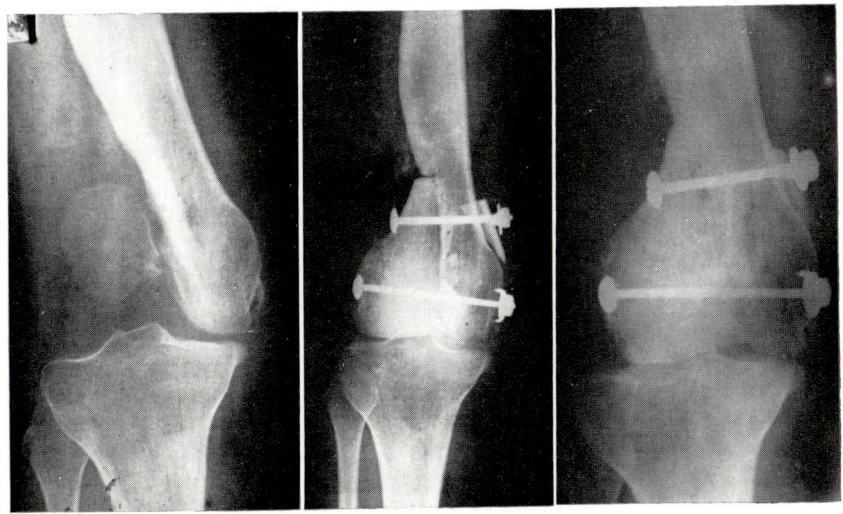

FIG. 41.   FIG. 42.   FIG. 43.

Patient N.A. whose lateral femoral condyle had been previously removed (Fig. 41); after replacement by a transplant (Fig. 42); appearance 4 years later (Fig. 43).

operation at which an osteoclastoma had been removed from the distal end of the left femur. She wore an external splint and used a crutch. The knee was abnormal in shape and the muscles wasted. There was no shortening. Extension of the knee was full and flexion to 150°. The leg could be abducted 25°–30° but was stable to adduction. The X-ray taken on 8th December is shown in Fig. 41.

On the 23rd December, 1958, the missing portion of femur was replaced by a transplant which fitted the femur closely and was secured with two screws. The articular surfaces were not perfectly matched (Fig. 42). Four months later the plaster was changed and the new one hinged at the knee. After a further five months the range of movement was 15°. She walked with a knee-hinged caliper and a stick.

An X-ray four years later (Fig. 43) shows that the transplant has retained its shape and structure. No line can be seen separating the transplant from the host: the distal end of the femur is one single bone. She takes full weight on the leg and has no limp. There is 40° of movement at the knee.

Proximal end of tibia. The most effective transplants were of the proximal end of the tibia. Out of seven operated on, in five sound union

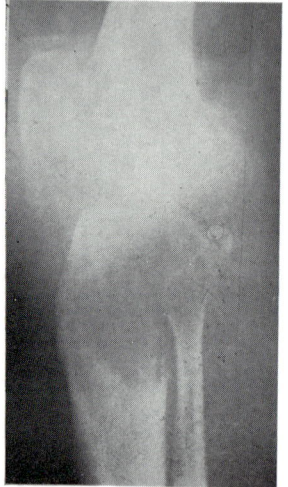
Fig. 44. Patient P.A. with an osteoclastoma of the upper tibia.

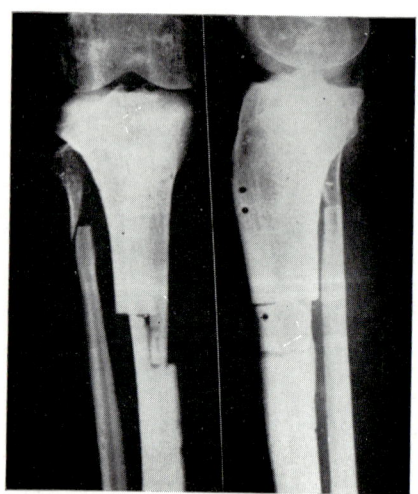
Fig. 45. After resection and transplant.

of the transplant with the host bone was secured, together with restoration of movement in the joint. These patients took full weight and had virtually normal limbs. These results are due to the compression technique of fixation; by using Gudushauri's compression apparatus we were able to begin movements after only one month.

Example 1. Patient P.A. had a recurrence of an osteoclastoma of the tibia (Fig. 44); the affected part of the bone was resected and a transplant substituted (Fig. 45). The ligaments were re-attached and the transplant fixed by Gudushauri's apparatus. Two months later, when the compression apparatus was removed, the tibia felt clinically solid. A knee-hinged plaster was applied and the patient discharged.

Figure 46 shows the patient at three years from operation when he had good function of the limb.

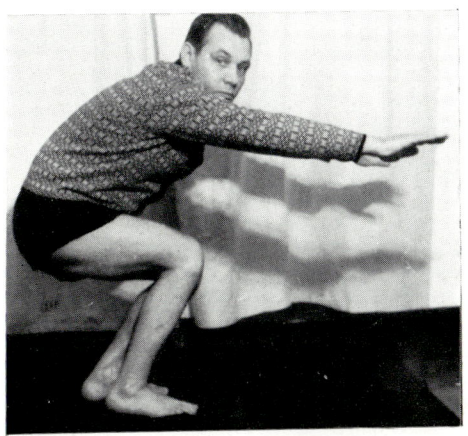

FIG. 46. Range 3 years later.

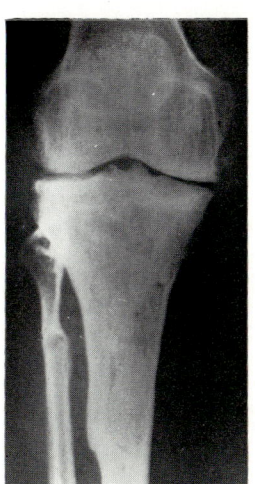 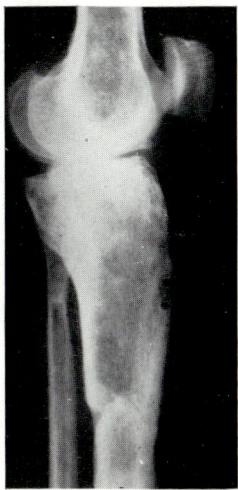

FIG. 47. Appearance 8 years after operation.

An X-ray after eight years (Fig. 47) shows that the transplant has retained its shape and structure, and is firmly united to the host bone.

Example 2. A woman L.S. came to C.I.T.O. on October 5th, 1960, with a large osteoclastoma of the left tibia (Fig. 48). The tumour had a soap-bubble appearance and was clearly demarcated from the rest of the bone; the lateral condyle looked crushed and the joint space reduced. On the 21st October, 1960, the proximal end of the tibia was resected and replaced by a transplant fixed by means of Gudushauri's apparatus.

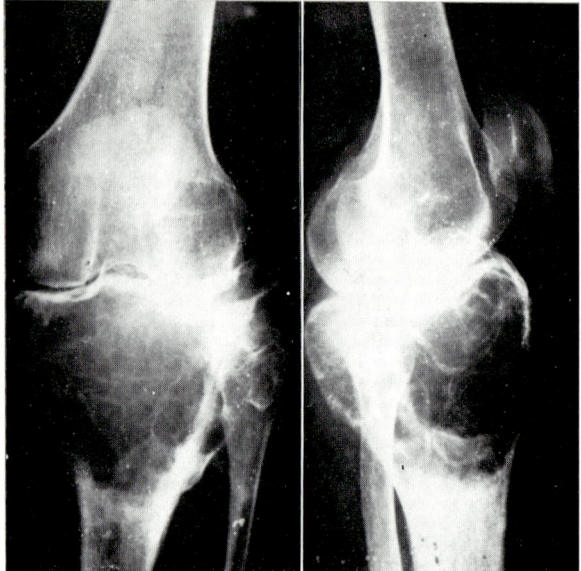

Fig. 48. Osteoclastoma of the upper tibia.

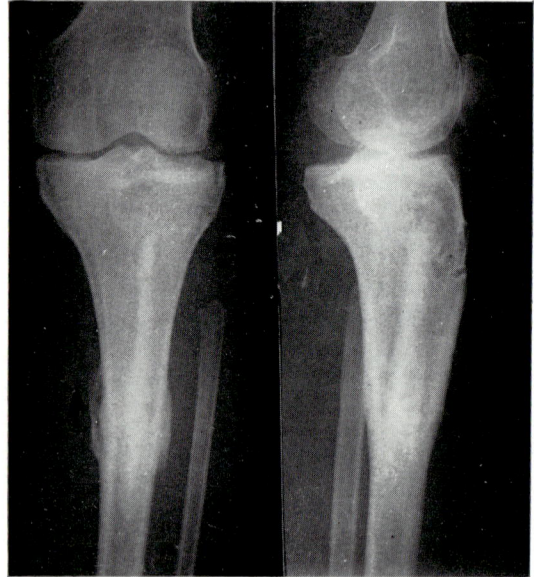

Fig. 49. The same patient 6 years after transplant.

The ligaments were re-attached. A plaster was applied extending up to the groin, and the compression wires cleaned daily with spirit.

Three months after operation the plaster was removed. The wound had healed by first intention, but alongside the scar where she had had X-ray therapy there was a radiation ulcer covered by a dry crust. For a

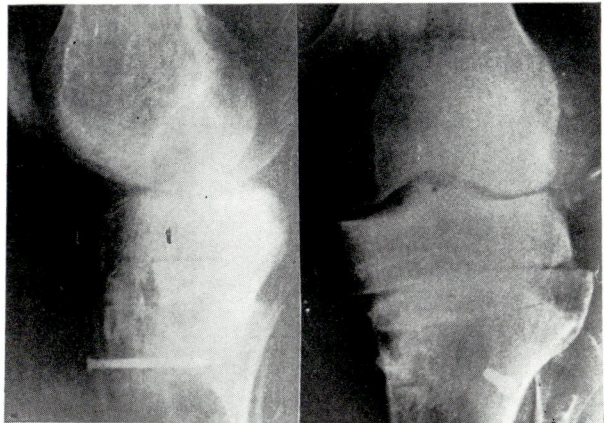

FIG. 50. Soon after upper tibial transplant.

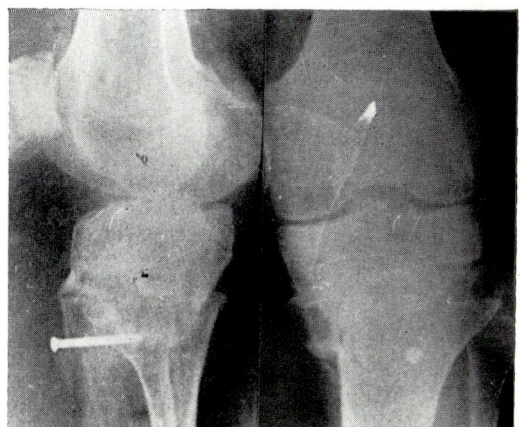

FIG. 51. The same patient 2 years later.

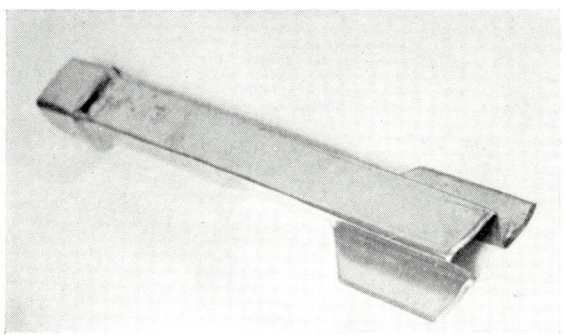

FIG. 52. The specially-designed chisel.

further month the compression was retained and knee movements continued; by now the range was 180°–140°. Gudushauri's apparatus was then removed, there being sound clinical union. A knee-hinged plaster was applied and she walked with crutches. The radiation ulcer was slowly healing; it now measured 2 × 2 cm. At 18 months from operation she was taking full weight on the leg. Movement at the knee was 180° to 90°.

An X-ray six years after operation (Fig. 49) shows that the transplant has retained its shape and structure, and is firmly united with the host bone. The joint space is normal.

Example 3. The patient, a miner aged 29, had sustained a compound fracture of the proximal end of the tibia with ligamentous damage. The

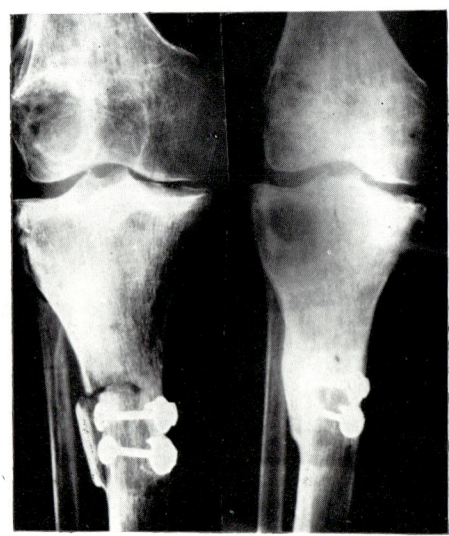

FIG. 53.   FIG. 54.

Eighteen months after operation (Fig. 53) the gap between transplant and host is still visible; at 3 years (Fig. 54) it has filled in completely.

fracture united with gross displacement, and the joint was so lax that he wore a leather splint. At C.I.T.O. the deformed articular end of the tibia was replaced by a transplant (Fig. 50), and the ligamentous connections restored. He began passive movements six weeks after the operation, and at three months was walking in a hinged plaster. At the end of a year he was back at light work with a fully stable limb, and Fig. 51 shows the X-ray at two years. In his case we used a 'swallow-tail' saw-cut; this was done with a special chisel, made by ourselves (Fig. 52). With it we were able to obtain accurate contiguity which resulted in good bony union.

In another transplant of the proximal end of the tibia, metal screws were used for fixation, together with a 'Russian lock' type of saw-cut. The transplant united with the host bone but a visible gap remained (Fig. 53), which took three years to fill in (Fig 54). The patient could

Fig. 55. Patient I.R. before operation.

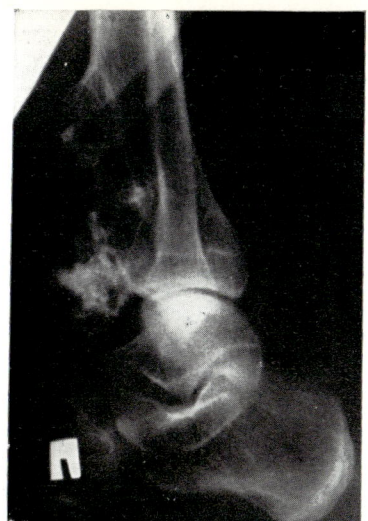

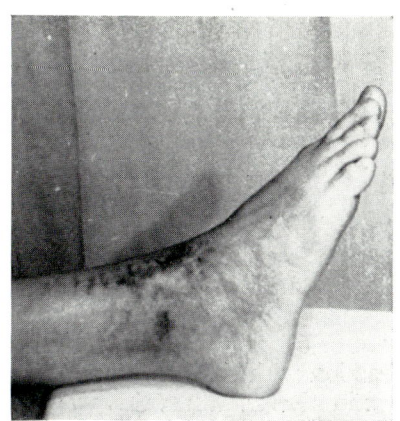

Fig. 56.

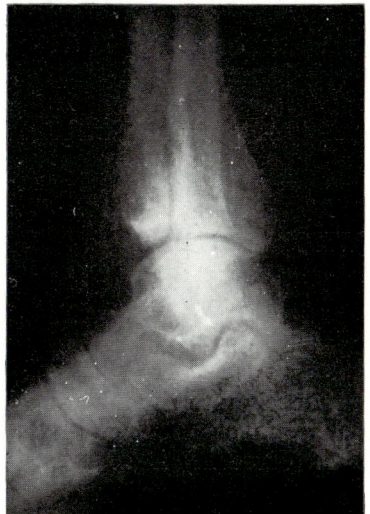

Fig. 57.
Range of movement (Fig. 56) and X-ray (Fig. 57) 2 years later.

use his limb but the knee range was only 20°–30° and we therefore excluded this case from the group of satisfactory results.

Distal end of tibia and fibula. On three patients we performed transplants of the distal end of the tibia. One with a transplant of only the medial side of the lower tibia has started work again. The other two also had good clinical and X-ray results.

Example. I.R. 37 years old, an office worker, came to C.I.T.O. on 9th June, 1959, with a tumour of the distal end of the right tibia. X-ray (Fig. 55) showed a broadly-based cauliflower-shaped tumour, with a well-defined outline and measuring 12·5 × 2·5 cm. It contained scattered islets of calcification, and the cortex was perforated. An osteochondroma was diagnosed. The tumour with part of the lower tibia was removed and the defect replaced by a transplant.

Two years later he could use the leg normally, taking full weight with no pain. Joint movements were satisfactory (Fig. 56). On X-ray (Fig. 57) the junction of transplant with host bone was invisible, the distal end of the tibia correctly shaped and the joint space normal.

THE FAILURE OF A FRESH TRANSPLANT

A patient S. aged 20, came to the C.I.T.O. polyclinic on 11th August, 1960, because of pain and stiffness of the left hip. The limb was wasted, and though hip movements were painless there was gross telescoping. She stated that six years earlier, in Kharkov, a resection had been done of the proximal part of the femur because of a tumour (Fig. 58a). The defective part had been made good by an articular transplant (Fig. 58b) taken from a cadaver a few hours before operation. The distal end of the transplant had been wedged into the medulla of the host femur, and a hip spica applied. Judging by the X-ray after 6·5 months (Fig. 58c) the transplant was being absorbed at the junction with the host bone.

For two-and-a-half years she got about in plaster. When this was removed, she gradually adapted herself to walking with a stick. Shortening was marked and she wore a surgical boot. An X-ray 3·6 years later (Fig. 58d) showed that the transplant had completely disappeared.

In this case we see that the fresh unfrozen articular transplant disappeared without trace. Absorption began at 5–6 months and was complete by the middle of the second year. This confirms what was demonstrated in our experimental work about the inadvisability of using fresh, unfrozen transplants.

TRANSPLANTATION OF WHOLE JOINTS

The data from our experimental research in transplanting articular bone ends preserved at low temperatures had been confirmed by clinically successful results; consequently we felt justified in performing the first transplant of a whole knee joint.

It is not our aim in this account to delve deeply into the theoretical question of transplanting whole joints: a group of doctors (M. V. Volkov, S. A. Imamaliev, Tatishvili, V. I. Varcobin) is at present

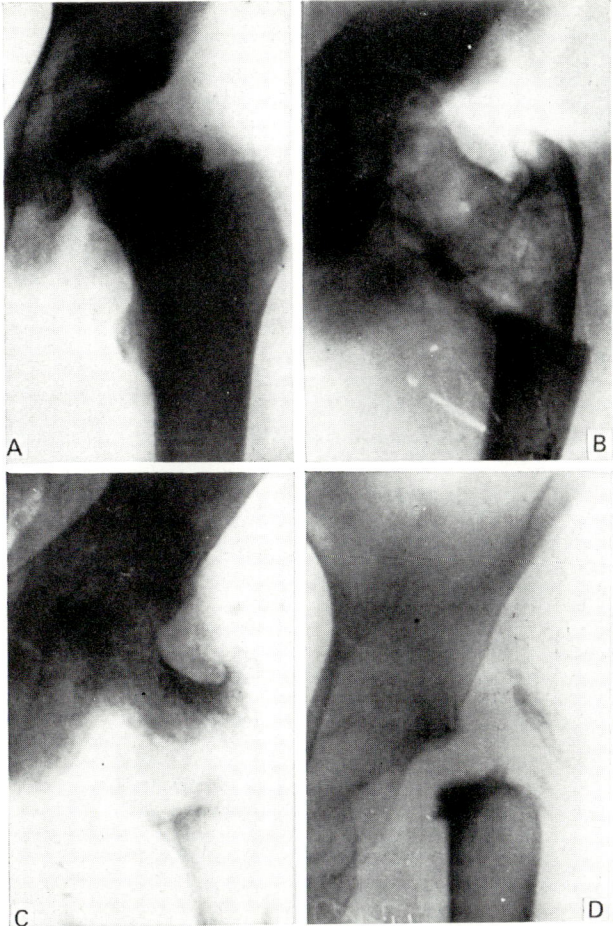

Fig. 58. (A) The original appearance; (B) a fresh articular transplant had been inserted; (C) 6½ months later absorption is occurring, and (D) at 3½ years the transplant has absorbed completely.

studying the problem. We have had both successes and failures in this field and here only certain aspects are discussed.

Techniques

In C.I.T.O. various techniques for transplanting whole joints were suggested; all were aimed at producing complete immobilization between the transplant and the recipient, while preserving movement in the transplanted joint. X-rays of the cadaveric joints permit careful matching of the dimensions of the donor's joint with the recipient.

Knee joint. The cadaver's knee is exposed through a curved anterior incision. The entire joint capsule is excised. The patellar ligament is cut, leaving a stump of 1·5 cm. attached to the tibia. The collateral ligaments are preserved; the lateral ligament is divided near its attachment to the fibula and at transplantation is sewn to the recipient's fibula. The bones are cut transversely with a Gigli saw. The transplant, sealed in a sterile vessel, is placed in a refrigerator at $-70°C$. It is stored for not less than a month and not more than six months. Before use it is placed in a physiological solution saturated with antibiotics.

The transplant operation is performed under general anaesthesia. The joint is exposed and the capsule (as far as the underlying disorder permits) is carefully preserved. The femur and tibia are cut through with a Gigli saw. The femur just proximal to the saw cut is held up with a bone hook and, with the help of a bone elevator, first the distal femur then the proximal end of the tibia are exposed. The elevator must hug the bone to

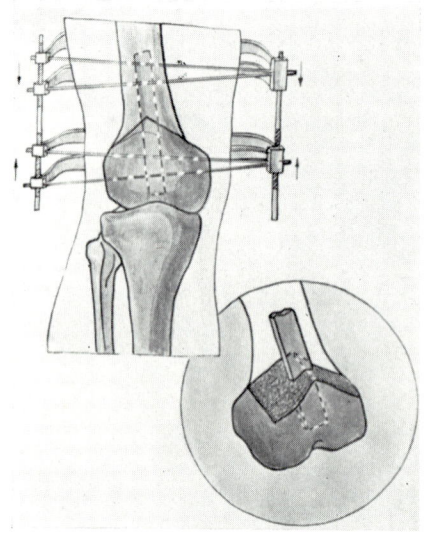

FIG. 59. Gudushauri's compression apparatus and a bone peg.

avoid damaging vessels. The patella is displaced, complete with its ligament which is carefully preserved; this step is important in the subsequent restoration of joint movement. After resecting the joint the cut ends of the femur and tibia are shaped with an electric saw to the form of a 'swallow tail'. The transplant, cut in a similar way so that it matches for shape and size, is fitted into position in the recipient. The patella is then replaced in its correct position, and the capsule and skin are sutured. In some cases the head of the fibula hindered correct positioning of the joint; if so the head was resected, carefully preserving the lateral popliteal nerve.

Fixation of the bones can be achieved in various ways. Figure 59 shows Gudushauri's compression method combined with a bone peg, for proximal fixation of the transplant.

When compression fixation has been used the leg is placed in a functional splint after operation and movements are begun at the end of the first month. The appliance is removed after 2-3 months, but the limb must be protected with a knee-hinged caliper for at least a year from operation.

Hip joint. The cadaver's hip is exposed by an incision along the femur and up to the iliac crest. The capsule is removed. With a wide chisel the pelvic bone is cut about 1·5–2 cm. proximal to the acetabular margin. The muscles attached to the greater and lesser trochanters are separated from the bone, and the femur is cut with a Gigli saw. The separated joint is placed in a sterile container and preserved as already described.

The recipient's hip joint is exposed using Kocher's incision. The greater trochanter is cut with a chisel and, with its attached muscles, is

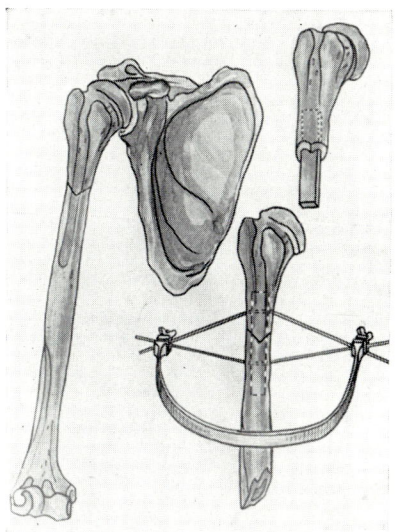

Fig. 60. Griffenstein's technique.

retracted upwards. The region of the hip joint is freed from soft tissues and the femoral shaft exposed for a length of 12–15 cm.; it is divided by a long oblique saw-cut. The acetabulum is cleared of pathological tissue and its margins defined. At about 1·2–1·5 cm. from the margin, square cuts are made with a broad chisel; the shape and size must correspond to those of the donor hip. Taking great care not to damage pelvic structures the recipient's hip is removed and the transplant placed in the prepared site. The proximal end of the transplant is sutured in position and, at its distal end it is fixed to the recipient's femur with two transverse screws or with bone pegs. The greater trochanter with its muscles is attached to the transplant. The wound is sutured in layers and drained for 3–5 days. A plaster spica is worn for 3–4 months.

Shoulder joint. The method of fixation is similar to that used for the knee. Figure 60 shows Griffenstein's technique; if a thoraco-brachial cast is used for $2\frac{1}{2}$ to 3 months after operation, then a stout intra-medullary bone peg may provide adequate fixation.

Illustrative Case Histories

Case 1. A female patient, Kh. N., 20 years old, came to C.I.T.O. with complete absence of the knee joint, which eight years previously had been resected because of a synovioma. She could not use the leg but walked with a crutch. The limb was 9–10 cm. short, the knee region flail, and the muscles grossly wasted.

At operation a crescentic incision was used to expose the affected area. The bone ends were freshened and the defect made good with a whole knee transplant. As the patient's patella was absent, its ligament was imperfect, but a new one, made from fascia lata was attached to the tibial crest. The transplant bone and the host bone were fixed together

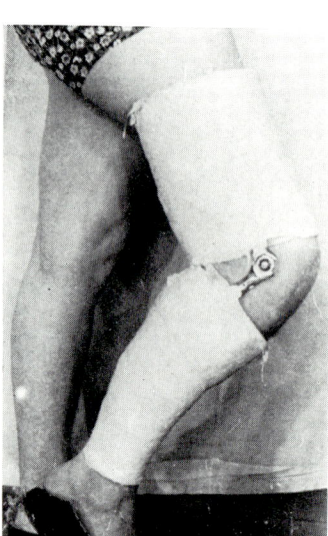

FIG. 61. Hinged plaster.

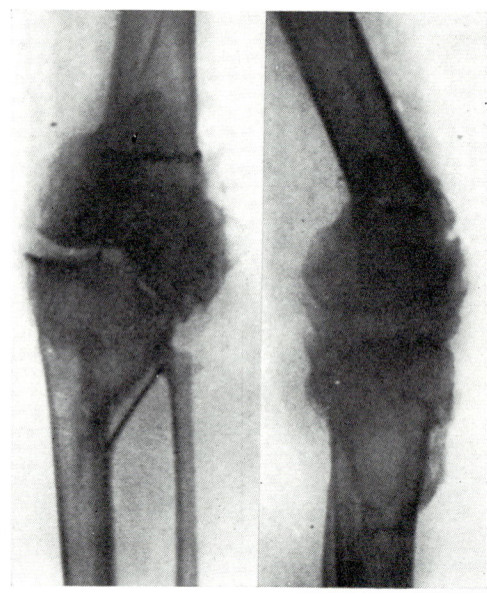

FIG. 62. Three years after whole knee transplant.

with two of Gudushauri's apparati, and the leg cradled in a Böhler splint.

At two weeks the stitches were removed; healing was taking place by first intention. Movements were started in the knee joint. After three months the apparati were removed and a hinged plaster applied (Fig. 61). After eight months the patient was walking and taking weight on the limb without auxiliary support.

Three years have passed: the patient has finished at technical school and works on production. The knee joint has $45°–50°$ of movement. There is 4 cm of shortening but no pain. X-rays show that the transplant has retained its shape and structure (Fig. 62).

Case 2. In the Volokolam hospital a patient had a tuberculous knee resected and replaced by a whole knee joint transplant (G. G. Tatishvili).

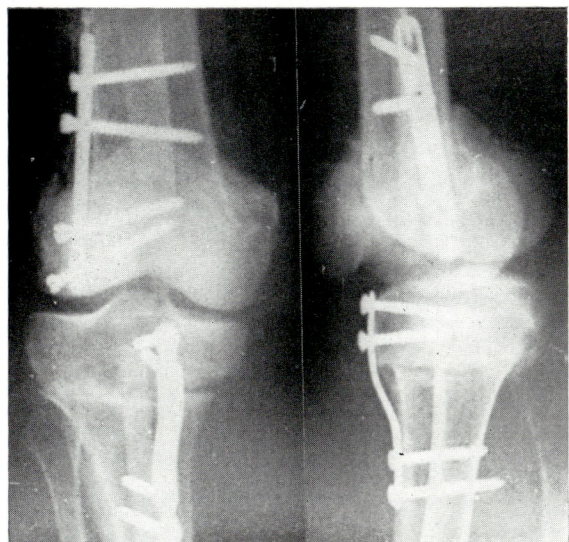

Fig. 63. Whole knee transplant fixed with plates and screws.

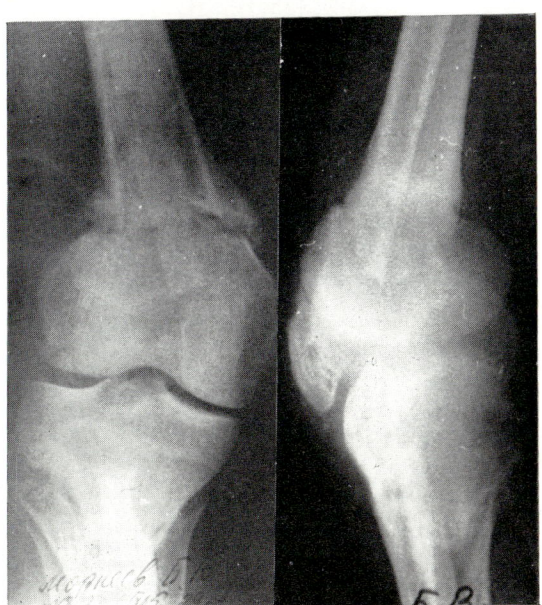

Fig. 64. Whole knee transplant fixed with intramedullary bone peg.

In this instance fixation was achieved by bone pegs augmented by compression produced by four metal wires with tension on two arcs.

Case 3. This patient, aged 23, had had a whole knee transplant following resection for tubercular infection; in this case fixation was achieved by plates and screws (M. V. Volkov. Fig. 63).

Case 4. V. I. Varsobin (at the Volokolam hospital) suggested fixing whole knee transplants with only intra-medullary bone pegs and plaster, as was done in the case of patient G.T. aged 32 (Fig. 64).

The above cases illustrate differing methods of fixation. In this new field the search for better methods is continuing and as yet we are undecided which is best.

Case 5. A female aged 33 had been operated on five years earlier for a tuberculous hip. The femoral head was removed and arthrodesis attempted using a trifin nail. The arthrodesis failed and the patient had

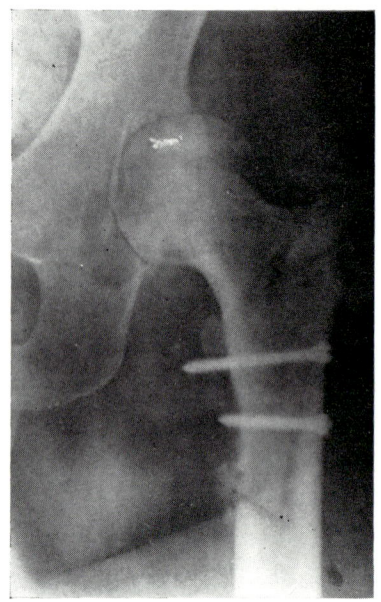

FIG. 65. Whole hip transplant.

pathological movement at the hip, could not use her leg, and walked with crutches. A total hip transplant was performed using the method already described (Fig. 65).

These are of course only individual cases, without a prolonged follow-up; but they do represent the first experiments in transplantation of whole joints which have been preserved at low temperatures. We wish to share with other specialists some of our data on this very important problem.

ERRORS AND COMPLICATIONS

This section contains an analysis of the errors and complications which arose in 88 patients who had articular bone end transplants performed at C.I.T.O. between 1957 and 1965.

A limited amount of literature on the subject is available in publications by E. L. Krupko, S. S. Tkachenko, A. A. Korj, R. R. Talishinsky and others. They, however, highlight one complication or another, giving no full appraisal of the problem as a whole. In order to present a more detailed picture we have divided the errors and complications into groups.

Group I. *Pre-operative mistakes.* This comprises those patients who were incorrectly assessed and in whom there was some definite contra-indication to transplantation.

Group II. *Operative mistakes and complications.*
(1) Incorrect choice of transplant (wrong size or shape, wrong age of donor, etc.)
(2) Inadequate fixation.
(3) Fracture.
(4) Imperfect restoration of ligaments.

Group III. *Post-operative complications.*
(1) Suppuration.
(2) Displacement of the transplant.
(3) Fracture of the fixing apparatus.
(4) Absorption of the transplant (immunological reactions).
(5) Laxity of the joint.
(6) Deforming arthrosis.
(7) Recurrence of the tumour.

Group I. Pre-operative errors. These stem from operating in the presence of contra-indications, such as: an inflammatory process in the region of the proposed operation (or a possible latent infection, e.g. a foreign body); extensive ulceration or scarring; injuries to peripheral nerves and muscles; the condition of soft tissues after massive irradiation (more than 12,000 r.); and the patient's age (which, for success, should be over 14 and under 50 years). One patient, for example, had a transplant following a gunshot wound of the hip, with shot still lodged in the soft tissues. Suppuration ensued, evidently due to lighting up a latent infection, and the transplant was rejected. Two other patients had transplants after X-ray therapy (27,000 and 12,000 r.); six to eight days later necrosis occurred, followed by secondary infection which led to rejection of the transplant.

In yet another patient, a woman, we have been battling with an ulcer after radiotherapy; this ulcer took six months to heal. Despite this complication, the result of the transplant was satisfactory in that the patient has a useful weight-bearing leg; but knee movements are restricted, the range being 30°–35°. The infection was confined to the soft tissues (which made it possible to retain the transplant), but because of the ulcer, knee movements were started very late.

A malignant tumour is a contra-indication to joint transplantation; only if amputation is categorically refused should transplantation be considered. One operation failed because of incorrect histological diagnosis. A suspected osteoclastoma of the femur was removed and a transplant substituted. The post-operative period was uneventful, but after four months a swelling appeared in the soft tissues and amputation was performed. Renewed histological investigation revealed malignancy; the patient died after a few months.

We had the opportunity of examining the X-rays of a 16-year-old patient from the Kirov Hospital who had the distal end of his femur replaced by a transplant from a 14-year-old donor. A year later the structure of the transplant was faulty and part of it had completely absorbed; arthrodesis proved necessary. Our experimental work with dogs (already described) and the work of M. G. Prives (1938) had demonstrated that young donors with incompletely ossified epiphyses should not be used for transplants.

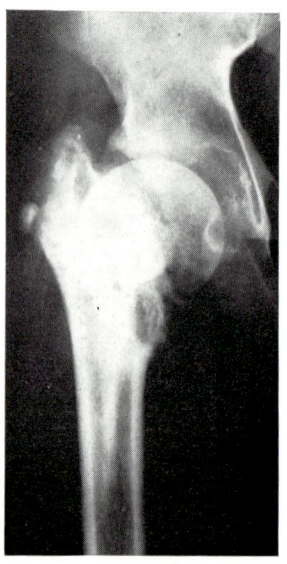

Fig. 66. Fracture and displacement after an ill-fitting transplant.

Group II. Mistakes and complications occurring at operation.
It is important that the transplant should match the host for shape and size. The patient M., for example, had a transplant following resection of the proximal end of the femur for osteoclastoma. The dimensions of the transplanted femoral head did not match those of the socket and as a sequel the neck fractured and became displaced (Fig. 66). It is also important that the transplant should be slightly smaller than the part removed; if it is too long tension in the surrounding soft tissues damages the articular cartilage.

Lack of correspondence between the articular surfaces of transplant and recipient (because of inaccurate bone cuts) leads to deforming arthrosis with severely limited movement. One patient, for example, with an osteoclastoma of the lateral tibial condyle, had this condyle replaced by a transplant at C.I.T.O.; the saw-cuts were inaccurately adjusted so that there was lack of correspondence between the articular surfaces. Seven years after operation, the patient could walk but the knee was painful and has only 20° of movement; the X-rays showed deforming arthrosis.

To avoid joint laxity it is important to pay careful attention to the capsule and ligaments. If the host capsule cannot be retained a new one can form from the surrounding tissues in 1–2 months. With regard to the

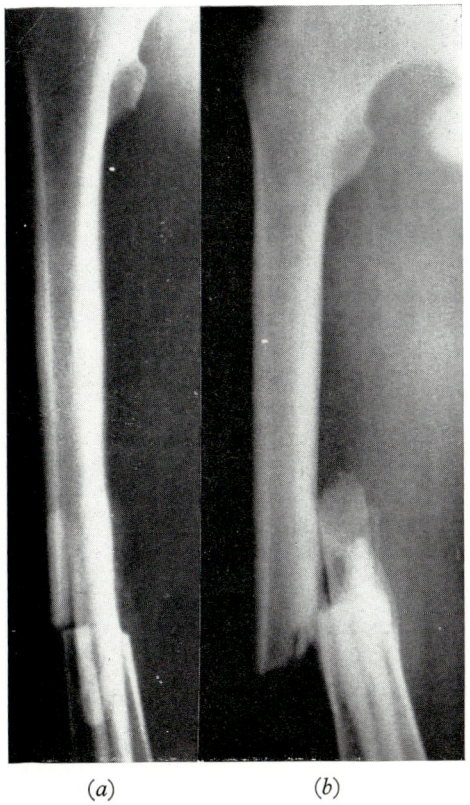

(a)   (b)

FIG. 67. (a) Transplant of the upper femur fixed with a bone peg, which (b) has subsequently fractured.

ligaments, those of the transplant are, as our experimental work showed, quite adequate to preserve joint stability.

Serious complications arise from inadequate fixation of the transplant to the host bone; sound union is essential. At the same time, for restoration of joint function it is imperative to begin movements early. Inadequate fixation may result in a pseudarthrosis at the bony junction; moreover, with inadequate fixation external splintage needs to be prolonged, with consequent failure to regain joint movement. These complications develop when an intramedullary bone peg breaks, especially as the fracture is liable to occur just when joint movement should be encouraged, i.e. 2–4 months after operation. The patient M., for example, had the proximal half of the femur replaced by a transplant with fixation by an intramedullary bone peg. As can be seen in Fig. 67 the peg broke and displacement followed. The intramedullary bone peg fractured in 13 cases; in these splintage had to be prolonged and this led to poor joint movement (and sometimes to union in poor position); reconstruction of the transplant in these circumstances was significantly delayed. Out of these 13 patients, the results in six were bad and only seven were satisfactory.

Group III. Post-operative complications. These may be early (during the first two months) or late (months, or even years after operation).

An important post-operative complication is an infected haematoma (8–9 per cent); the idea that haematoma leads to infection is confirmed

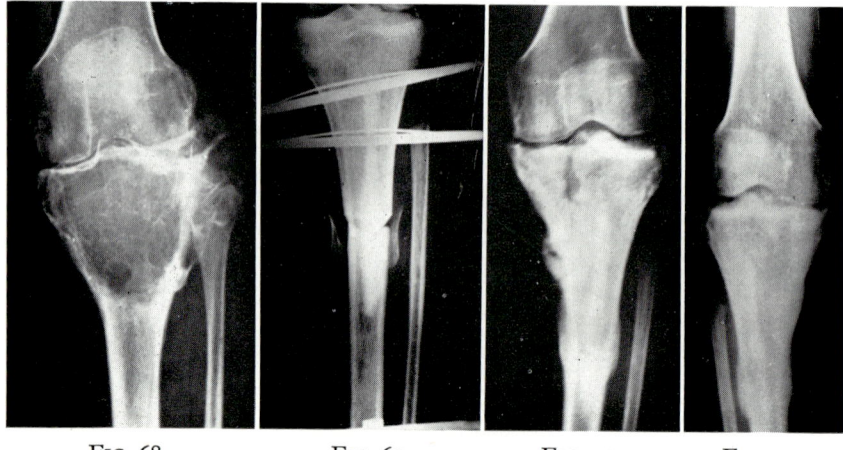

Fig. 68.   Fig. 69.   Fig. 70.   Fig. 71.

Patient S. (Fig. 68) the original osteoclastoma; (Fig. 69) soon after transplant, showing the fixation; (Fig. 70) fracture sustained 3 years later; (Fig. 71) complete healing subsequently occurred.

by the fact that six out of eight cases of infection occurred at the hip or the distal end of the femur; in both sites the bulk of muscle predisposes to haematoma. (Hence the value of drainage for 1–2 days.) All eight cases of infection had traceable causes. These included a flare following an old gunshot wound, infection following prolonged use of Gudushauri's apparatus and secondary infection of an irradiation ulcer. The subject of infection in bone and joint transplants is a separate and complicated problem, which should be specially investigated because the cause of late infection is not yet understood.

In one case a transplant fractured three years after operation. It was peculiar in that the transplant fractured vertically at a distance from the host bone. After immobilization complete bony union occurred and joint movements were regained, demonstrating that even after three years the transplant had retained its osteogenic qualities. This patient, S., a female, came to C.I.T.O. in 1960 with an osteoclastoma of the tibia (Fig. 68). The proximal tibia was resected and replaced by a transplant (Fig. 69). A year later she could take full weight and had good knee movement. Then, at three years from operation, she fell from a train, sustaining the fracture shown in Fig. 70. After three months in plaster she regained full use of the leg. Now, seven years after operation, she uses the leg normally and has full knee range. The X-ray (Fig. 71) shows restoration of the upper tibia, healing of the fracture without trace, and a reasonable joint space.

Absorption of the transplant was observed when the surgical technique was faulty or the preservation period too short. Experimentally we had found that the optimum period of low-temperature storage was 4–5 weeks.

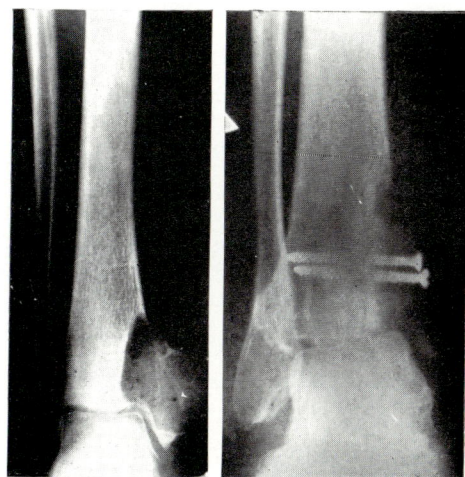

Fig. 72.   Fig. 73.

Patient E.Z. (Fig. 72) original appearance; (Fig. 73) after transplant partial absorption is occurring.

When it was as short as two weeks the transplants underwent absorption at 6–8 months; substitution did eventually follow, but it was only partial. Clinically these findings were confirmed in three patients, two of whose case histories are quoted below.

One patient, E.Z., had the lesion shown in Fig. 72. He was given a transplant which had been preserved for only 13 days. Satisfactory union with the host took place, and he could walk normally with good ankle movement; the X-ray, however (Fig. 73), shows partial absorption.

Another patient, L.V., had a transplant preserved for 14 days; not only was the preservation period too short, but in this case the surgical technique also was inadequate. She was a 46-year-old housewife who came to C.I.T.O. on 18th August, 1958, with a painful bony swelling of the left fifth metacarpal (Fig. 74). On the 10th September, 1958, a transplant was substituted for the diseased bone. The saw-cut in the host bone was Z-shaped, and the transplant was attached to it by two catgut stitches. X-ray after operation (Fig. 75) shows that the tumour was completely removed and the defect filled by the transplant which fits the host bone accurately. Two weeks later, when the plaster was changed, a check X-ray showed lack of contact between host and transplant. The X-ray a year later (Fig. 76) shows the transplant partly absorbed.

A transplant is, of course, eventually absorbed, and substituted by material from the host; but the processes of absorption and substitution must be synchronous. This synchrony is of paramount importance, and

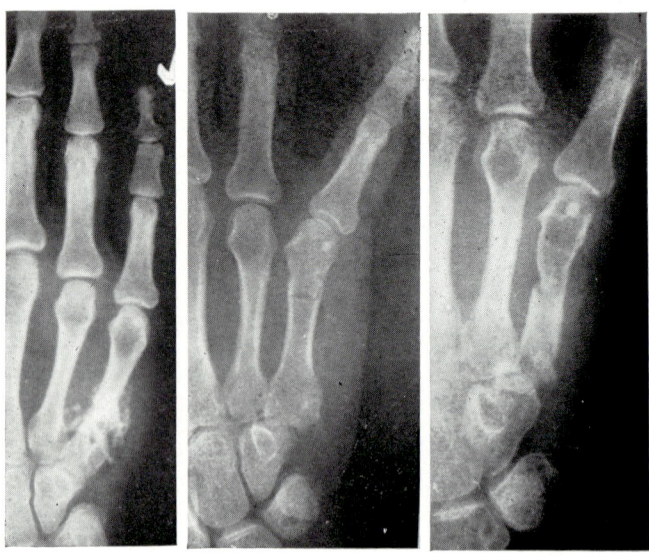

FIG. 74. FIG. 75. FIG. 76.

Patient L.V. (Fig. 74) original appearance; (Fig. 75) after replacement by a transplant; (Fig. 76) partial absorption at 1 year.

one cause of premature absorption is faulty preservation; our experiments on dogs taught us that, for articular bone ends, the optimum was 25–30 days at a temperature of $-70°C$.

Joint laxity, leading to subluxation or dislocation has already been referred to; it follows inadequate restoration of ligaments, and may also occur if movements and weight-bearing are started too early.

Joint stiffness is often the sequel to prolonged immobilization; if bony fixation is inadequate then external splintage may have to be prolonged and joint mobilization not started till very late. In fact, out of 88 transplants, some stiffness occurred in 24 cases.

Mal-union is sometimes a problem. Thus, a transplant of the proximal end of the tibia was performed on patient B after the removal of an osteoclastoma (Fig. 77). The intramedullary bone peg subsequently fractured (Fig. 78); after prolonged immobilization the bones united, but in this faulty position (Fig. 79). Angulation continued during the process of substitution of the transplant, and the patient ended up with deformity and limited movement of the knee.

When compression methods were used to fix transplants of the proximal tibia the results were much better; the firm fixation permitted early joint movement. Compression techniques are indicated in transplants of the tibia and the upper humerus, but not for the femur where its use may predispose to infection.

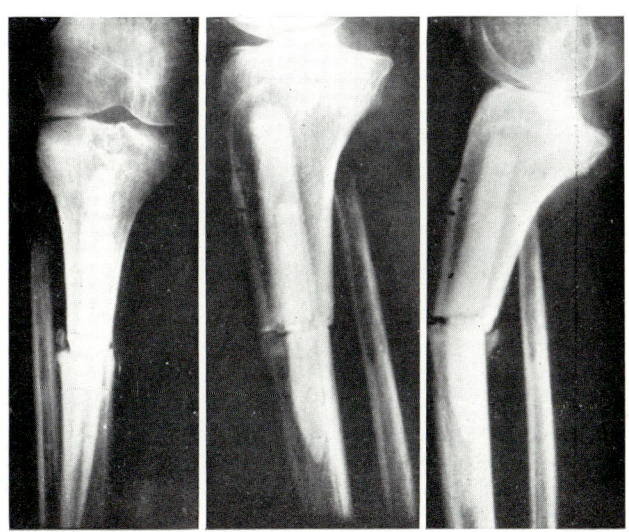

FIG. 77.   FIG. 78.   FIG. 79.

Patient B. (Fig. 77) transplant of upper tibia; (Fig. 78) the intramedullary peg has broken; (Fig. 79) shows the angulation which followed.

Conclusions

(1) All the errors and complications in transplanting articular bone ends can be divided into three groups: (a) Pre-operative; (b) Operative; and (c) Post-operative.

(2) These complications arise in connection with: (a) technical errors; (b) wound infections; and (c) incompatibility between donor and recipient.

Technical errors have been discussed; we feel strongly that strict adherence to the correct technique significantly reduces complications.

Infections also have been considered. They may arise early (in the first 2–3 weeks), or late; late infection is a complex problem needing further research.

Incompatibility is of special interest. Modern techniques enable surgeons to perform complicated transplant operations, but the secret of success lies in overcoming tissue incompatibility. Our work with dogs demonstrated that transplants of articular bone ends were accepted providing they had been preserved at a temperature of $-70°C$, ideally for 25–30 days.

(3) Out of 88 patients who received transplants of articular bone ends, the results were: 17 poor, 25 satisfactory and 46 good.

References*

ABALMASOVA, E. A. (1956). Experimental transplantation of bone homoio-transplants preserved at low temperatures. *Diss. Cand. M.*

BARKOV, YU, I. (1955). On the organisation, preparation and preservation of homoioplastic osseous and cartilaginous transplants at low temperatures. *Vestnik Khirurg.* i/n Grekov.

BAXTER, H. and ENTIN, M. A. (1951). Clinical Study of Fate of Autografts in Man. *Amer. J. Surg.*, **81,** 285.

BLOKHIN, V. N. (1955). Skin plastic surgery.

BREDIKHIN, I. A. (1862). On the revival of bone out of the periosteum generally and in particular after resection. Moscow.

BUSH, L. (1947). The use of homogenous bone grafts. *J. Bone Jt. Surg.*, **29,** 3 620–628.

CHAKLIN, V. D. (1961). Physiological and clinical bases and methods in bone plastic surgery. *Tez. dokladi:* 2nd All-union Conference of surgeons, traumatologists, etc. Moscow, 44.

CHASE, S. and HERNDON, C. (1955). The fate of autogenous and homogenous bone grafts. *J. Bone Jt. Surg.*, **37A,** 4, 809–841.

FEDOTENKOV, A. G. (1959). Mass organisation for preparation and preservation of cattle cartilage for use in plastic surgery. *Vestnik Khirurg.*, **81,** 10.

FILATOV, A. N. (1958). The problem of the transplantation of tissues and organs at the present time. *Vestnik Khirurg.*, **10,** 3.

FILATOV, V. P. (1933). Transplantation of cornea. *Sovet. vestnik oftal.*, **2,** 136.

GINSBURG, I. S. (1925). Bone surgery of the spine. Baku.

GINSBURG, R. L. (1946). Pseudo-arthroses of the long tubular bones and their treatment. *Diss. Doct. M.* **t,** 1–3.

GOLOVIN, G. V. (1956). Bone homoioplastic surgery. *Vestnik Khirurg.*, **9,** 100.

HERBERT, J. (1949). Les possibilites de greffes homogenes et la conservation doess. *Sem. Hôp. Paris*, **6,** 2776.

IMAMALIEV, A. S. (1959). Problems of semi-joint transplantation. *Ortop. travm. protez.*, Moscow, **19,** 5, 62.

IMAMALIEV, A. S. (1962). Hemi-articular transplants in experimental and clinical conditions. *Ortop. travm. protez.* **23,** 9, 15.

IMAMALIEV, A. S. (1962). Homoioplastic surgery of articular bone endings. *Diss. Doct.* 1–2 M.

INCLAN, A. (1942). The use of preserved bone graft in orthopaedic surgery. *J. Bone Jt. Surg.*, **24,** 1, 81–96.

JUDET, H. (1908). Essai sur la greffe des tissues articulaires. *C. R. Acad. Clerm.-Ferrand*, **146,** 193–196; 600–603.

JUDET, J. and JUDET, R. (1954). Animal bone grafts in human surgery. *Acta Orthop. Belg.*, **19,** 4, 135.

KOVALENKO, P. P. (1953). Preserved cadaveric cartilage and its application to restorative surgery. *Diss. Cand.*, Rostov on Don.

KRUPKO, I. L. (1960). The effect of preserved cadaveric bone on the regeneration of bone tissue. *Trudi IV Vseukrainsk Sezda Traumatolog., Ortoped. Kiev.*, 209.

KÜTTNER, H. (1913). Einige Dauerresultate der Transplantation aus der Leiche. *Arch. klin. Chir.*, **102,** 48–56.

LEXER, E. (1908). Über Gelenktransplantation. *Arch. klin. Chir.*, **90,** 2, 263–278.

NADEIN, A. P. and SAVCHIK, A. B. (1960). Preservation of homoio-tissue in sterile paraffin. Short extracts from proceedings of conference on the use of articular transplants in surgery. Leningrad, 23.

NOVACHENKO, N. P. (1946). Vascularisation of transplanted bone. Kiev-Kharkov.

OLLIER, Z. (1867). Traite experimental et clinique de la regeneration des os et de la production artificielle du tissu osseux. Paris.

ORELL, S. (1931). Experimental chirurgische Studie über Knochentransplantate und ihre Anwendung in der praktischen Chirurgie (Vorläufige Mitteilung). *Dtsch. Z. Chir.*, **232,** 701–713.

PANOVA, M. I. (1960). On the preservation and transplantation of homoio-tissues. *Khirurg.*, **6,** 84–88.

Pavlov-Silvanski, V. N. (1914). The problem of free plastic surgery of joints. *Khirurg.*, **36,** 211, p. 62.

Penski, Yu. R. Experiments in transplantation of articular surfaces of the epiphyses. Kharkov, 1893.

Pepper, F. J. (1954). Studies on the viability of mammalian skin autografts after storage at different temperatures. *Brit. J. Plastic Surg.* **6,** 4, 241.

Petraschews, K. A case of free transplantation of half a joint. *Abstr. Intern. Surg.*, 1913, **17,** 525.

Priorov, N. N. Bone plastic surgery. *Trudi Tsentraln. Inst. Traumatalog. i. Ortoped.* T. 1 – 2 M., 1946.

Priorov, N. N. (1960). Theory and practice of transplantation of bones and joints. *Trudi IV Sezda Ukrainsk. Traumatolog. i. Ortoped. Kiev.*, 103.

Prives, M. G. (1938). The blood supply of the long tubular bones in man. *Vestnik Khirurg.*, **20,** 175.

Pstrov, N. N. (1913). Free plastic surgery of bones. *Diss. SPB.*

Reynolds, F. and Oliver, D. (1950). Experimental evaluation of homogenous bone grafts. *J. Bone Jt. Surg.*, **32A,** 2, 283–297.

Rob, C. (1954). Preservation and transplantation of human tissues. *Lancet*, **ii,** 225.

Rob, C. (1955). *Surg., Gynec., Obstet.*, **100,** 5, 515.

Sauerbruch, F. *Die Chirurgie der Brustorgane.* 2. Aofl. Bd. 1–2, Berlin, Springer, 1920–1925). Die Erkrankungen der Lunge. XVI, 9319, 111.

Shamov, V. N. and Kostyukov, M. Kh. (1929). The study of homoio-plastic surgery from the cadaver: transfusion of blood from the cadaver. *Novi Khirurg, Arkhiv*, 69–71, **18,** 184.

Shulutko, L. I. (1948). Clinical notes on bone plastic surgery. *Trudi Kazansk nauchno issledovatal. inst. ortoped. i vosstanovitel. Khirurg. Kazan*, 165.

Sicard, A. and Binet, J. P. (1950). La conservation des transplants, osseux et leur emploi en chirurgie. *Pr. med.*, **25,** 443–444.

Timashkevitch, K. D. (1966). A comparative study of bone homografts by various methods. *Byull. eksp. Biol. Med.*, **62,** 93.

Volkov, M. V. (1962). Primary bone tumours in children. Moscow.

Wilson, P. D. (1947). Experiences with a bone bank. *Ann. Surg.* **126,** 932.

Yumashev, G. S. (1957). The clinical use of lyophilised bone homoio-transplants. *Vestnik Khirurg.*, **4,** 65.

Zaichenko, I. L. (1940). The substitution of bone defects by various types of plastic material. *Trudi 2nd Ukrainsk. S. ortoped. Kiev.*, 86.

Zatsepin, S. T. (1961). A method of fixing united bone pieces without the use of metal appliances. *Khirurg.*, **9,** 116.

---

* Some of the names mentioned in the early sections of this chapter are of purely historical interest and were therefore not included in the author's list of references.

Chapter 8

THE ORTHOPAEDIC SURGERY OF CEREBRAL PALSY AND SPINA BIFIDA

W. J. W. SHARRARD

ORTHOPAEDIC SURGERY IN CEREBRAL PALSY

Cerebral palsy comprises all those conditions in which interference with the motor system arises as a result of lesions within the brain. Recent years have seen a better understanding of the multiple handicaps of hearing, sight, speech and mental and emotional function that may accompany the locomotor handicaps of a child suffering from cerebral palsy. Combined management by paediatrician, physiotherapist and orthopaedic surgeon, working together, can achieve more than any one specialist working alone. In the early part of this century, ill-advised, over-enthusiastic and indiscriminate surgery on nerves and tendons, without proper analysis of the paralysis, deformity and function in the affected limb often did as much harm as good. A better understanding by the orthopaedic surgeon of the neurological and paediatric aspects of cerebral palsy has made it possible to rationalize the place of surgical treatment in co-operation with physical medicine specialist, physiotherapist and paediatrician.

The Pathophysiology of Locomotor Disability

The simplest classification of cerebral palsy is that which is based on the manifestations in the limbs, that is by spasticity, athetosis, ataxia, tremor or rigidity. The orthopaedic surgeon is likely to be concerned mainly with those suffering from spastic paralysis, the commonest form of cerebral palsy.

Paresis of voluntary action is an important part of the functional neurological picture in spastic paralysis. In a child with severe spasticity of the calf, for instance, the dorsiflexors of the ankles may be of normal strength in some individuals and of varying degrees of weakness in others. Variations in the pattern of weakness and spasticity in muscle groups in the limbs account for many of the typical problems of locomotion that arise in spastic paralysis.

In hemiplegic involvement, spasticity or weakness are seldom seen at the hip or knee, but spasticity in the triceps surae and weakness of the ankle dorsiflexors is common. In spastic diplegia, there is commonly spasticity in the triceps surae, particularly in the gastrocnemius, associated with weakness of the dorsiflexors of the ankle and spasticity in the adductors with weakness of the abductors of the hip. In spastic quadriplegia, there is commonly spasticity in the hip adductors and flexors, the hamstring muscles and the triceps surae and weakness of the dorsi-flexors of the ankle, the gluteal muscles and the quadriceps. In bilateral affection, the pattern of involvement is usually symmetrical, but the degree of it may differ on the two sides.

A child with cerebral palsy is born without deformity, but deformity may develop at any time from the early months of life. The development of deformity has often been assumed to be due to spasticity alone. An analysis of the relationship between spasticity in the triceps surae and the development of equinus showed that relative weakness of voluntary dorsiflexor power was more closely related to the development of equinus than was spasticity in the triceps surae (Sharrard 1964a); other authors have made similar observations. The relative shortening of muscles and tendons that gives rise to deformity in children suffering from spastic paralysis thus has something in common with deformities that may develop in the same way in poliomyelitis, peripheral nerve lesions and spina bifida (Sharrard 1967a). This finding makes it possible to forecast the liability to the development of deformity and offers a rational basis for the employment of peripheral orthopaedic surgical procedures in cerebral palsy.

Physiotherapy, Bracing and Surgery in Cerebral Palsy

There are few who would nowadays dispute the value of physiotherapy in the management of the limbs in cerebral palsy, though advocates of different systems of treatment abound. The precise effects of physiotherapeutic techniques are very difficult to assess. Children suffering from cerebral palsy who have been denied any kind of physiotherapy, take longer to develop motor function and are more likely to become deformed; but no controlled trial has yet been devised to determine how much of the improvement attributed to any particular treatment arises spontaneously as the result of growth and maturation of nervous function and how much arises from the treatment that has been given.

Correct postures in the control of abnormal reflex activity (Bobath 1961), graduated exercise therapy, hydrotherapy, education in balance and the use of appropriate aids to locomotion all contribute to improved motor function in some measure. Foley (1961) has shown that the stretching of spastic muscles alters the responsiveness of the stretch reflex for short periods and this finding lends support to the value of passive stretching in the management of spastic muscles. It may diminish but cannot completely eliminate the liability to the development of deformity.

Braces, calipers and other forms of external support are used extensively in some centres, but they have some important disadvantages. The weight of a conventional brace is an additional load for an already weak limb to carry. In the presence of severe muscle imbalance, deformity progresses however carefully splintage is applied. The patient comes to rely on the splint and develops habits of gait that may make it almost impossible to discard the brace in later years and a rigid external support does nothing to encourage activity in weak muscles which may become weaker still. If a combination of surgery and physiotherapy correctly applied allows a joint to support itself and eliminates deformity, there is seldom need for external support except for short periods in spastic paralysis or to control unwanted movements in athetoid paralysis.

The main indication for surgical treatment is in the correction of fixed deformity. Deformity that arises in association with paralysis, arises primarily in muscles and tendons and only secondarily involves other soft tissue and finally joints and bone. Progressive limitation of movement at any joint with relative shortening of musculo-tendinous structures should be corrected, if possible, by surgery, when it threatens to impair function and before significant secondary bony deformity or malalignment of joints has occurred.

Until recent years, it has been the usual practice to avoid surgery until the child was older and bone growth was nearing completion, the liability to deformity being controlled as far as possible by the use of plaster, splints and physiotherapy. Surgery in younger children between the ages of two and ten years has now been shown by several workers (Sharrard 1961, 1967a, Thompson 1966, Craig 1967) to give good results, provided that there is careful pre-operative assessment, appropriate and limited soft tissue surgery and good post-operative management and physiotherapy. Less extensive procedures are needed than if surgery is delayed and secondary deformities due to prolonged bad posture and gait do not develop. Thompson (1966) believes that spastic children may benefit from surgery even when there are no contractures, by altering the point at which the stretch reflex is elicited. He feels that the optimum time for surgery is when there is a reasonable expectation that surgery can free the child from external support.

The practice of early preventive surgery demands that care be taken in pre-operative neurological and functional assessment. Decisions to operate should not and need not be made in haste, but should be made on the results of serial observations from the early months of life and in consultation with paediatrician, physiotherapist and parents. Extensive tenotomy, myotomy, neurectomy or tendon transplantation can lead to the opposite deformity and it is better to do a little and be prepared to operate again should the deformity recur. Once a deformity is known to be progressing in spite of adequate conservative measures, it is likely to increase further and more rapidly with time because of the loss of mechanical advantage to the action of the weaker muscles. In these circumstances, neither the age of the child nor, within reasonable limits, lack of intelligence is a contra-indication to surgery.

Craig (1967) notes that lack of head control and lack of balance and equilibrium reactions in all positions are contra-indications to surgery in the lower limbs in a cerebral palsied child. The persistence of strong chronic pathological reflexes in severe spastic or athetoid patients may also be a contra-indication to surgery or diminishes the effectiveness of any surgery that can be offered. For the upper limb, peripheral surgery is much less often appropriate than in the lower limb. Fixed deformity is less liable to develop provided that adequate physiotherapy and occupational therapy are employed.

Pre-operative Assessment

From the time of the diagnosis of spastic paralysis, regular examination should be made of the range of passive movements, the presence of spasticity and the strength of voluntary activity at all joints. In the first two years of life, it may be difficult to make an accurate assessment of voluntary power, but, after this, it should be possible to assess the strength of voluntary action in terms of the Medical Research Council system of muscle grading. Particular attention needs to be paid to the ranges of abduction, extension, medial and lateral rotation of the hip, of extension of the knee and of dorsiflexion, inversion and eversion of the foot and ankle.

Some limitation of movements may be compatible with satisfactory limb function. At the hip, lack of the last 30° of abduction, medial or lateral rotation is not important, but once the range of abduction becomes less than 20°, dislocation is almost certain to develop. More than 25° of flexion deformity, even if compensated by lumbar lordosis, is not acceptable, unless there is severe mental retardation.

At the ankle, loss of up to 30° range of passive dorsiflexion is not important, but any fixed equinus, varus, or valgus should not be allowed to develop. At the knee, not more than 10° or 15° of fixed flexion is acceptable.

Account must always be taken of the effects of deformity at one joint upon other joints. If fixed flexion is allowed to develop at the hip, a child may walk with the knee flexed, but this does not necessarily mean that fixed flexion of the knee is present. Provided that the primary hip deformity is corrected sufficiently soon, secondary fixed flexion of the knee can be avoided.

Once a decision has been made that deformity or impending deformity needs surgical treatment, a precise assessment should be made of the muscles most involved in the deformity. Those that are particularly likely to be short are the psoas, adductor longus, gracilis, semitendinosus, gastrocnemii or peronei. In an older child, or where deformity has existed for two or three years, it may be difficult to differentiate between fixed deformity and severe spasticity. The final decision as to which muscles or tendons should be operated upon may have to be made after the child has been anaesthetized.

Principles of Early Surgical Treatment

The aim of surgery is to correct but not over-correct shortened tissues; to correct muscle imbalance; to improve function, gait and appearance; and to stabilize weak joints. In the early stages of development of deformity, the limitations of movement arise only from shortness of muscles and tendons. Careful elongation of musculo-tendinous structures alone is sufficient to eliminate deformity. Deformity that has been left uncorrected for too long may have resulted in secondary contracture of joint capsules and ligaments which may then also require division or elongation. After even longer, secondary bony deformity may develop and osteotomy be needed, but, with early surgery, operations on bone and joint are not often necessary. Similarly, with early correction of adductor shortening, subluxation of the hip can be corrected easily and dislocation is rare.

Correction of muscle imbalance in spastic paralysis is better achieved by weakening the stronger muscles than by attempting to strengthen the weaker muscles by tendon transplantation. Muscle or tendon elongation, in itself, reduces the power of a muscle by 1 M.R.C. grade. If there is need to diminish the power of the over-acting muscle further, partial neurectomy can be added. Occasionally transfer of a very strong muscle may be appropriate, but great care should be taken in deciding the site to which the tendon is to be transferred.

Sometimes, the main reason for surgery is cosmetic. Tendon elongation or transfer of wrist flexors to the dorsum may not necessarily give great improvement in hand function, but a considerable improvement in social acceptance of the deformity by others and the same considerations apply to arthrodesis of the wrist or thumb joints.

Operative Procedures in the Lower Limb

HIP

The operation most commonly needed at the hip is adductor tenotomy. Occasionally, in a child less than 18 months old, adduction deformity that is threatening to cause dislocation of the hip, may be corrected by subcutaneous adductor tenotomy. In most other patients, open adductor tenotomy should be performed through an incision 2 cm. below the groin crease and parallel to it. The tendons most likely to need division are those of adductor longus and gracilis. In most patients this should be combined with division of the anterior branch of the obturator nerve, leaving the posterior branch intact. Rarely, adductor brevis or magnus may need division and the posterior branch of the obturator nerve may need to be crushed but not divided. The author's experience agrees completely with that of Silver, Simon and Litchman (1966) that intrapelvic obturator neurectomy should not be done nor should both branches of the obturator nerve be divided extrapelvically because of the possibility of development of fixed abduction deformity.

Fixed flexion of the hip can nearly always be corrected in the early stages by elongation of the psoas tendon through the same incision as for adductor tenotomy. The tendon should be elongated by a Z incision, the ends of the tendon being sutured together. If the ends are not sutured, loss of hip flexion power may be excessive. Only in long-standing flexion deformity is it necessary to divide the muscles attached to the anterior superior iliac spine and, if this is still insufficient to give correction, a femoral osteotomy at the level of the lesser trochanter can be performed. With early psoas release the author has found the need for extension osteotomy to be very uncommon.

Medial rotation deformity of the hip may be present as part of a fixed flexion and adduction deformity, the adductors being powerful medial rotators of the flexed hip. If this is so, correction of the flexion and adduction will automatically correct the medial rotation. Sometimes, fixed medial rotation may be present even though an adduction and flexion deformity have been corrected. If so, anteversion of the upper end of the femur will be found to be present and this should be corrected by lateral rotation osteotomy of the femoral shaft.

If, in spite of adequate adductor tenotomy and obturator neurectomy, adduction deformity recurs, because of severe weakness of the gluteal abductors, with a threat of dislocation, iliopsoas transplantation laterally (Mustard 1952) or postero-laterally (Sharrard 1964b) may be indicated to prevent dislocation. Varus osteotomy has, in the author's experience, been less often needed to treat subluxation of the hip if adequate correction of the soft tissues has been obtained in the earlier years of life. Valgus of the femoral neck does not, of itself, cause dislocation provided that adduction deformity does not develop and balance between adductor and abductor action is maintained.

In a long-standing and irreducible dislocation, associated with severe flexion and adduction deformity, degenerative change in the head of the femur may develop very rapidly even though the child is unable to walk, and the hips become painful. Excision of the head and neck of the femur may be needed to relieve pain and to allow the child to sit in comfort.

Fixed extension deformity at the hip is extremely rare in cerebral palsy, but limited flexion of the hip, due to shortness of the hamstring muscles, is not uncommon. It gives rise to a diminished stride, exaggerated rotation of the pelvis in walking and inability to sit with the knees extended. Proximal release of the hamstrings by releasing the tendon of origin from the ischial tuberosity gives very satisfactory improvement (Seymour and Sharrard 1968).

KNEE

It has been the author's experience that if fixed flexion of the hip and equinus of the ankle is corrected sufficiently early in life, the child does not develop a flexed knee gait and fixed flexion of the knee is not common. If it does develop, simple tenotomy of the gracilis, semitendinosus and possibly biceps femoris may be sufficient to correct deformity. In the occasional patient who has primary weakness of the quadriceps or where fixed flexion of the knee has been allowed to develop in association with fixed flexion of the hip, correction of the hip deformity may need to be followed by hamstring transfer as described by Eggers (1952). Eggers originally described transfer of all the hamstrings with division of the medial and lateral patellar retinacula. Evans and Julian (1966) emphasize that this extensive transfer may lead to over-correction and they advise transfer of the tightest muscles, usually semitendinosus and/or biceps femoris, and either elongating the semimembranosus or leaving it intact. The number of tendons that need to be transferred is related to the strength of the quadriceps as assessed pre-operatively. The author believes that the tendons should be transferred into bone at the lower end of the femur or they are very likely to become detached from their new insertion.

If there is a tendency to medial rotation at the hip, the medial hamstring muscles should be transferred into the lateral femoral condyle as recommended by Craig (1967).

ANKLE

Equinus deformity initially arises more frequently from contracture of the gastrocnemii than from shortness of the whole triceps surae. Correction of gastrocnemius shortening is best achieved by separation of the gastrocnemius tendons from the soleus as described by Strayer (1950) and Pollock (1953). Release of the origins of the gastrocnemii as described by Silfverskiold (1924) is more difficult and is likely to lead to a back-knee gait. Where there is marked weakness of voluntary dorsiflexion of less than M.R.C. grade 3, division of the upper nerve to the soleus may be combined with the gastrocnemius slide. If there is shortening of the whole triceps surae, elongation of the tendo calcaneus is needed, but over-lengthening should be avoided by suturing the elongated tendon with the foot at a right angle to the leg.

FOOT

Spasticity of the abductor hallucis muscle gives rise to adduction deformity of the forefoot and hallux valgus in adolescence. Bleck (1967) advised excision of the abductor hallucis tendon and capsulectomy of the first metatarso-cuneiform joint with satisfactory results. If hallux valgus persists, arthrodesis of the first metatarso-phalangeal joint should be performed rather than arthroplasty.

Valgus and varus deformities of the hindfoot, usually associated with equinus deformity, may arise from over-action of the peronei or tibialis posterior respectively. Elongation of the short tendon may be sufficient to correct deformity, but if not, or if the deformity recurs, transfer of the tendon through the interosseous membrane to the dorsum of the foot, together with extra-articular arthrodesis of the subtaloid joint (Grice 1952) or calcaneal osteotomy (Dwyer 1959; Silver *et al.* 1967) gives good results.

Pollock and English (1967) note that operative correction of foot deformities should not be done before knee flexion deformity has been corrected. If there is deformity at the hip, knee and foot, they should be corrected in descending order. There is no contra-indication to correction of two joints at the same time and simultaneous gastrocnemius slide and adductor tenotomy has been found to be the commonest combination of operations needed in the lower limb (Fig. 1).

Operative Procedures in the Upper Limb

Surgery for the upper limb is much less often indicated than in the lower limb. The fact that normal function can never be obtained whatever is done has generated unwarranted pessimism about the results of surgical treatment. Recent contributions by Goldner (1955), Mortens (1965), Samilson and Morris (1962) and Swanson (1960) show that surgery has a definite place.

Careful assessment is essential as it is for the lower limb. As Samilson (1967) emphasizes, signs such as non-appearance of the parachute reaction and persistence of the tonic neck reflex are signs of a bad prognosis which make functional improvement in the upper limb

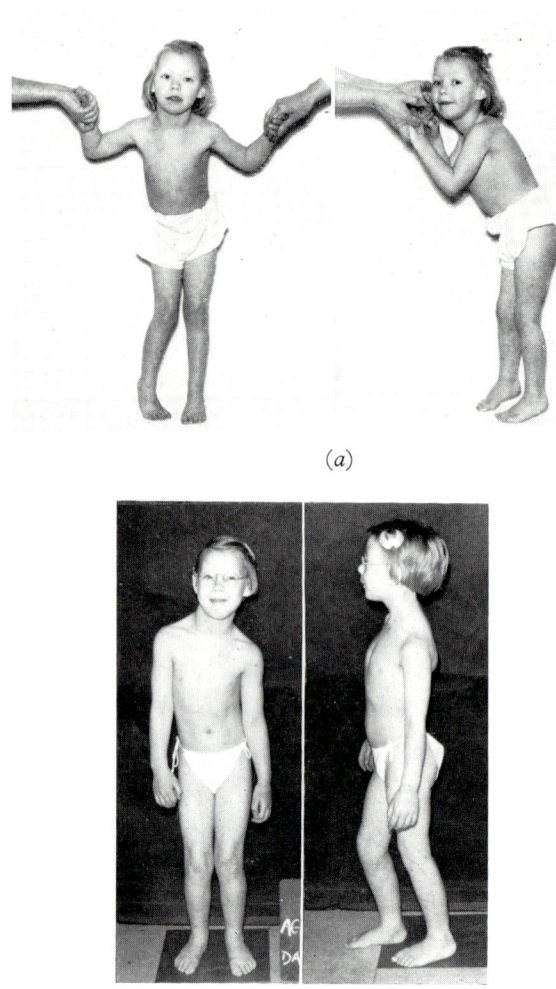

Fig. 1. (a) Bilateral equinus and adduction deformity in spastic cerebral palsy. (b) Improved stance and gait following gastrocnemius recession and adductor tenotomies.

unlikely even with the best surgical intentions. As in the lower limb, fixed deformity should be treated by soft tissue release, which may be followed by an appropriate tendon transfer.

WRIST

At the wrist the commonest deformity that may develop is flexion, sometimes associated with ulnar deviation. If there is adequate action in the finger extensors and no significant shortening of the long flexor tendons, transfer of the flexor carpi ulnaris to the radial wrist extensors is indicated. If there is weakness of supination the transfer may be performed round the ulnar border of the forearm after releasing any pronation contracture. Arthrodesis of the wrist is appropriate after the age of ten if there is fixed flexion deformity of the wrist, even if the only improvement may be cosmetic; if there is shortening of the long flexors of the fingers, arthrodesis should be combined with some shortening of the forearm at the arthrodesis.

THUMB

Adduction and flexion of the thumb so that it lies in the palm is the commonest cause of disability in the hand in spastic paralysis. Contractures of the adductor pollicis, flexor pollicis brevis and the first dorsal interosseous should be released. Goldner (1961) recommends transfer of the flexor carpi radialis to the extensor pollicis longus to supplement extension and abduction of the thumb. Arthrodesis of the first metacarpo-phalangeal joint and sometimes of both this joint and the carpo-metacarpal joint of the thumb is of value.

FINGERS

The flexor digitorum superficialis tendon may be tenotomized and transferred through the interosseous membrane to the finger extensors if the latter are weak. Swanson (1960) recommends tenodesis of the superficialis tendons to the palmar aspect of the proximal phalanges for swan-neck deformity of the fingers.

Operative Procedures for the Spine

Deformities of the spine are fortunately rare in cerebral palsy, though when they do occur they are likely to be severe and incapacitating. Conservative treatment by plasters or braces can seldom prevent the progressive deformity arising from strong and spastic asymmetrical trunk musculature.

Lumbar lordo-scoliosis can be improved considerably by extensive mobilization of the erector spinae on the concave side of the deformity, the aim being to correct soft tissue shortening and to denervate the lumbar portion of the erector spinae. In a child over the age of ten, the spine may be fused and Harrington rods help to give additional support during the process of fusion. If spasticity is severe in the lateral abdominal muscles, it may be helpful to perform anterior rhizotomy of alternate motor roots from the 11th thoracic to the 3rd lumbar.

Spasticity Without Deformity

In a young child, severe spasticity, for example, in the triceps surae, may make attempts to obtain independent walking difficult, in spite of adequate physiotherapy and relaxation techniques. Clinical examination may show no fixed deformity, and in this circumstance tendon elongation or myotomy may be contra-indicated because of the presence of strong active opponents of the spastic muscles. Local anaesthetic agents or alcohol can give satisfactory relief of spasticity without affecting motor power. Two ml. of 45 per cent alcohol into the motor point of the muscle preceded by 2 ml. of 1 or 2 per cent lignocaine is a useful technique that may sometimes be employed when a muscle is severely spastic but there is no contracture. The effects of this last for four to six months only. For more permanent chemical neurectomy, injection of phenol is available, but it is probably advisable that such techniques be done at open operation, rather than by blind injection. Such techniques have a limited but useful part to play in the management of spastic cerebral palsy.

ORTHOPAEDIC SURGERY IN SPINA BIFIDA

The last ten years has seen a completely new approach to problems associated with developmental abnormalities of the spine and neuraxis. Such abnormalities are much more common than was previously thought and it is probable that at least 1500 such children are born alive each year in Great Britain.

The variety and complexity of abnormal development may result in spinal defects varying from a skin dimple or a split spinous process to complete failure of closure of skin, posterior elements of vertebral and dural coverings of the spinal cord and failure of tubulation and development of part of the spinal cord. The important lesions, in practice, are of two kinds—closed lesions covered with intact skin and open lesions, in which the spinal cord or nervous tissues present on the surface of the body.

Closed lesions include meningocele, dermal cysts, lipomata of the cauda equina, diastematomyelia, congenital absence of sacrum or sacrum and lumbar vertebrae and myelodysplasia with or without abnormal vertebral formation. Of these, only meningocele is likely to have no orthopaedic consequences, provided it is operated upon sufficiently early in life. All the other abnormalities are likely to be associated with deformity and paralysis in the lower limbs, either at birth or presenting during the course of growth. Children with this type of abnormality have always been seen from time to time in orthopaedic work, but the significance of the spinal lesion and its relationship to lower limb abnormality has only recently been appreciated and the need for combined action by neurosurgeon and orthopaedic surgeon emphasized.

Open lesions, that is myelomeningocele and myelocele, have previously been regarded as untreatable, because of the high incidence of meningitis and the presence of associated congenital hydrocephalus in over 80 per cent of patients. The introduction of satisfactory control of hydrocephalus by ventriculo-cardiac shunts, the use of antibiotics to treat meningitis and the recognition of the value of operative closure of the spinal lesion on the first day of life (Sharrard et al. 1963, Sharrard, Zachary and Lorber 1967a) has completely altered the prognosis for life and lower limb function. Even if the spinal defect is severe and the hydrocephalus marked, adequate and early surgical treatment can result in survival of more than 75 per cent of patients, and in hydrocephalic patients, normal intelligence in 85 per cent and intelligence as adequate as in spastic children in the remainder. It follows, therefore, that up to 1000 children a year in Great Britain are potentially capable of survival with sufficiently adequate mental ability to benefit from orthopaedic surgery for any paralysis and deformity that they may have in their lower limbs. Even if immediate surgery on the spinal lesion has not been performed, and the almost inevitable severe paraplegia in the lower limbs is present, more than 30 per cent of patients survive and may need orthopaedic help (Sharrard, Zachary and Lorber 1967b).

The Mechanism of Paralysis and Deformity in the Lower Limbs

The lower limb paralysis in a child born with neurological abnormality in the spine may be primary or secondary. The primary paralysis is the result of aplasia or dysplasia of nervous tissues in utero. It may take several forms, a common example being that in which some or all of the sacral neural segments are functionless and lumbar neural segments are intact. For example, a child with normal activity in the first four lumbar neural segments will show strong action in the hip flexors, adductors, quadriceps and tibialis anterior, with complete paralysis of the other lower limb muscles. Innervation down to and including the fifth lumbar segment will result in the same muscle activity together with action in the dorsiflexors of the foot and ankle and paretic activity in the gluteal abductors (Sharrard 1962, 1964b). In some the position may be made more complex by the persistence of caudal islands of reflexly acting neural tissue, so that a child may present with normal activity in the first four lumbar neural segments, absent activity in the fifth lumbar and first sacral segments and reflex activity in the second and third sacral segments (Stark and Baker 1967). In most children, the distribution of the paralysis in the two limbs is remarkably symmetrical, but this is not always so, as is shown by the neurological picture in children with hemimyelomeningocele in which the spinal cord lesion is confined to one half of the spinal cord and the lower limb paralysis affects only one limb. The paralysis also affects the spinal muscles and in these patients unilateral paralysis gives rise to congenital scoliosis (Duckworth, Lister and Sharrard 1968).

Although some degree of primary lower limb paralysis is extremely common in children with open myelomeningocele, it is possible for there to be a normal neural content in a spinal cord that is widely open and exposed, even from the mid-thoracic level to the sacrum and, in these children, lower limb function can be normal if surgical closure of the spinal lesion is undertaken within the first 12 hours of life.

Secondary paralysis may arise in one of several ways. In closed lesions, such as lipoma of the cauda equina or diastematomyelia, increasing paralysis may result from stretching of tethered nerve roots associated with growth of the lumbar vertebrae, or by compression of neural tissues within the confines of the spinal canal. In open lesions, secondary paralysis may develop if the spinal lesion is treated conservatively, as a result of infection or drying of the exposed neural tissue or by the traction on the nerve roots that results when the myelomeningocele fills with cerebro-spinal fluid and bulges away from the surface of the body during the first week of life. In this way, a child born with potential for partial or even full innervation of the lower limbs may become secondarily paralysed during the first four days of life by attempts to treat the spinal lesion conservatively or by inadequate surgery.

Deformity in the lower limbs may also be primary or secondary. At birth, between 60 and 70 per cent of myelomeningoceles show some primary deformity in the lower limbs. The degree of deformity may vary between clawing of the toes, and multiple deformity with dislocation of the hips, recurvatum of the knees and severe varus deformities of the feet. Studies of the relationship between intra-uterine paralysis and birth deformity has shown a strong correlation between the extent and type of deformity that is present at birth and the primary intra-uterine paralysis (Sharrard 1967b). This suggests that many and possibly all of the deformities in the lower limbs in these children are intra-uterine paralytic deformities, rather than associated congenital deformities. The recognition of this has important consequences in the surgical management of the limbs.

Secondary deformities are those which develop after birth, and they are usually the result of secondary paralysis. A myelomeningocele child born without deformity in the lower limbs and therefore with potential for normal lower motor neurone innervation may, for instance, lose function in the sacral nerve roots. In the course of growth with unbalanced muscle activity, dislocation of the hip and paralytic deformities of the feet may develop.

Assessment of Paralysis and Deformity

As in other paralytic disorders, an assessment of the extent of the deformity at each joint and of the activity of the various muscle groups must be made before treatment is begun. Assessment of muscle activity is never easy in children and can never be very precise in a child below the age of five or six years. Nevertheless, the attempt should be made to grade muscle action at least as paralysed, paretic or normal and, if possible, as normal voluntary action, reflex action or a combination of the two. A knowledge of the segmental innervation of the lower limbs often makes it possible to define the distribution of the lower limb paralysis in terms of spinal cord or root involvement (Sharrard 1964c). Ideally, the first assessments should be made by the orthopaedic surgeon on the first day of life, before the spinal lesion is treated, or, if not, as soon as the spinal lesion is healed. There is need for continued neurological assessment as the child grows so that secondary deformities may be anticipated or prevented. Percutaneous faradic stimulation of the nerves and muscles of the lower limbs gives additional support to clinical assessment of paralysis (Stoyle 1966, Sharrard 1967b), as may electromyography (Duckworth and Sharrard 1968). Electrical techniques are especially valuable if deformity occurs fairly rapidly after adequate surgical correction. In such instances, it may be found that muscles that show no clinical activity, voluntary or reflex, may indicate their presence by a response to electrical stimulus or the presence of action potentials on electromyography and it may be that some of these muscles have motor but no sensory innervation.

In some children the deformities may be extreme and such deformities have sometimes, mistakenly, been referred to as arthrogrypotic. The child shown in Figure 2 has fixed flexion of the hip of more than 90°, fixed adduction of 30° and fixed external rotation of 90°. As a result, the patella faces laterally, but its position is masked by the fact that there is 40° of fixed recurvatum of the knee. The feet are grossly adducted and inverted and the forefoot faces in the opposite direction to that of the knee. Deformities of this degree have previously been thought to be incorrigible, but experience has shown, that with a sufficiently energetic approach, deformity can be corrected and the limbs made capable of bearing weight.

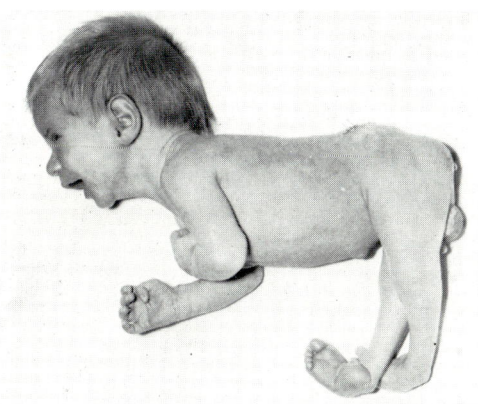

FIG. 2. Birth deformities in spina bifida. Fixed flexion, adduction and lateral rotation deformities of the hips with dislocation, recurvatum of the knee and calcaneovarus deformities of the feet.

Assessment of sensory loss other than by very rough testing by pin-prick and observing the reaction of protest or movement of the limb, is not possible in a very young child. Observations in older children suggest that the sensory loss usually corresponds segmentally with the motor loss. Wherever there is doubt, it is wise to assume that there is sensory loss that precludes the use of forcible means of correcting deformity by rigid splintage or plaster.

Principles of Orthopaedic Treatment

The aim of orthopaedic treatment is to correct deformity, to maintain correction and to obtain the maximum function in the lower limbs. As in all paralytic deformity, shortness of the soft tissues, particularly of tendons, is the most important element in the maintenance of deformed position. Deformity in the osteo-cartilaginous structures is less marked, provided that the deformity has not been allowed to persist for more than two years. Most of the time-honoured methods of correcting congenital deformity or deformity in early childhood by rigid splinting or serial plasters are contra-indicated in spina bifida because of sensory loss and the liability of the skin to develop pressure sores. Traction by frames, such as might be appropriate for congenital dislocation of the hip, should only be used with great caution and, even if pressure sores are avoided, there is danger of producing fractures in the thin porotic bones of paralysed limbs. Careful correction of foot deformity by elastic strapping can be successful (Walker 1968) and daily passive manipulation by parents or physiotherapists has a place in minimizing deformity or its recurrence. In general, it is safer, especially where there is extreme deformity and rigidity of soft tissues, to correct deformity by open operative division of tight muscles, tendons, tendon sheaths, ligaments and joint capsules. The division and elongation of soft tissues must be much more radical than is usually necessary in the management of ordinary congenital deformity or other paralytic deformity, because failure to obtain correction cannot be compensated by forcing the position of the limb in plaster or rigid splinting post-operatively. If division of soft tissues alone is not sufficient to produce complete correction of the deformity, it may then be justifiable to complete the correction by an osteotomy of the appropriate bone.

When deformity has been corrected, action must be taken to restore muscle balance by appropriate muscle or tendon transplantation or by denervation of over-active muscles. Sometimes this can be done at the same time as the operation for correction of deformity or it may be done as a second operation. There may sometimes be difficulty in deciding which tendon to transplant and where to transplant it. Whenever there is doubt, the tendon whose action corresponds to the direction of the deformity should be at least one of those transferred. If subsequent events show, by recurrence of deformity or by the development of a new deformity, that the original transplant was not entirely satisfactory, there is nothing to be lost by performing a second tendon transfer or moving the original transferred tendon to a new position.

All forms of fixation and splintage need to be used with great care in spina bifida. Plaster casts can be used post-operatively with safety, provided that no attempt is made to force further correction by pressure from the plaster. Night splints should not be used, because they are a very potent cause of pressure sores; correction of deformity can equally well be maintained by daily passive movements. The child should not be allowed to bear weight on an insensitive foot until any deformity has been corrected and satisfactory footwear has been made that does not cause pressure on toes or bony points. Where these principles have been followed, pressure sores in the feet have rarely developed (Sharrard and Grosfield 1968).

Spontaneous fractures are commonly seen in the lower limbs. They occur most frequently where paralysis is severe or after a period of immobilization in bed or in plaster. The most common site for fracture is in the juxta-metaphyseal region, particularly at the lower end of the femur or the upper end of the tibia. There is a characteristic history of fairly sudden onset of a painless warm swelling in the limb. Abnormal mobility may be demonstrable for a few days, but, more commonly, the child is not referred for radiographic examination until the fracture has already started to unite, which it does with very abundant callus formation. If the child already has calipers, immobilization is best achieved by continuing the use of the calipers, day and night, until the fracture has united. In other circumstances, fixation should be applied for the minimum length of time to avoid further osteoporosis. Supplementary calcium, vitamin D and vitamin C may be helpful when fractures repeatedly occur in severely porotic bones.

The timing of procedures to correct deformity is often critical. When deformities are present at birth, it is natural for an orthopaedic surgeon to wish to correct them as soon as possible. Splints that would be appropriate for the treatment of congenital dislocation of the hip or congenital talipes equino-varus in an otherwise normal child, are not effective and may even be dangerous in the early weeks of life. They embarrass the management of the spinal defect and the hydrocephalus during this period. It is better to wait until the child is thriving, his spine is well healed, hydrocephalus is controlled and renal function is satisfactory, before attempting any orthopaedic measures, apart from the very simplest, such as elastic strapping to the foot. Operative correction of some deformities may be feasible before the sixth month, but in many instances, if the deformity is not progressive it may be better to wait until the child is old enough and large enough to make surgery practicable and effective. This means that most orthopaedic procedures should be undertaken between the age of six months and three years, with the aim of correction of all deformities so as to allow the child to walk before he starts school.

Before even the most minor orthopaedic surgery is done, a check should be made on renal function. A child, who superficially appears well, may be precipitated into uraemia, even by such a minor procedure as adductor tenotomy. In general, multiple deformities in the lower limbs should be corrected proximo-distally and, when a programme of correction is worked out, correction should not be made at one joint, unless there is the intention to correct all the deformities in both lower limbs, the ultimate aim being to make it possible for the child to walk or at least to sit without danger of developing pressure sores.

Hip Deformities

Subluxation or dislocation of the hip is present at birth or develops during the first three years of life in more than half of all children suffering from myelomeningocele. Dislocation is very frequently associated with normal innervation from the first three or four lumbar neural segments and paralysis caudal to this level (Sharrard 1964*b*). Subluxation is likely to be present when there is innervation down to the fifth lumbar segment, because there is then some activity in the gluteal abductors; dislocation always results eventually if the adductors and hip flexors are normally innervated.

The acetabulum is often well preserved if the hip dislocates rapidly and remains dislocated, but if the hip dislocates in and out of joint for a period, there may develop a deficiency of the acetabular roof. Dislocation and subluxation are almost always associated with relative shortness of the adductor muscles. The dislocation can be reduced in 9 out of 10 instances if a sufficiently radical open adductor tenotomy with division of all the adductor muscles, including the adductor magnus, is performed. The aim should be to obtain 90° of abduction. The obturator vessels and nerve should be preserved. This operation may be performed at any time from the third month of life onward and successful reductions of dislocations have been obtained in several patients more than nine years old. Reduction of the dislocation can be maintained by splintage in the frog position of abduction, flexion and neutral or medial rotation, but this position should not be maintained constantly for longer than four weeks,

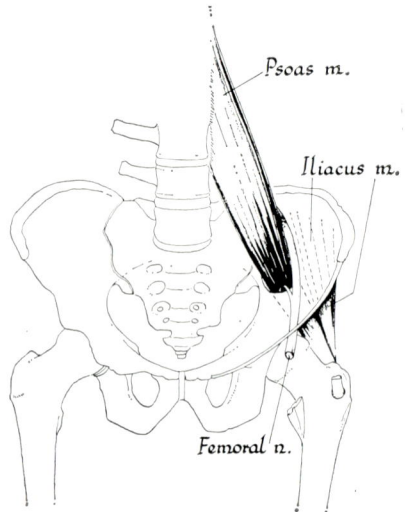

FIG. 3. Diagram of posterior ilio-psoas transplantation.

because the hip flexors will become converted into flexors and abductors and it may be extremely difficult to bring the hips down again later.

If there is complete paralysis of all gluteal musculature or paresis of the gluteal abductors and paralysis of gluteus maximus, the situation that is usually present when the hip is dislocated, muscle balance can be restored by posterior transplantation of the iliopsoas muscle (Sharrard 1964b), as shown in Fig. 3. This operation should preferably be done one or two weeks after adductor tenotomy. If the hip has not been fully reduced following the adductor tenotomy, it will usually reduce once the psoas tendon has been divided. Only rarely is there need to perform an open reduction of a dislocated hip. In children over the age of five in whom the acetabulum proves to be inadequate, an innominate osteotomy (Salter 1961) or acetabuloplasty (Pemberton 1965) can be performed at the same time as the iliopsoas tendon is transplanted.

The transplanted iliopsoas muscle will prevent further dislocation and allow walking without the need for any splintage at the hip level in a high proportion of patients, and, unless acetabular reconstruction has been performed, it is unnecessary to immobilize the hip in abduction and extension for longer than four or five weeks. In the small number in whom dislocation has recurred, this is usually found to have been due to an inadequate adductor tenotomy, poor fixation of the iliopsoas tendon to the greater trochanter or fixation of the tendon to the trochanter under inadequate tension. Occasionally excessive new bone formation in the region of the transplant may vitiate the result. Most dislocated and subluxated hips show abnormal valgus and anteversion of the neck of the femur. When it is extreme, varus osteotomy may be required after the psoas has been transplanted and the need for this may be indicated by failure of the hip to regain adduction within two or three months of the removal of plaster fixation following psoas transplantation. More usually, the neck of the femur recovers its normal angle within one to

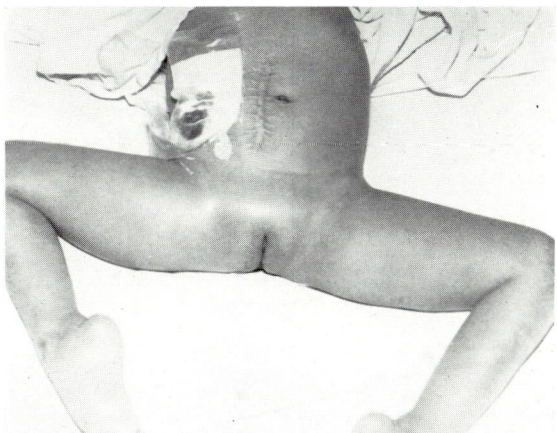

FIG. 4. Fixed flexion and abduction of the hips, fixed flexion of the knees and equinus deformity of the feet in spina bifida.

two years of psoas transplantation as the result of the pull of the tendon on the greater trochanter. Persistent anteversion should not necessarily be corrected by lateral rotation osteotomy such as might be appropriate in a normal child following reduction of a congenital dislocation of the hip. If rotary osteotomy of the femur is performed, the aim should be to correct a medially or laterally rotated position of the hip, independent of the radiological appearances of anteversion or retroversion.

Fixed flexion deformity of the hip, without adduction deformity or subluxation, may develop when the hip flexors are the only active muscles in the region of the hip or when the adductor and abductor muscles are balanced, but there is weakness of hip extension due to paresis of the gluteus maximus. In either case, the deformity is best corrected by elongation of the iliopsoas tendon and, if necessary, mobilization of the hip flexor muscles attached to the anterior superior iliac spine. The iliopsoas tendon should not be transplanted posteriorly if there is paralysis of all other hip muscles. Occasionally, in a child who has been allowed to sit in a wheelchair for a considerable period of time, soft tissue division alone may not allow the deformity to be corrected or short femoral vessels and nerve may prevent complete correction. Extension osteotomy at sub-trochanteric level with removal of up to an inch of length of shaft of femur, may be needed to obtain correction (Figs. 4 and 5). The osteotomy usually needs to be fixed internally by a plate or nail-plate.

It is sometimes found that even after a hip has been reduced and muscle action of the hip balanced as regards flexion/extension and abduction/adduction, there may be a predominance of lateral rotation,

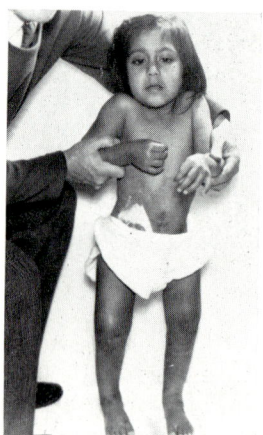

Fig. 5. Same child as in Fig. 4 following multiple osteotomies and tenotomies.

so that the child walks with the foot turned outwards even though there is no fixed lateral rotation deformity. Transfer of the insertion of the sartorius muscle to the outer side of the knee, will give sufficient active medial rotation to correct the gait.

Knee Deformities

Fixed extension deformity or recurvatum of the knee may be present at birth or may develop later, when there is normal action in the quadriceps and paralysis of the hamstring muscles. When recurvatum is severe, the sartorius and gracilis muscles are displaced anteriorly to become secondary extensors of the knee. Elongation of the quadriceps may be required, but it should be done with care to avoid weakening the quadriceps too much. In most children, limited flexion of the knee will correct itself under the influence of gravity and with the help of physiotherapy.

Flexion deformity of the knees may arise in children who develop spasticity in the lower limbs, or who have been allowed to sit for long periods without attempts to maintain passive extension of the knee joints. Hamstring tenotomy, posterior capsulectomy of the knee, transfer of one or more hamstring muscles to the posterior aspect of the lower end of the femur and occasionally supracondylar extension osteotomy of the lower end of the femur may be appropriate to correct such deformity. The choice of methods will depend on the level of activity of the flexors and extensors of the joint and the degree of fixed deformity present.

Foot Deformities

Every possible variety of foot deformity has been seen in children with spina bifida. The commonest deformities are calcaneo-varus, equino-varus and calcaneus. Most of these deformities are associated with activity in corresponding muscle groups, the activity either being under voluntary control or reflex. Correction of the deformity is made more difficult by the almost invariable absence of sensibility in the foot. Although repeated manual passive stretching and sometimes very careful elastic splintage may give some correction of deformity, operative division of short soft tissues is almost always needed to obtain complete correction and some form of tendon transfer is likely to be needed in almost every case. Where the deformity is severe, there is often shortness of skin on the inner side of the ankle and foot in varus deformities and on the dorsum of the foot in calcaneus deformities.

Correction is best obtained between the ninth month and second year of life. The skin incision should be a V-Y or other plastic surgical manoeuvre so as to allow comfortable skin closure when the deformity has been corrected. If pre-operative clinical and electrical evaluation has shown that a muscle is paralysed, it may be divided if it is short, and allowed to retract. In varus deformities the common finding is that the tibialis anterior and posterior muscles are acting in the presence of paralysis of all other muscles below the knee. Extensive division of the tendo calcaneus, the tibialis posterior tendon and the tendons of both the long toe flexors just above the medial malleolus, division of the medial ligament of the ankle, the medial and posterior capsule of the ankle joint and the medial and posterior capsule of the subtaloid joint will allow correction of all but the most severe varus deformities. The tendon of the tibialis anterior is divided close to its insertion and may be transferred laterally to the region of the base of the fourth metatarsal. If correction sufficient to allow the foot to be plantigrade is not obtained by soft tissue division alone, even if the ankle joint it allowed to subluxate in the process, further correction by osteotomy of the calcaneum may be needed, either at the same time as the soft tissue division or at a second operation. Whatever else, the varus deformity must be corrected so as to avoid pressure on the outer border of the foot when the child bears weight.

Calcaneus deformities are usually more easy to correct. They are associated with activity in all the dorsiflexors in the presence of paralysis of all plantarflexors except possibly the peronei. Correction is usually obtained fairly easily by division or elongation of all the extensor tendons and transfers of the tibialis anterior and peroneus tertius tendons through the interosseous membrane into the tendo calcaneus.

Paralytic vertical talus, in which there is calcaneo-valgus deformity of the forefoot and equino-valgus deformity of the hindfoot, is an extremely complex and severe deformity that is often seen when there is innervation down to the first sacral segment and paralysis below this level. Extensive division of tight structures on the outer and inner sides of the foot may be needed to correct the deformity and to reduce the mid-tarsal dislocation. Multiple tendon transfers are needed to restore balance of action at the hindfoot and forefoot.

Severe or recurrent equino-varus deformity may occasionally arise when there is paralysis of all muscles below the knee, except the triceps surae and intrinsic muscles of the feet. This situation presents when there is isolated action of the second and third sacral segments and the muscle activity is usually reflex. For this reason, the presence of active muscle may not be appreciated unless electrical testing is made before operation. Simple tenotomy of the tendo calcaneus may not be sufficient to correct this deformity and, if the equinus is corrected by division of the tendo calcaneus, it will usually be found that the long toe flexors are also tight and need to be divided or the toes will be extremely likely to develop pressure sores at their tips. Moreover, the continued action of the intrinsic muscles will produce cavo-varus deformity and, even if a very adequate tenotomy of the tendo calcaneus has been done, it may show remarkable powers of repair with the development of equinus deformity again within a year of adequate correction. In the absence of any other muscle that can be transferred, this situation is best treated by hemi-transplantation of the tendo calcaneus to the dorsum of the foot (Sharrard and Grosfield 1968), combined with selective plantar denervation of the intrinsic muscles (Garceau and Brahms 1956).

In children who have almost normal innervation in the lower limbs, there is a danger that fixed clawing of the toes may develop because of relative weakness of the intrinsic muscles of the feet. This is particularly likely to occur in children with closed spinal lesions. Shoe pressure easily leads to pressure sores, infection and the need to amputate one or more toes. Transplantation of the long flexor tendons to the extensor surfaces of all the lesser toes is indicated before fixed deformity develops.

Spine Deformities

It is fortunate, that in spite of the abnormality of the posterior elements of the lumbar spine, spinal deformity presents no problem in over 80 per cent of patients with spina bifida. Congenital kyphosis of the lumbar spine is, however, a serious deformity when it presents in association with myelomeningocele (Hoppenfeld 1967). The neural tissues are tightly stretched over the backs of the deformed vertebral bodies and closure of the skin defect, which is usually very wide, is usually impossible even with the help of relaxing incisions in the flank. Correction of the deformity on the first day of life by excision of one or two vertebral bodies with preservation of the spinal cord and nerve roots is feasible and makes the closure of the skin defect possible without excessive tension. In spite of the severity of the operation in a newborn child, survival has been the rule and, in more than half, neural function has been preserved in the lower limbs (Sharrard 1968). In those in whom the deformity has not been corrected at birth, but who have survived in spite of the break-down of skin cover, complete paralysis in the lower limbs is the rule. The application of calipers to allow walking, is usually prevented by the prominent kyphotic lumbar spine. Transverse spinal osteotomy or osteotomy excision can be done to allow caliper fitting, provided that renal function is sufficiently adequate to permit an operation of considerable magnitude.

Education in Walking

Whatever the level of paralysis, it is almost always possible to train a child to walk independently. The only exception to this is where serious and uncorrected hydrocephalus or incorrigible spinal deformity has been

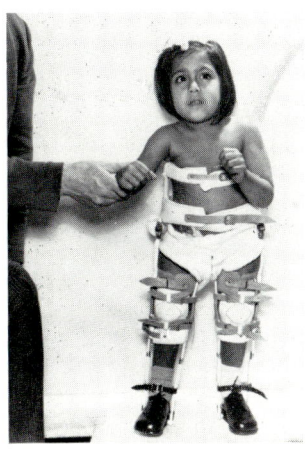

FIG. 6. Calipers with trunk support and semi-mobile hip hinges.

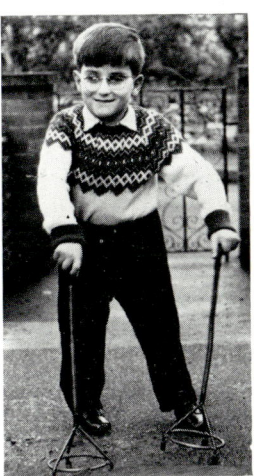

FIG. 7. Same child as in Fig. 2 following multiple reconstructive procedures. No external splintage required.

allowed to develop. Children with spina bifida usually have normal upper limbs and partially or completely normal trunk musculature. Even if there is no muscle activity in either lower limb, a spinal brace with double long calipers hinged to allow a small range of free hip flexion and abduction (Fig. 6) makes walking possible (Herzog and Sharrard 1966). It is surprising how well completely paraplegic children can become able to walk with the aid of elbow crutches or tripod sticks in the home or at school for distances of several hundred yards on level ground. The amount of bracing required when there is some voluntary activity in lower limb muscles will depend on the extent of that innervation. Following posterior iliopsoas transplantation, splintage at hip level may often be discarded when the quadriceps is also sufficiently powerful; light below-knee bracing is all that is needed (Fig. 7). Physiotherapy to strengthen residual muscle action and to teach walking with progressively diminishing external support, follows the same lines as those employed in patients with poliomyelitis or cerebral palsy.

Future Prospects

With closure of the spinal defect on the first day of life, adequate and early correction of hydrocephalus and correct management of the renal tract, more than 60 per cent of children born with open myelomeningocele can be expected to survive in future into adult life. One in five will have minimal paralysis and will be able to attend normal school; the remainder will need schools for the physically handicapped, most will need measures to manage partial or complete urinary and bowel incontinence. For the relief of back pressure on the kidneys and for social reasons, urinary diversion by means of an ileal conduit has proved effective. Nevertheless, the hazards of recurrent hydrocephalus should the shunting system block, and renal damage due to infection or back pressure, are likely to persist throughout life and to present problems similar to those encountered in patients with traumatic paraplegia.

Acknowledgements

Figures 1 and 6 are reproduced by kind permission of the Editor and publishers of the *Journal of Bone and Joint Surgery*.

For Figures 2 and 7 we are similarly indebted to the Editor and publishers of the *Postgraduate Medical Journal*.

References

BLECK, E. E. (1967). Spastic abductor hallucis. *Developm. Med. Child Neurol.*, **9**, 602.

BOBATH, K. (1961). The nature of the paresis in cerebral palsy. In "Child Neurology and Cerebral Palsy". Little Club Clinics in Development Medicine, No. 2, p. 88. London: Medical Advisory Committee of the National Spastics Society.

CRAIG, J. J. (1967). Cerebral palsy. In "Modern Trends in Orthopaedics", Fig. 5. p. 44. Ed. by W. D. Graham. London: Butterworths.

DUCKWORTH, T., LISTER, J. L. and SHARRARD, W. J. W. (1968). Hemimyelomeningocele. Paper presented at the 12th Annual Meeting of the Society for Research into Hydrocephalus and Spina Bifida, Lund.

DUCKWORTH, T. and SHARRARD, W. J. W. (1968). Personal communication.

DWYER, F. C. (1959). Osteotomy of the calcaneum for pes cavus. *J. Bone Jt. Surg.*, **41B**, 80.

EGGERS, G. W. N. (1952). Transplantation of the hamstring tendons to femoral condyles to improve extension and decrease flexion in cerebral spastic paralysis. *J. Bone Jt. Surg.*, **32A**, 827.

EVANS, E. B. and JULIAN, J. D. (1966). Modifications of the hamstring transfer. *Developm. Med. Child Neurol.*, **8**, 539.

FOLEY, J. (1961). The stiffness of spastic muscle. *J. Neurol. Neurosurg. Psychiat.*, **24**, 125.

GARCEAU, G. J. and BRAHMS, M. A. (1956). A preliminary study of selective plantar denervation for pes cavus. *J. Bone Jt. Surg.*, **38**, 553.

GOLDNER, J. L. (1955). Reconstructive surgery of the hand in cerebral palsy and spastic paralysis resulting from injury to the spinal cord. *J. Bone Jt. Surg.*, **37A**, 1141.

GOLDNER, J. L. (1961). Upper extremity reconstructive surgery in cerebral palsy and similar conditions. In "Instructional Course Lectures". American Academy of Orthopaedic Surgeons. St. Louis: Mosby, **18**, 169.

GRICE, D. S. (1952). An extra-articular arthrodesis of the subastragalar joint for the correction of paralytic flat feet in children. *J. Bone Jt., Surg.*, **34A**, 927.
HERZOG, E. G. and SHARRARD, W. J. W. (1966). Calipers and brace with hip locks. *Clin. Orthop.*, **46**, 239.
HOPPENFELD, S. (1967). Congenital kyphosis in myelomeningocele. *J. Bone Jt. Surg.*, **49B**, 276.
MORTENS, J. (1965). Surgery of the hand in cerebral paralysis. *Acta orthop. Scand.*, **36**, 441.
MUSTARD, W. T. (1952). Iliopsoas transfer for weakness of the hip abductors. *J. Bone Jt. Surg.*, **34A**, 647.
PEMBERTON, P. A. (1965). Pericapsular osteotomy of the ilium for treatment of congenital subluxation and dislocation of the hip. *J. Bone Jt. Surg.*, **47A**, 65.
POLLOCK, G. A. (1953). Lengthening of the gastrocnemius tendons in cases of spastic equinus deformity. *J. Bone Jt. Surg.*, **35B**, 148.
POLLOCK, G. A. and ENGLISH, T. A. (1967). Transplantation of the hamstring muscles in cerebral palsy. *J. Bone Jt. Surg.*, **49B**, 80.
SALTER, R. B. (1961). Innominate osteotomy in the treatment of congenital dislocation and subluxation of the hip. *J. Bone Jt. Surg.*, **43B**, 518.
SAMILSON, R. L. (1967). Surgery of the upper limbs in cerebral palsy. *Developm. Med. Child Neurol.*, **9**, 109.
SAMILSON, R. L. and MORRIS, J. M. (1962). Surgical improvement of the cerebral palsied upper limb. Electromyographic studies and results of 128 operations. *J. Bone Jt. Surg.*, **44B**, 899.
SEYMOUR, N. and SHARRARD, W. J. W. (1968). Bilateral proximal release of the hamstrings in cerebral palsy. *J. Bone Jt. Surg.*, **50B**, 274.
SHARRARD, W. J. W. (1961). The mechanism of deformity in cerebral palsy. *Proc. R. Soc. Med.*, **54**, 1016.
SHARRARD, W. J. W. (1962). The mechanism of paralytic deformity in spina bifida. *Developm. Med. Child Neurol.*, **4**, 310.
SHARRARD, W. J. W. (1964a). The nature and management of spasticity. The peripheral surgery of spasticity. *Proc. R. Soc. Med.*, **57**, 724.
SHARRARD, W. J. W. (1964b). Posterior iliopsoas transplantation in the treatment of paralytic dislocation of the hip. *J. Bone Jt. Surg.*, **46B**, 427.
SHARRARD, W. J. W. (1964c). The segmental innervation of the lower limb muscles in man. *Ann. R. Coll. Surg. Engl.*, **35**, 106.
SHARRARD, W. J. W. (1967a). Paralytic deformity in the lower limb. *J. Bone Jt. Surg.*, **49B**, 731.
SHARRARD, W. J. W. (1967b). Methods of assessment and their relation to treatment by early closure. *Proc. R. Soc. Med.*, **60**, 767.
SHARRARD, W. J. W. (1968). Spinal osteotomy for congenital kyphosis in myelomeningocele. *J. Bone Jt. Surg.*, **50B**, 466.
SHARRARD, W. J. W. and GROSFIELD, I. (1968). The management of deformity and paralysis of the foot in myelomeningocele. *J. Bone Jt. Surg.*, **50B**, 456.
SHARRARD, W. J. W., ZACHARY, R. B. and LORBER, J. (1967a). The long-term evaluation of a trial of immediate and delayed closure of spina bifida cystica. *Clin. Orthop.*, **80**, 197.
SHARRARD, W. J. W., ZACHARY, R. B. and LORBER, J. (1967b). Survival and paralysis in open myelomeningocele with special reference to the time of repair of the spinal lesion. In "Research into Hydrocephalus and Spina Bifida". *Developm. Med. Child Neurol.*, Suppl. No. 13, p. 35. London: The Spastics Society Medical Education and Information Unit in Association with William Heinemann Medical Books Ltd.
SHARRARD, W. J. W., ZACHARY, R. B., LORBER, J. and BRUCE, A. M. (1963). A controlled trial of immediate and delayed closure of spina bifida cystica. *Arch. Dis. Childh.*, **38**, 18.
SILFVERSKIOLD, N. (1924). Reduction of uncrossed two-joint muscles of the leg to one-joint muscles in spastic conditions. *Acta chir. scand.*, **56**, 315.
SILVER, C. M., SIMON, S. D. and LITCHMAN, H. M. (1966). The use and abuse of obturator neurectomy. *Developm. Med. Child. Neurol*, **8**, 203.

SILVER, C. M., SIMON, S. D., SPINDELL, E., LITCHMAN, H. M. and SCALA, M. (1967). Calcaneal osteotomy for valgus and varus deformities of the foot in cerebral palsy. *J. Bone Jt. Surg.*, **49A,** 232.

STARK, G. D. and BAKER, G. C. W. (1967). The neurological involvement of the lower limbs in myelomeningocele. *Developm. Med. Child Neurol.*, **9,** 732.

STOYLE, T. F. (1966). Prognosis for paralysis in myelomeningocele. *Developm. Med. Child Neurol.*, **8,** 755.

STRAYER, L. M. (1950). Recession of the gastrocnemius. An operation to relieve spastic contractures of the calf muscles. *J. Bone Jt. Surg.*, **32A,** 671.

SWANSON, A. B. (1960). Surgery of the hand in cerebral palsy and the swan-neck deformity. *J. Bone Jt. Surg.*, **42A,** 951.

THOMPSON, S. B. (1966). Indications for surgery in the lower limbs of the cerebral palsied child. *Developm. Med. Child Neurol.*, **8,** 437.

WALKER, G. F. (1968). A combined early physical and surgical approach to deformed feet in spina bifida. Paper presented at the 12th Annual Meeting of the Society for Research into Hydrocephalus and Spina Bifida. Lund.

Chapter 9

ANTERIOR SURGICAL APPROACHES TO THE SPINAL COLUMN

A. R. HODGSON and A. C. M. C. YAU

Tuberculosis of the spine is very common in Hong Kong. Prior to 1955, these cases were treated by the standard method of immobilization in plaster beds, drainage of cold abscesses and posterior spinal fusion in addition to anti-tuberculous drug therapy. This method of treatment was unsatisfactory on two counts: (*a*) the lesion was not attacked directly, and (*b*) a long period of hospitalization was the rule rather than the exception, and yet there was no way of telling for certain that the lesion was healed. In 1955 Hodgson and Stock (1956) embarked on a programme of treatment utilizing two principles: (*i*) radical excision of all diseased tissue, and (*ii*) stabilizing the spine thus left unstable by means of anterior interbody bone grafts. Consequently, various anterior approaches to the spine were sought for and developed.

The concept of approaching the spine anteriorly is not new. It dates back to Geraud (1750), Maisonneuve (1852) and Rodolfi (1859); and in the present century papers have been written by Burns (1933), Mercer (1936), Iwahara (1944), Jaslow (1946), Gjessing (1951), Cauchoix and Binet (1957), Cloward (1958), Dommisse (1959), Bailey and Badgley (1960), Sacks (1960), Harmon (1961), Robinson *et al.* (1962), and here in Hong Kong, Hodgson and Stock (1956), Hodgson and co-workers (1960), Fang and Ong (1962).

The purpose of this paper is to describe in detail the various surgical approaches to the spine.

The Transoral Approach to Cervical One and Two Vertebrae

It is difficult to approach the atlanto-axial joints from the side of the neck as numerous structures get in the way, such as the mandible, parotid salivary gland, internal carotid artery and vein and cranial nerves, whilst there is hardly any anatomy overlying these joints anteriorly; otolaryngologists (Thomson and Negus 1947) have used the peroral route to evacuate retropharyngeal abscesses, and through the same route excision of an osteoma of the axial body has been described by Southwick and Robinson (1957). As tuberculosis of the upper two cervical vertebrae, subluxation of the atlanto-axial joint and fracture-dislocation of the same joint are not uncommon in Hong Kong, this method of approach was adopted by Fang and Ong (1962).

Preoperatively, oral and nasal infections are dealt with, and an anterior plaster shell to include the head in extension is made for nursing the patient on his face; while for nursing him on his back a short mattress reaching up to his shoulders suffices.

Position: Supine with the head in hyper-extension on a head rest.

Procedure: Preliminary tracheostomy is performed after induction of anaesthesia, and a mouth gag of the Boyle-Davies type is inserted. The soft palate is folded back on itself and stitched so as to give adequate exposure. The uvula and soft palate may be bisected in the sagittal plane to improve the exposure or to permit visualization of the atlanto-occipital joint. Instead of splitting the palate longitudinally, it can be divided transversely. This trans-palatal approach has been described by Wilson (1951) for the removal of growths arising in the region of the basiocciput or basisphenoid. However, we have had no experience of the latter two procedures as there were no cases necessitating the exposure of the atlanto-occipital joint. The hypopharynx is packed and the posterior pharyngeal wall is palpated to locate the anterior tubercle of the atlas. An incision about 5 cm. long is made along the median raphe with its centre about 1 cm. below the anterior tubercle (Fig. 1); it should not extend too low down because subsequent closure will have to be carried out blindly. The incision is made down to bone and flaps are raised by blunt dissection to just short of the outer border of the lateral masses; to go beyond endangers the vertebral vessels. If these vessels are damaged, gelfoam (spongiostan) is used to control the bleeding. Dissection in this region is relatively avascular, though in children abundant lymphoid tissue may cause more oozing. In long standing atlanto-axial subluxation or dislocation, dense scar tissue is encountered akin to that found in spondylolisthesis in the lumbo-sacral region.

Long stay sutures are used to retract the soft tissue flaps, thus exposing the underlying anterior arch of the atlas, the body of the axis and the atlanto-axial joints on each side (Fig. 2). To fuse these joints, slots are made across them more medially than laterally to safeguard the vertebral vessels, and autogenous iliac grafts are inserted (Fig. 3). Onlay grafts should not be used as this makes closure of the pharyngeal wound difficult, especially when the subluxation is unreduced.

With atlanto-axial dislocation, the anterior aspect of the displaced atlantal masses and scar tissue overlying them are nibbled off, the joints cleared and the atlas is gently levered back into place by obtaining a purchase with a blunt hook around the unfractured odontoid process and pushing the arch of the atlas upwards and backwards. Sometimes the anterior arch is also nibbled off as well as the fractured odontoid process and this may further aid reduction. Strenuous efforts at reduction must not be persisted in as this may lead to tearing of vertebral veins bound down by scar tissue in a long standing dislocation. Fusion can be achieved in the subluxated or dislocated position.

Tuberculosis of this region is not uncommon: when encountered the lesion is debrided and reduction of the dislocation, when present, is achieved by hyper-extending the head; the bone grafting procedure is similar to that described above.

With fine atraumatic catgut, interrupted sutures are used to close

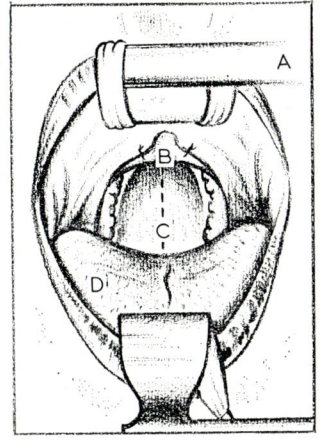

FIG. 1.

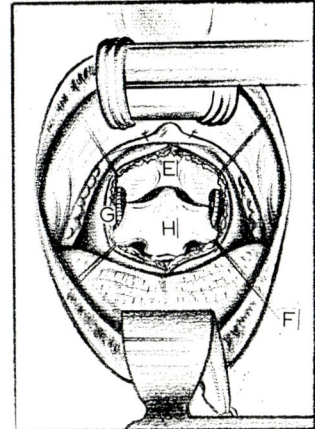

FIG. 2.

FIG. 1. A. Boyle Davies mouth gag. B. Uvula and soft palate folded back with stitches. C. Midline incision. D. Tongue.

FIG. 2. E. Anterior tubercle of Atlas. F. Stay suture for retraction of posterior pharyngeal wall and associated structures. G. Vertebral vessels. H. Axis.

FIG. 3. I. Anterior arch of Atlas and odontoid process removed. J. Bone graft spanning atlanto-axial joint.

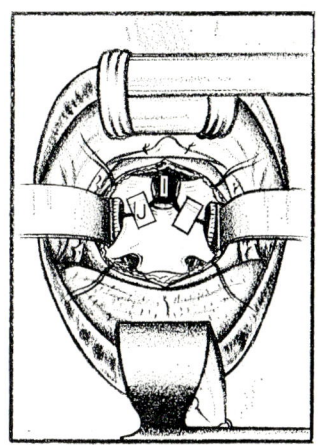

FIG. 3.

successively the anterior longitudinal ligament, the bucco-pharyngeal fascia and constrictor muscles, and finally the pharyngeal mucosa.

Post-operative Management

The patient is given intravenous fluids for one to two days followed by a fluid diet until the pharyngeal wound is well healed. The tracheostomy tube is left in place until bronchial secretions are reduced to normal amounts, usually for a few weeks. It is routine to keep patients on antibiotics to prevent wound infection. Patients are nursed alternately on the plaster shell and short mattress and are kept at rest until there is evidence of bony consolidation, which takes about three months.

Complications. *Operative:* Damaged vertebral vessels.
Postoperative: (1) Wound infection. Since Ryle's tubes have been dispensed with no further infections have occurred; (2) Development of

a nasal tone. (3) Spinal cord complications are possible, but have not occurred to date.

Transthyrohyoid Approach to Cervical Two, Three and Four Vertebrae

These vertebrae can be approached through the side of the neck with not too much difficulty and probably this should be the route of choice. However, for the sake of completeness the transthyrohyoid approach is described. Malgaigne and Langenbeck quoted by Kocher (1911) described this approach for resection of laryngeal tumours and Fang and Ong (1962) have worked it out for the spine.

The pre-operative management and position on the operation table is similar to that for the transoral approach.

Incision: A collar incision between the hyoid and thyroid cartilages extends from one carotid sheath to the other.

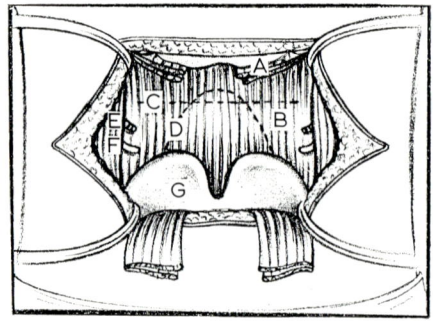

FIG. 4. 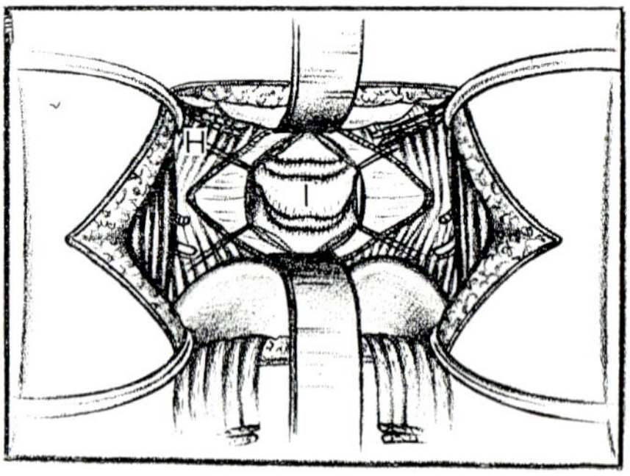   FIG. 5.

FIG. 4. A. Hyoid bone with cut ends of sternohyoid and thyrohyoid muscles. B. Thyrohyoid membrane. C. Incision. D. Epiglottis. E. Internal laryngeal nerve. F. Superior laryngeal artery. G. Thyroid cartilage.

FIG. 5. H. Stay suture for retraction of posterior pharyngeal wall. I. Cervical three body and adjacent discs.

Procedure: The platysma is divided in the line of the skin incision. The sternohyoid and thyrohyoid muscles are identified and divided close to their hyoid origins; this exposes the underlying thyrohyoid membrane together with the internal laryngeal nerve and the superior laryngeal vessels (Fig. 4). These structures are found piercing the postero-inferior part of the thyrohyoid membrane and, to avoid damaging them, the membrane is cut transversely near its superior attachment from one lateral thyrohyoid ligament to the other; this is done with care as the epiglottis is an immediate median and posterior relation. Fibro-fatty tissue is encountered; working through this and cutting the mucous membrane lining the vallecula, the hypopharynx is entered. By means of self-retaining retractors of the Jackson-Burrows variety, the hyoid and the epiglottis are retracted apart and this brings into view the posterior pharyngeal wall. A vertical midline incision is made and this exposes the bodies of C2-4 (Fig. 5). The vertebral lesion is dealt with as at other levels and the posterior pharyngeal wall is closed with atraumatic catgut in three layers as in the trans-oral approach. The anterior mucous membrane, thyrohyoid membrane and strap muscles are closed successively. Before approximating the platysma and skin, a soft drain is left in the wound and removed in twenty-four to forty-eight hours.

Post-operative management. This is similar to that for the transoral approach, with the exception that a short mattress is not necessary as the head need not be in the fully extended position.

Complications. *Operative:* There were none.

Postoperative: Complications of tracheostomy have been encountered, such as the development of fibrous polypi.

Approach to the Cervical Spine C2-C7

This region of the cervical spine can be approached through either the posterior triangle of the neck or the anterior triangle. Tuberculous pus from diseased cervical vertebrae often tracks and points in the posterior triangle of the neck and this has led us to develop the approach to the diseased vertebrae via the posterior triangle (Hodgson 1965).

If a limited exposure is required, a unilateral collar incision as described for the approach to disc lesions suffices. If more exposure is required the sterno-cleidomastoid muscle may be divided along the line of the incision in its posterior half or *in toto*. An incision paralleling the posterior border of the sternocleidomastoid muscle gives a much wider exposure, though an unsightly scar.

The approach through the anterior triangle has been described by Southwick and Robinson (1957): the incision follows the anterior border of the sternocleidomastoid muscle (Fig. 6) and a plane of cleavage is developed between this muscle and the carotid sheath on one side and the strap muscles together with the thyroid gland, larynx and trachea, pharynx and oesophagus on the other. This gives a good exposure of the cervical bodies. We have used this approach, utilizing a hemi-collar incision for limited lesions but we feel that the route along the posterior triangle is relatively easier and there is less anatomy to deal with.

Approach Through the Posterior Triangle

Position: As for thyroidectomy with a low flat sandbag between the shoulder blades. The neck should not be hyperextended as this puts the sternocleidomastoid and strap muscles on stretch, making retraction difficult.

Incision: A unilateral collar incision is made on either the left or right side. We prefer the right side because there is one structure less to encounter, namely the thoracic duct, although Southwick and Robinson (1957) prefer the left, their reason being that a recurrent laryngeal nerve palsy is more likely to result from retraction on the right side than the left, but we have not met with this complication.

The skin incision is centred over the level of the lesion and extends from the midline to the anterior border of the trapezius (Fig. 6). The cricoid cartilage is a useful surface landmark, it overlies C6 vertebral body.

Procedure: The incision goes through skin, superficial fascia and platysma. The external jugular vein, if in the way, is ligated and divided. A supraclavicular nerve may encroach on the operative field; it is mobilized and retracted. If the sternocleidomastoid muscle is particularly broad, it is divided in its posterior third or half and this brings the

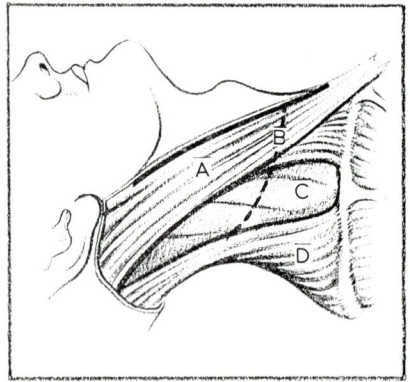
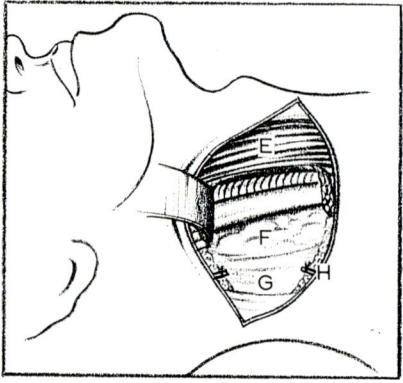

Fig. 6. Fig. 7.

Fig. 6. A. Sternocleidomastoid muscle and incision along its anterior border. B. Hemi-collar incision. C. Floor of posterior triangle. D. Trapezius.

Fig. 7. E. Sternocleidomastoid muscle partially cut and carotid vessels exposed. F. Pad of fat behind carotid vessels. G. Floor of posterior triangle. H. Ligated and divided external jugular vein.

common carotid sheath into view. By blunt dissection in the fat pad behind the sheath, a plane is developed overlying the prevertebral fascia of the posterior triangle (Fig. 7). This plane is further developed cranially and medially across the vertebral bodies to the left side. The carotid sheath and its contents, the pharynx, trachea and oesophagus and the overlying thyroid gland, are retracted forwards and to the right by Shuck-Smith retractors (smaller sizes). This exposes the cervical bodies

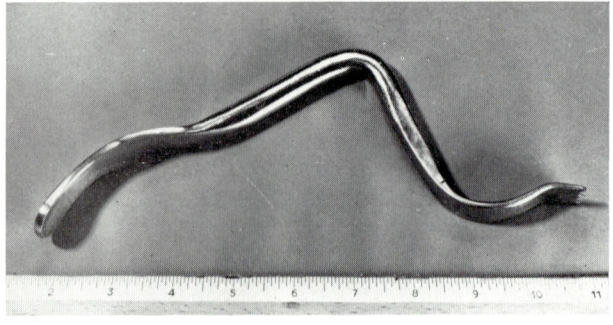

Fig. 8. S-shaped cervical retractor.

and to make for easier retraction, an 'S' shaped retractor (Fig. 8) is slipped into the place of the Shuck-Smith retractor. This 'S' shaped retractor has blunt teeth which grip the far side of the vertebral bodies. With the insertion of one or two more retractors cranially and/or caudally, the bodies are exposed (Fig. 9). The sympathetic chain is the only structure lying on the prevertebral fascia alongside the vertebral bodies. If manipulated or inadvertently cut, a Horner's syndrome will develop. We have felt that in some cases the symptoms of cervical spondylosis are sympathetic in origin and have therefore cut this chain deliberately; the resulting syndrome takes a year or two to disappear. Sometimes at the lower end of the wound the inferior thyroid artery or a muscular branch arising from the second part of the vertebral artery may hinder the exposure and is dealt with accordingly.

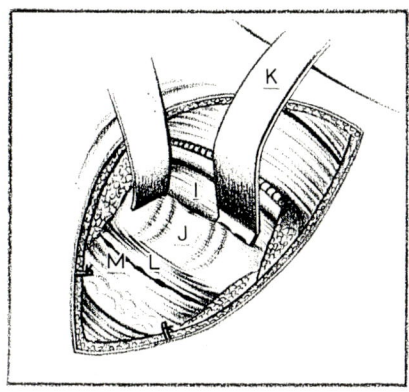
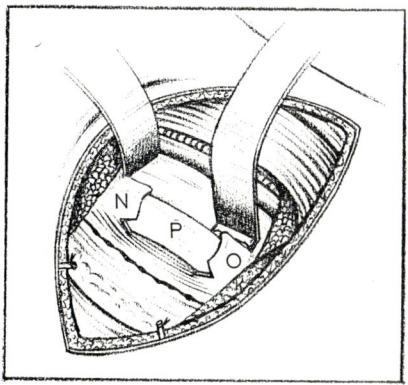

FIG. 9.   FIG. 10.

FIG. 9. I. Pharynx. J. Cervical five body and adjacent discs. K. S-shaped retractor. L. Longus cervicis muscle. M. Sympathetic chain.

FIG. 10. N and O. Cervical four and six vertebrae. P. Bone graft.

To identify the vertebra, a palpable anterior osteophyte corresponding to that on the X-ray will give the correct level. If no osteophytes are present, the anterior tubercle of the transverse process of the sixth cervical vertebra is a useful landmark. If operative discograms are contemplated in cases of cervical spondylosis, then there will be no problem in judging that level; otherwise, a needle is inserted into the disc space and an X-ray taken.

The level of the lesion in tuberculosis can usually be found without difficulty. Sometimes, the disease process has not involved the anterior longitudinal ligament which looks normal on inspection. However, palpation of the ligament in its length will reveal an area of bogginess and when incised in the midline, caseous material will often well out under pressure. All diseased tissue is removed as described for other levels, the only difference being that the vertebral bodies are small and therefore the bone graft must be mortised in with exactness (Fig. 10). If chisels are used to cut out diseased bone, the direction of the cut must not be backwards but sideways to ensure that the spinal cord is not damaged. The anterior longitudinal ligament is approximated, if possible, with a few interrupted catgut sutures. The rest of the closure is similar to that described below.

Complications. In spinal tuberculosis, all tissue planes may be matted together and there is the possibility of damaging a supraclavicular nerve and/or the sympathetic chain. Other complications are similar to those described for tuberculosis in general.

INTERBODY FUSION FOR CERVICAL DISC LESION

Having identified the disc space to be fused, more of it is exposed by dissecting back the cervicis longus muscle on the side of the approach. The disc space is entered by de-roofing it with a small-bladed scalpel

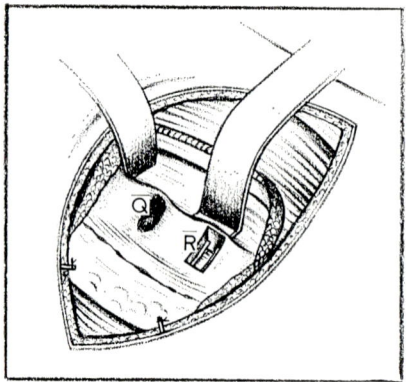 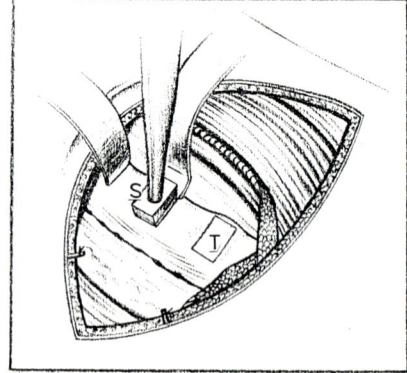

Fig. 11.   Fig. 12.

Fig. 11. Q. Intervertebral disc de-roofed and nucleus pulposus removed. R. Graft bed prepared. Note little ledge of bone left posteriorly.

Fig. 12. S. Bone graft being punched home. T. Graft well in.

and all the nucleus pulposus is removed with a pituitary rongeur. If osteophytes obstruct the view they are chiselled off. The depth and width and any pathology in the space is noted before proceeding to remove the adjacent cartilage, otherwise subsequent bone oozing obscures the view. It is best to leave a little rim of bone at the back when preparing the bed for grafting (Fig. 11). The size of the cavity is measured and it is then packed with gelfoam while the bone graft is obtained from the patient's iliac crest. The vertical height of the graft should be 2–3 mm. wider and this will jam the bodies apart, widen the intervertebral foramina and thus relieve pressure on the issuing nerve roots.

Before the bone graft is punched home, the gelfoam is removed and the cavity inspected for any remaining cartilage. As the graft is driven in the anaesthetist hyperextends the neck to facilitate insertion. Two disc spaces can be done in one sitting (Fig. 12) but not three as the spine will be too unstable and grafts will tend to slip. In such a case a trough should be made in the bodies spanning the three disc spaces to be fused and a long autogenous iliac graft mortised in carefully.

Before closure of the wound, a little drain is left in it leading up to the spine. The sternocleidomastoid muscle, the platysma and skin are closed successively. Blood loss during the procedure for disc lesions is insignificant and transfusion has never been found to be necessary.

Postoperatively the drain is removed in twenty-four to forty-eight hours. Tuberculous cases are nursed in previously prepared plaster shells while disc cases are left free in bed and they are allowed up as soon as they are able.

Complications. These are the same as those met with in dealing with tuberculosis of the cervical spine.

Split Sternal Approach to the Cervico-dorsal Spine

When one or two vertebrae are involved in a disease process in this region, it can be dealt with relatively easily through the neck or through

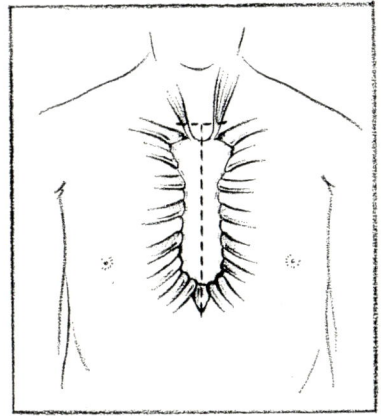

FIG. 13. Skin incision for split sternum approach.

the chest. However, when more vertebrae are involved as in tuberculosis, neither route gives adequate exposure but the sternal split approach exposes cervical 4 to thoracic 4 vertebrae and even one or two more bodies if there is a mild kyphosis. Essentially the approach is similar to that for thymectomy and it has been described by Cauchoix and Binet (1957).

Position: As that for thyroidectomy with a sandbag between the shoulder blades so as to thrust the sternum forwards.

Incision: A 'T' shaped incision (Fig. 13) is made with the transverse component along the lower neck crease two fingers' breadth above the supra sternal notch from the medial border of one sternocleidomastoid muscle to the medial border of the other, and the vertical component along the mid line of the sternum extending to just beyond the xiphisternum.

Procedure: Skin flaps are mobilised for a short distance and the transverse incision is deepened through the platysma and investing cervical fascia. Both sternohyoid and sternothyroid muscles are mobilized by blunt dissection and divided in the line of the skin incision. The inter-clavicular ligament is exposed; an occasional vessel may be found running transversely and it has to be secured before this ligament is incised down to the bone. Attention is next directed to the xiphisternum which is dissected free and excised. Fingers are inserted at either end of the sternum and soft tissue is gently freed from the under surface of the sternum and the adjacent costal cartilages. It is now safe to split the sternum in the mid line with a Sauerbruch's sternotome or a Gigli saw. Strong self-retaining retractors are inserted and the two halves of

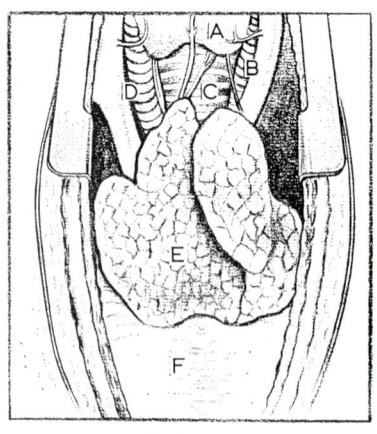
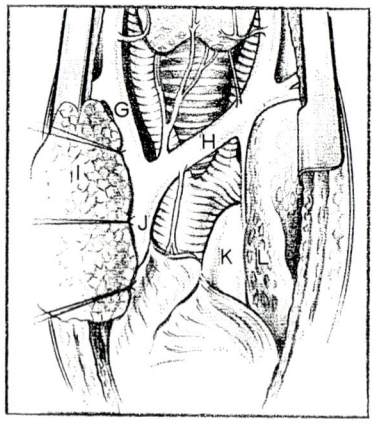

FIG. 14.   FIG. 15.

FIG. 14. A. Thyroid gland with draining veins. B and D. Left and right carotid vessels. C. Trachea. E. Thymus gland. F. Pericardium.

FIG. 15. G. Right brachiocephalic vein. H. Left brachiocephalic vein. I. Thymus gland retracted to right with stay sutures. J. Superior vena cava. K. Pulmonary artery. L. Lung.

the sternum spread apart exposing the mediastrium (Fig. 14). The pleura, now under vision, is swept further laterally and connective tissue is dissected off the thymus and pericardium. The self-retaining retractors are spread still further apart before proceeding to strip the pleura from the left edge of the thymus. This edge is raised from the underlying pericardium by dividing entering vessels and the whole lobe is retracted towards the right by means of stay sutures (Fig. 15). Dissection proceeds upwards to free the cornu of the left lobe which may extend to the thyroid gland. While freeing the under surface of the gland, draining vessels to the left brachiocephalic vein will have to be ligated and divided; similarly for those entering the right vein if the whole gland is to be excised.

The next step is to mobilize the left brachiocephalic vein which may be ligated with transfixion stitches and divided or may be divided between non-traumatizing clamps with a view to re-anastomosis at the end of the operation. In 17 cases ligation and division was carried out and subsequent oedema of the arms was noted, an increase of 3 to 5 cm. in girth. In the following ten cases this vessel was re-anastomosed but the increase in arm girth was no different.

The left inferior thyroid artery is next sought on the immediate medial aspect of the left carotid artery and divided between ligatures. Dissection proceeds in the interval between the left carotid artery on one side and on the other, the right brachiocephalic trunk, trachea, oesophagus and thyroid gland, taking care not to damage the thoracic duct which passes to the left, and the left recurrent laryngeal which runs in the opposite direction. After developing this interval, the careful placement of retractors will bring into view the spinal segment cervical four to

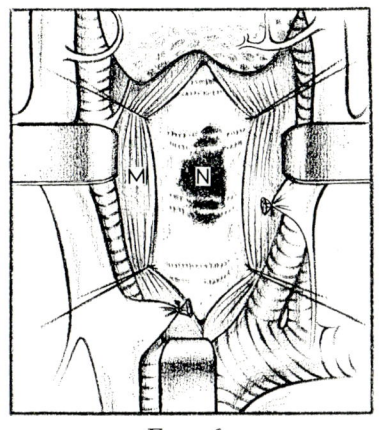 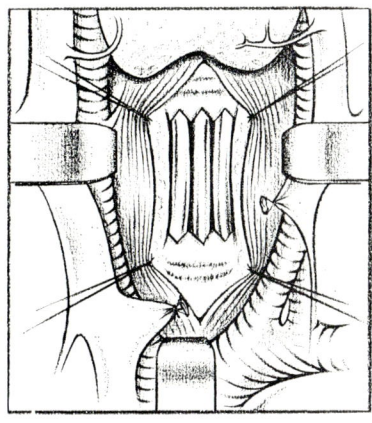

FIG. 16.   FIG. 17.

FIG. 16. M. Anterior longitudinal ligament and abscess wall retracted by stay sutures. N. Vertebral lesion.

FIG. 17. Lesion excised and three strut grafts inserted.

thoracic four (Fig. 16). A vertical incision is made in the anterior longitudinal ligament to expose the diseased area which is dealt with as described in the transthoracic approach. As in the cervical region, the chisel cuts directly backwards and care must be exercised not to inflict any damage on the spinal cord or to concuss it. In this region, grafting is more difficult because the thoracic curve changes direction as it joins the cervical spine and as the bodies are small probably only two homogenous rib strut grafts may be placed in securely (Fig. 17). Closure of the anterior longitudinal ligament is achieved with a few interrupted catgut sutures and the left brachiocephalic vein is re-anastomosed if so desired. For approximation of the two halves of sternum, the inter-scapular sandbag is removed, both shoulders of the patient brought forward on assistant's fists, awl holes made in the sternum with a protective spatula on the under surface and interrupted strong stainless steel wires are used to bring the two halves together. The divided strap muscles are repaired with interrupted catgut sutures and similarly with the periosteum over the sternum. A drain is left in the anterior mediastium leading out at the lower end of the wound and is attached to a suction bottle. This is withdrawn after a few days or when little or no drainage is seen. The pleura or pericardium may be breached inadvertently; in the latter case no repair is necessary and in the former the breach is repaired and a chest film is taken in the theatre and if need be chest drains are inserted.

Post-operative Management

Patients are nursed on anterior and posterior plaster shells which include the head. Sedation is required to control pain and coughing initially and deep breathing exercises are instituted as early as possible. Once there is evidence of clinical union, patients are mobilized gradually in an ordinary bed. This period varies from six to twelve weeks or more, depending on the age of the patient and on the length, type and stability of the grafts. When the patient is ambulatory the decision whether to use any external support or not will be left to the discretion of the individual surgeon. The above regimen applies in general to all spine cases.

Complications. The operative complications and post-operative brawny swelling of the arm have already been mentioned. In the follow up of children, a mild degree of pigeon chest has been found to develop after the split sternum procedure.

Transthoracic Approach for Cervical Seven to Lumbar Two Vertebrae

The following description is that for tuberculosis of the spine, but the surgical approach is essentially the same for any other spinal condition.

The chest is usually opened on the left side where the aorta forms a definite landmark, while on the right the inferior vena cava may be incorporated in a tuberculous abscess and is liable to be damaged. A right thoracotomy is indicated where radiography shows a very large abscess on the right side, with little or nothing on the left, or when there are pulmonary complications such as an empyema or penetration of the lung by a tuberculous paravertebral abscess.

Position: The right or left lateral position is used according to the side of the pleural cavity to be entered. The surgeon stands on the spinal side of the patient and a better view of the vertebrae is obtained if the patient is tilted slightly towards the surgeon. A sandbag or bridge under the involved vertebrae not only helps to spread the ribs apart but also to impact the bone grafts on the near side of the vertebrae, when the sandbag is removed or the bridge lowered.

Incision: An incision is made along the rib, which, in the mid-axillary line, lies opposite the point of maximum convexity of the kyphus or the centre of the lesion. This is usually two ribs higher than the centre of the vertebral lesion. It is desirable to enter the chest near the upper border of the disease process, for owing to the slope of the ribs it has been found easier to work downwards beneath the lower ribs than upwards beneath the upper ones. In a patient with severe kyphosis, the ribs are packed closely together: the operative view is better if another rib is removed subperiosteally above or below as the case may be. When the lesion is situated between cervical seven and dorsal seven or eight a 'J' shaped parascapular incision is required. The scapula can then be lifted off the chest wall after dividing the scapulo-thoracic muscles. The appropriate rib is selected and the procedure follows that described below.

Procedure: Left Thoracotomy Approach. The skin incision extends forwards to the costochondral junction and backwards to the lateral border of the erector spinae muscle. With a diathermy needle, the muscles are cut in layers, and finally the periosteum of the chosen rib likewise. With a periosteal elevator, the rib is freed from the periosteum completely. It is cut as far forwards and as far backwards as possible and is removed and kept sterile for use as a bone graft later. The remaining spinal end of the cut rib may bleed profusely and if so is packed with gelfoam or Horsley's wax.

With a scalpel a small incision is made in the rib bed and the parietal pleura. If there are no adhesions, the lung falls away from the parietal

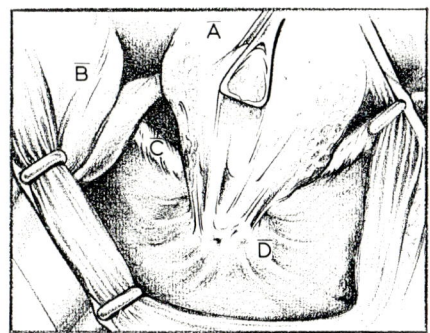

FIG. 18. Left thoracotomy. A. Lung adherent to abscess. B. Diaphragm. C. Aorta. D. Abscess wall.

pleura, but often adhesions are present; a finger is then inserted into the chest and the visceral and parietal pleura are separated by blunt dissection. As dissection proceeds, the parietal pleura is cut along the line of the rib bed. Before inserting a self-retaining retractor, with the aid of a sponge stick and fingers, more of the lung is stripped away from the wound edges, so that the retractor can be inserted and the ribs spread apart. The lung is freed as completely as possible. Adhesions are usually avascular, but not always. Thick and dense adhesions should be diathermied before cutting (Fig. 18). This type of adhesion is commonly found between the paravertebral abscess and the lung, indicating that there has been lung involvement (Yau and Hodgson 1968). The lung abscess is opened (if division of the adhesion has not already opened it), all caseous material is removed, the remaining cavity is insufflated with streptomycin powder and the pleura closed with atraumatic catgut. Care must be taken in dissecting the lung off the aorta, for in one case the paravertebral abscess had not only penetrated the lung but was also eroding the aortic wall. In such a case, it is easier and safer to free the aorta from below and from above and to isolate the dense adhesion, which can then be cut after careful palpation. Occasionally an empyma will be encountered. A decortication will have to be carried out resulting in a great deal of oozing from both the chest wall and lung surfaces, which will also have numerous air leaks.

Having freed the lung, it is retracted forwards and this displays the bulging paravertebral abscess and the aorta. In long standing cases, the abscess will be just a mass of dense scar tissue, often a centimetre in thickness. A vertical incision is made in the groove between aorta and abscess as long as is necessary to expose the diseased vertebrae. It is important that this incision is made close to the aorta, for if made more laterally the pleura is densely adherent to the abscess wall. With a pair of long scissors and non-toothed dissecting forceps and by blunt dissection a plane is developed between the aorta and the abscess. Strands of areolar tissue will be found crossing this plane; thick ones should be

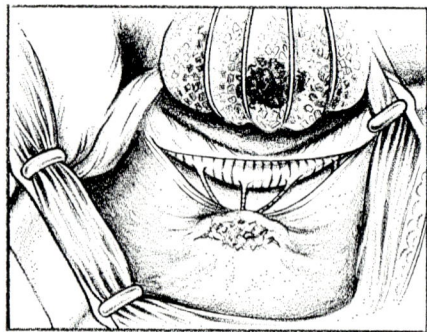

FIG. 19. Lung freed from abscess, parietal pleura incised along aorta exposing intercostal arteries converging at kyphus.

diathermied before they are cut. As the dissection proceeds towards a deeper plane by spreading the tissues apart with scissors, the intercostal vessels come into view. A good length of these vessels must be exposed for either ligation and division, or coagulation and division. Exposure of these vessels is made easier by pushing the aorta forwards and medially. In the presence of a marked kyphosis with destruction of more than three vertebral bodies, the aorta is kinked to almost the same degree as the kyphus and the intercostal vessels supplying the destroyed vertebrae are found bunched together at the apex of the curve (Fig. 19). This makes mobilization of the aorta tedious but not difficult. The number of intercostal vessels that need to be divided depends on the extent of the disease. As many as eight have been divided on one side, including the important tenth intercostal artery of Adamkiewicz but we have not seen any evidence of impairment of the blood supply to the spinal cord. During division of these vessels, branches of the hemiazygos vein and elements of the splanchic nerves will also be divided. When mobilization of the aorta is complete, it is displaced forwards and medially away from the spine with a Morriston-Davies raspatory, and the abscess is palpated across the front of the vertebral bodies.

Sometimes the abscess is tense and bulging and the aorta is stretched over it under considerable tension making mobilization of the aorta difficult without first incising and draining the abscess.

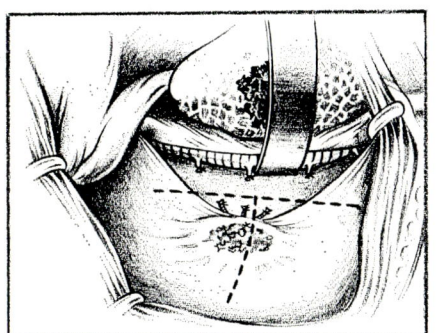 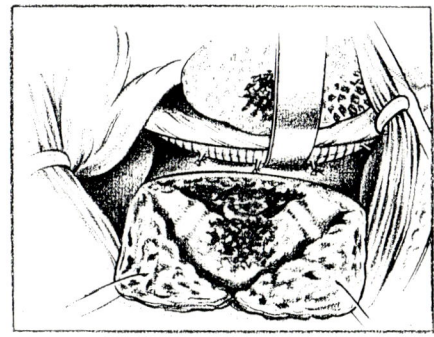

Fig. 20. Fig. 20a.

Fig. 20. Aorta mobilized and dotted lines indicate the incision for exposure of diseased vertebrae.

Fig. 20a. T-shaped flaps raised exposing underlying pathology.

The abscess is opened by a 'T' shaped incision, made first transversely opposite the centre of the disease process in the spine and completed by a vertical incision medial to the laterally placed ligatures on the intercostal vessels (Fig. 20). Two triangular flaps are raised with a diathermy needle (Fig. 20a) and to improve the exposure, especially when more

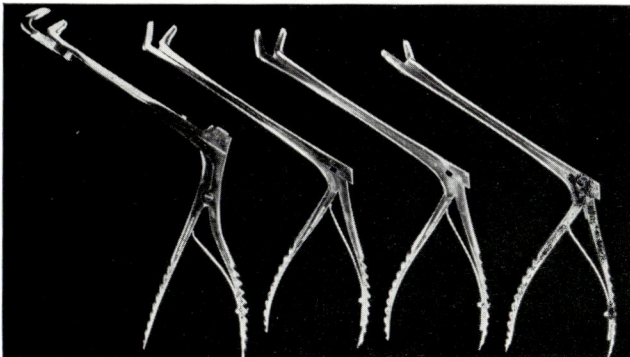

Fig. 21. Hodgson's rongeurs.

than two vertebrae are diseased, the 'T' shaped incision is converted into an 'H'. Intercostal vessels will again be encountered and bleeding is controlled by diathermy. At times it is difficult to catch bleeding points in a fibrotic abscess wall and a useful technique is to diathermy these points through a fairly fine tipped metal sucker which is kept moving around in a circular fashion over the bleeding point. The flaps are retracted by means of stay sutures attached to the muscle along the wound edges. Granulation and fibrotic tissue is cleared away from the vertebral bodies by means of Hodgson's rongeurs (Fig. 21).

The next step is to remove the diseased bodies, bony sequestra and sequestrated discs, but leaving the discs adjacent to normal vertebra to a

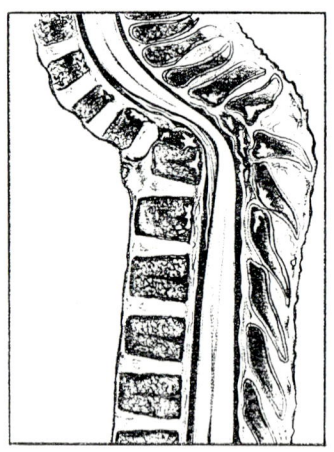

Fig. 22.

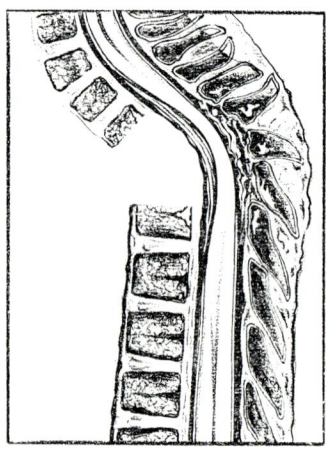

Fig. 23.

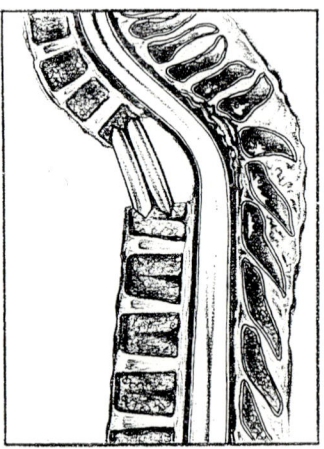

Fig. 24.

Fig. 22. Postmortem specimen showing spinal cord compressed by and stretched over the internal kyphus.

Fig. 23. Diseased tissue excised and yet the spinal cord is not free.

Fig. 24. Pachymeningitis externae of Michaud excised and cord has prolapsed forwards. Bone grafts in position.

later stage, so as to minimize bone bleeding. Diseased bone is usually avascular. Alternate use of chisels and rongeurs will clear all diseased tissue and this will lead one down to the contralateral abscess, the contents of which are evacuated by suction and by pituitary rongeurs. Care must be taken when chiselling backwards into the spinal canal, so as not to damage the spinal cord, more so when there is an acute kyphus (Fig. 22). In such a case it is prudent to visualize the spinal canal, above or below the kyphus first and then work towards the kyphus. At this stage, the posterior limit of the cavity is the posterior longitudinal ligament, which is covered by granulation tissue and is frequently separated from healthy vertebral bodies above and below by small collections of pus or sequestra and occasionally by a sequestrated disc. Often indentations can be seen and felt in the posterior longitudinal ligament (Fig. 23). This is the result of prolonged pressure on the ligament by subluxated vertebra, sequestra or sequestrated discs. Linear cuts, using a small-bladed scalpel, are made in this ligament and it is removed piece-meal by means of pituitary rongeurs. The shiny dura behind it is then displayed. In cases of acute kyphosis, the dura and cord prolapse forward and become less kinked (Fig. 24) and more often than not it starts pulsating (if it was not pulsating previously). If there is no pulsation despite complete decompression and if there is any persistent indentation or if the paraplegia has been of long duration, the dura is opened to allow the spinal cord to be inspected. Cerebro-spinal fluid will gush out and the cord will

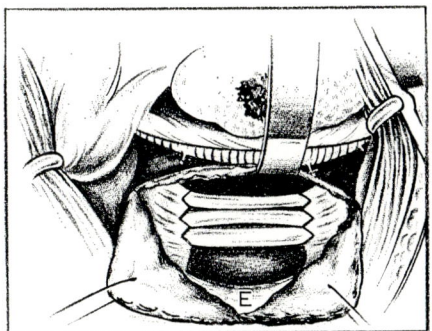

FIG. 25. Bone grafts in position. Note the distance between the posterior graft and the spinal cord labelled E.

then start pulsating. Less commonly, there are intradural adhesions and these are gently broken down by a McDonald dissector which can then be passed up and down the spinal canal to detect any further obstructions. The opening in the dura is sutured if possible; if not a piece of gelfoam is placed over it. On three occasions in our series a fistula developed between the subarachnoid space and the pleural cavity. One was closed by swinging a pleural flap; in the second the fistula sealed off spontaneously, though it took three months; the third patient died of tuberculous meningitis. However, we feel that it is imperative that the cord should be explored (Hodgson *et al.* 1964). It is useful to run one's finger along the length of the exposed cord to detect any induration or nodule in the cord and this will indicate cord penetration by the disease and can be confirmed by opening the dura. In such a case, complete recovery of the paraplegia is not expected. Rarely the cord will be felt to be just a thickened fibrotic band and these cases invariably present with severe paraplegia in flexion.

The final step is to excise the discs adjacent to normal vertebrae and to cut grooves in the normal bodies in the coronal plane at about the middle. By pressure on the kyphus, the spine is sprung open and the distance between the grooves measured with calipers. A bone graft from the excised rib is cut to the required length. It is inserted while the kyphus is sprung and when pressure is released from the kyphus, the graft will be very firmly impacted. Usually two grafts can be inserted side by side (Fig. 25). Additional grafts may be inserted in front or behind the initial ones; the required lengths are measured without springing the kyphus and during insertion the spine should not be sprung as this might dislodge the first two grafts.

The abscess cavity is instilled with two grams of streptomycin and 200 milligrams INH and the pleura and abscess wall closed with atraumatic catgut sutures. Occasionally closure is difficult because there has been a marked correction of the kyphosis; however, it is not necessary to have complete closure.

An intercostal drain is inserted before the chest is closed in layers. The drain is connected to a three-bottle suction apparatus and can usually be removed in forty-eight hours when drainage has tapered off to less than 100 c.c. in twenty-four hours and when a chest film shows complete expansion of the lung.

Right Thoracotomy Approach. The procedure is similar to that of the left-sided approach. During exposure of the lower thoracic vertebrae, care is taken to identify the inferior vena cava and to retract it out of harm's way, or else the abscess is opened at its outer limit, thus avoiding this great vein. Intercostal vessels are dealt with *pari passu* as the abscess is incised.

Upper Thoracic (C7-D3)

This is a difficult area to approach, especially so when more cervical vertebrae are involved. In such a case we favour a split-sternal approach as described by Cauchoix and Binet (1957).

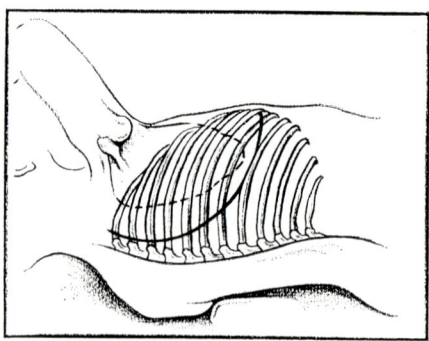

FIG. 26. Right thoracotomy position and parascapular incision marked out by heavy thick line.

For lesions between C7 and D3 vertebrae we prefer to use a standard left or right thoractomy incision (Fig. 26). The scapula is lifted off the chest wall and third rib excised. To improve exposure, the insertion of the scalenus medius muscle is ablated and the second rib excised.

The rest of the procedure is as already described. Before opening the abscess it is wise to catch the first, second and possibly the third intercostal arteries as they come off the aorta, so as to diminish the amount of subsequent bleeding. When the disease is approached from the left side, we have not seen the thoracic duct because of the thickened parietal pleura. The lowest part of the brachial plexus is seen in this approach but does not interfere with evacuation of diseased tissue. The main difficulty is not the exposure but the subsequent fusion, for the spine at this area is reversing its normal thoracic curvature and the bodies are relatively smaller. In addition there is always an element of scoliosis and rotation in these cases and it is not easy to maintain adequate fixation of the bone graft by compression.

Approach to Dorso-lumbar Disease

If the disease extends from D10 or D11 downwards to L1 or L2, the best approach is through a left thoracotomy taking out the ninth rib. The left sided approach is better than the right, for the left dome of the diaphragm is lower and it is easier to retract the spleen away from the operating field, but we have used the right approach on many occasions without difficulty.

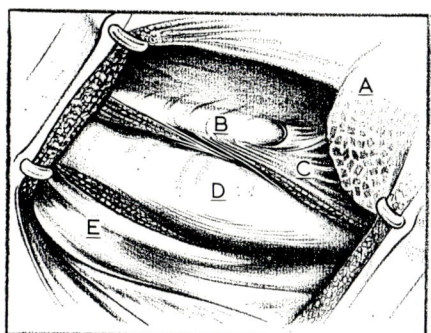

FIG. 27. Combined thoraco-abdominal approach. A. Lung. B. Aorta. C. Diaphragmatic crus. D. Thoracic twelve body. E. Psoas muscle.

The position is the same as for a left thoracotomy approach and a bridge or sandbag is centered over the vertebral lesion.

The skin incision follows that of the ninth rib, which is excised and the pleural cavity entered.

The lung is retracted and the aorta mobilized as before. The diaphragm is cut in line with the aorta and along its periphery but leaving an adequate amount of muscle for subsequent repair. By means of Deaver retractors, the diseased vertebrae are exposed after raising soft tissue flaps from the abscess wall. The lesion is dealt with as for lesions at other levels.

At the end of the operation, the diaphragm is reconstituted with catgut sutures and the pleural cavity drained as in a standard thoracotomy approach. Figure 27 depicts another method of approach to dorso-lumbar lesions. The left tenth rib is excised and both body cavities are entered, the abdominal extraperitoneally, the thoracic intrapleurally. The rest of the procedure is similar to that already described.

Correction of Fixed Spinal Curves

Having gained considerable experience in the correction of tuberculous kyphoses, we embarked on the operative correction of fixed scoliotic curves (Hodgson 1965) whether idiopathic, congenital or paralytic in origin. The surgical approach is essentially the same as that for tubercular spines with a few modifications.

When looking at the lateral X-ray film of a severe scoliotic one sees a kyphotic deformity which is usually not a true kyphosis but the result of rotation of the vertebral bodies. Our aim is to correct the scoliosis by spinal osteotomy; the rotational deformity will, to some extent, then be corrected automatically. Two methods are used to achieve correction; either a wedge is resected and closed on the side of convexity, or a wedge

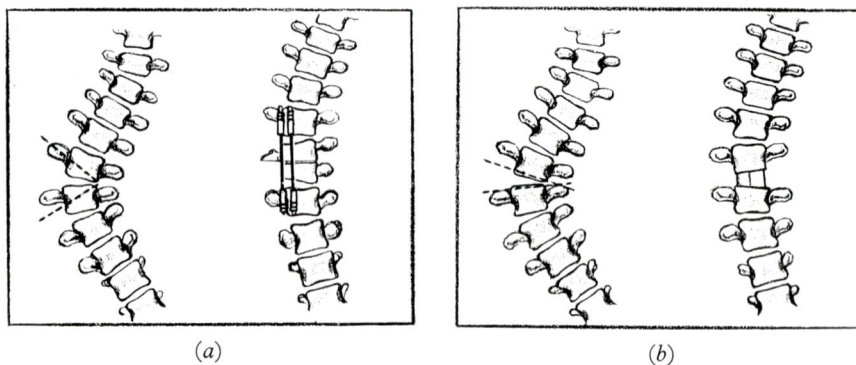

FIG. 28. (a) Closing a wedge in scoliosis. (b) Opening a wedge with bone grafts.

is opened on the concave side (Fig. 28a and b). Opening a wedge should be reserved for young individuals with dorso-lumbar curves of moderate degree (30° to 60°). Pre-operative investigations should always include cardio-pulmonary function tests and myelograms. We have not had a case in which cardio-pulmonary function was so poor as to preclude operation. In severe scoliosis there is always deformation of the spinal canal and sometimes even pressure on the cord by deformed and rotated posterior spinal elements such as the laminae. If the myelodil column does show deformation, then this should be the site of the osteotomy, otherwise the apex of the curve is selected.

Operative Procedure for a Transthoracic Approach

The patient is placed in the lateral position with the convex side uppermost on an operating table that breaks at the apex of the curve so that the head end and tail end can be elevated to help close the osteotomy site.

Incision: The appropriate rib is selected as previously described; the incision extends further backwards to the spinous process or a little beyond so that the erector spinae muscle on the near side can be divided and that on the far side elevated as in a standard laminectomy (Fig. 29).

Procedure: The rib is excised and disarticulated at the vertebral end. It is deformed and lies hard up against the rotated vertebral body and may have to be removed in segments. The pleural cavity is entered through the rib bed and rib spreaders inserted. It will be noted that the pleural cavity is deformed and that the vertebral bodies are more superficial than expected, practically under the skin (Fig. 30). The osteotomy is done through a disc space and this is identified by counting ribs or by taking an X-ray. No mobilization of the aorta or vena cava is necessary as they have moved to the far side. The intercostal vessels lying on the

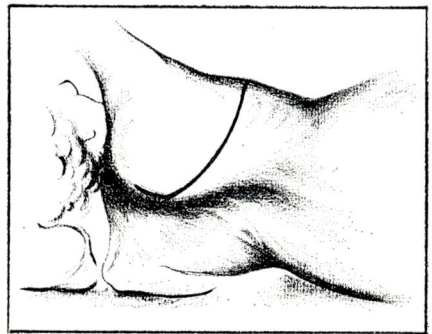 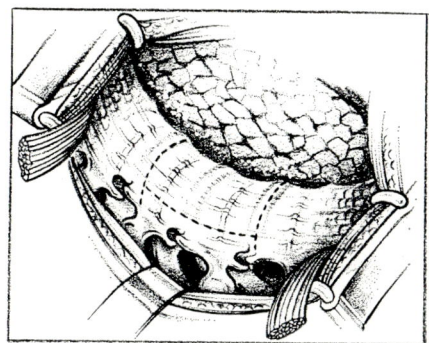

Fig. 29.   Fig. 30.

Fig. 29. Right thoracic scoliosis. Incision. See text for details.

Fig. 30. Right thoracotomy. From top to bottom: Lung; vertebrae—dotted lines mark incision for elevating parietal pleura; transverse and spinous processes exposed after elevating erector spinae muscles.

adjacent vertebral bodies are diathermied, the parietal pleura turned back to expose the disc (Fig. 31) and this is removed in its entirety with the exception of the annulus fibrosus on the far side. While working backwards in the direction of the spinal canal, care must be exercised as the spinal cord is not in its usual anatomical position; otherwise the posterior annulus is left intact and the corresponding lamina removed, exposing the dura. With the cord in view, one can then work forwards nibbling off the pedicle and the posterior annulus. While working in the vicinity of the cord, Batson's plexus of veins may be damaged and the bleeding will have to be controlled by gelfoam packs or patties; also for the sake of exposure, one or two nerve roots will have to be sacrificed.

Attention is next turned to cutting a wedge in the vertebral bodies; the base of the wedge is situated postero-laterally and includes the bodies, pedicles and the associated laminae: a soft tissue bridge consisting of annulus and a little bone is left at the apex situated antero-laterally on the far side (Fig. 32). The size of the wedge depends upon the amount of correction required and is worked out on the X-ray film. Possibly not

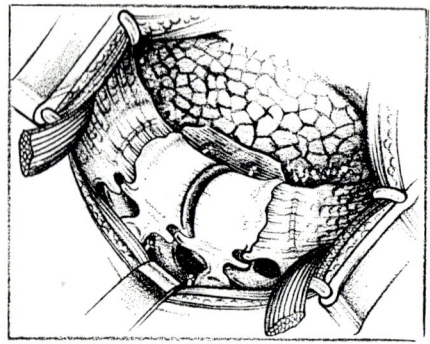 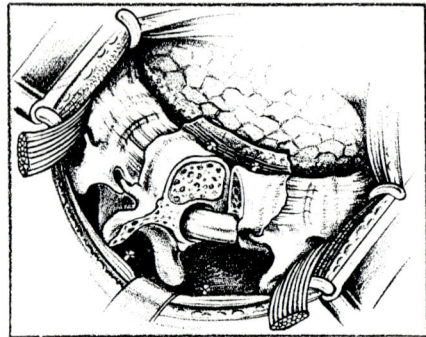

FIG. 31.   FIG. 32.

FIG. 31. Intercostal vessels ligated and parietal pleura turned back to expose disc and adjacent vertebrae.

FIG. 32. Disc excised, appropriate sized wedge cut in vertebrae and spinal cord exposed after excision of transverse and spinous processes.

more than 45° should be taken at one sitting, further correction can always be attained at a second operation. We have tried to get more correction by cutting two wedges at consecutive discs at the same operation, but this prolongs the procedure, making it more difficult without achieving the desired result. When bone is being removed from the vertebral bodies there is apt to be brisk bleeding and this is controlled by packing while the posterior elements are tackled. Thus attention is directed alternately to the anterior and posterior elements until the required wedge is cut and the cord exposed. When excising hemivertebrae, we have found thick scar tissue in front of the spinal canal and even thick strands of undifferentiated connective tissue straddling the cord.

The next step is to get an adequate exposure for the insertion of Harrington's rods to close the wedge. This may entail excision of the posterior 10 cm. of the ribs above and below if this has not already

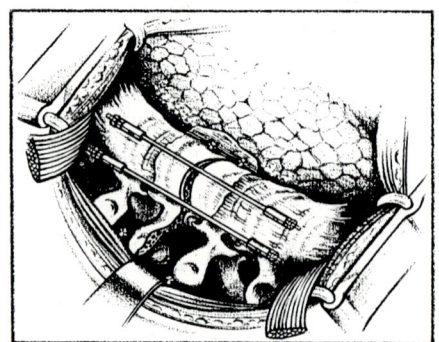 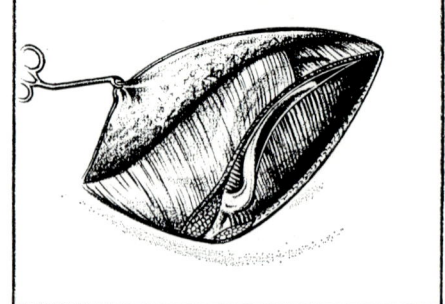

FIG. 33.   FIG. 34.

FIG. 33. Harrington rods in position and wedge almost completely closed.

FIG. 34. Right sided J-shaped incision exposing eleventh and twelfth ribs.

been done when getting the necessary exposure for wedge resection. Two rods are used, one situated posteriorly at the pedicle or its root, and the other at the antero-lateral aspect of the bodies. Hooks are inserted into the body of the vertebra adjacent to that in which the wedge was cut just above the intervertebral disc so that the hook gets a firm purchase on dense bone bordering the cartilage plate (Fig. 33). As the hooks are approximated with the rods *in situ*, the head and tail ends of the operating table are raised to assist in closing the gap. While this is in progress a strict watch is kept on the cord, for any bony pressure on it; if there is pressure, the appropriate amount of bone is nibbled off. Wound closure is similar to that already described.

The technique of wedge resection for dorso-lumbar differs from that described above in only two ways. Firstly, the skin incision is 'J' shaped (Fig. 34) and a skin flap is turned headwards to expose both the eleventh and twelfth ribs. The abdominal musculature is cut along the twelfth rib, which is excised and the lumbar spine is exposed extraperitoneally. To gain better exposure of lumbar one and thoracic twelve bodies, the eleventh rib is resected subperiosteally to give easier retraction. Working in the twelfth rib bed, the diaphragmatic origin is cut to expose parietal pleura which is pushed away by blunt dissection and more diaphragm and crus cut to expose the bodies. Thus, this is a combined extra-peritoneal and extra-pleural approach. Secondly, the lumbar nerve roots are isolated and retracted out of harm's way, unlike intercostal nerves which can be sacrificed with impunity.

Opening a Wedge

In thoracic scoliosis, the approach is transthoracic and is similar to that described for closing a wedge (except, of course, that it is done on the concave side). If the apex of the curve is at dorsal twelve or lumbar one

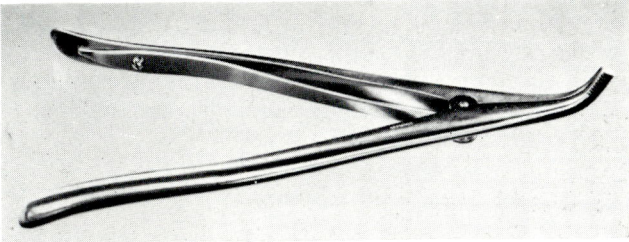

FIG. 35. Vertebral spreaders.

vertebra, then the approach is subdiaphragmatic by resecting the eleventh or twelfth rib (vide infra) but the incision extends to the midline for subsequent exposure of lamina and spinous process. The disc space to be wedged open is cleared of all nuclear material and the cartilage plates are shaved off carefully to preserve the underlying cortical bone for strength when autogenous grafts are inserted. As before, posterior elements are removed on the near side and the cord can be seen. Vertebral spreaders (Fig. 35) are inserted and adjacent vertebral bodies spread apart. Sometimes, the soft tissue hinge, comprising slightly less than half the annulus fibrosus on the far side, stretches too, resulting in a trapezoidal wedge. The kidney bridge of the operating table centred at the apex of the curve is raised to help open the wedge which is also held open temporarily by wooden blocks inserted while the bodies are kept apart by spreaders. Massive autogenous iliac grafts, usually two, are cut to the correct shape and size to replace the wooden blocks. Empty spaces around the grafts are packed with cancellous iliac bone (Fig. 36). Wound closure is tedious but can be achieved with patience.

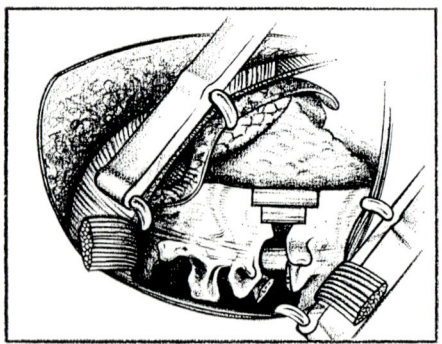

FIG. 36. Wedge opened on concave side of scoliosis and grafts in position.

Post-operative management. Patients are nursed on previously prepared anterior and posterior plaster shells or on a Stryker turning frame. By eight to twelve weeks post-operatively, the osteotomy site is firm and the patients can be mobilized on an ordinary bed. They are allowed up wearing some form of support until there is radiological evidence of consolidation.

Complications. While opening a wedge, the thoracic duct was ruptured in one case, and in another there was transient weakness of one lower limb. In closing wedges, there was one case of paraesthesia in one lower limb, one case in which the Harrington's hook slipped and one in which the rod migrated through the wound.

Upper Lumbar Approach (D12 to L2)

The most satisfactory approach is through the eleventh rib, as described by Fey (1925). This approach can be kept extrapleural and extraperitoneal. The patient lies on his right side, if the left eleventh rib is to be removed. The skin incision is along the line of this rib. The abdomen is entered extraperitoneally. The origin of the diaphragm is dissected off the rib and vertebrae and care taken not to damage the parietal pleura. (If it is damaged the defect is repaired with atraumatic catgut sutures and the last stitch tied while the anaesthetist keeps the lung inflated.) To expose the vertebral bodies the psoas muscle is detached at its upper end and turned downwards. The lumbar vessels are found lying close to the midpoint of the vertebral bodies and are dealt with accordingly. At the close of the operation catgut sutures are inserted into the detached part of the diaphragm and the surrounding soft tissues.

Lumbar Approach (L2 to L5)

If access to L2 vertebra is required, it is best to go through the twelfth rib as described by Digby (1941); alternatively, the normal nephrectomy/ureterostomy incision will suffice.

The description which follows is of an approach to the lumbar spine for tuberculosis.

Position: We prefer to approach the spine from the left because it is easier to deal with the aorta than with the inferior vena cava. The patient is placed in the right lateral position with a bridge centred over the kyphus. This increases the distance between the lower rib margin and the iliac crest. If the kyphosis is severe, this distance is greatly narrowed or non-existent when the bridge is lowered.

Incision: The incision resembles that for a nephro-ureterectomy, extending backwards to the lateral border of the erector spinae muscle and forwards to the linae semilunaris.

Procedure: With diathermy, the layers of the abdominal musculature are incised in the line of the skin incision. The peritoneum is stripped off the posterior abdominal wall and the ureter and kidney with it. This manoeuvre may be difficult because of adhesions. Care must be taken to identify the ureter lest it be damaged. If a large psoas abscess is present, this simplifies matters for often it has achieved the soft tissue dissection and, when opened, leads directly to the diseased vertebrae. The abscess may be opened in line with the fibres of the psoas muscle or across it transversely. It is to be noted that the abscess is intramuscular rather than under the sheath as commonly described. When the contents are evacuated, thick strands of soft tissue will be found running transversely across the abscess cavity. These strands contain lumbar vessels; they are diathermied and divided. The lumbar nerve plexus is rarely encountered as it lies in a more posterior plane. If no abscess is present, the psoas muscle will be fibrotic and may either be divided transversely and the cut ends turned up and down, or its origins from the vertebral bodies are detached and reflected laterally (Fig. 37). Where there are missing vertebral bodies, the origins will be found crowded together as are the lumbar vessels. The Morriston-Davies rib raspatory is a useful instrument with which to strip the muscular origins and soft tissue from the front of the vertebral bodies. Lumbar vessels are dealt with when encountered and unlike the thoracic region, they are difficult to secure beforehand. The aorta and the inferior vena cava are displaced to the right side of the vertebral bodies and the psoas muscle to the left. The sympathetic chain may be reflected with one or other structure. At times this chain is not identifiable, owing to the disease process.

Diseased vertebrae are dealt with as before and a massive autogenous iliac graft inserted. In children, bank bone may be used instead. With the lowering of the bridge, the graft will be firmly impacted; this will also make it easier to close the abdominal musculature.

To expose the body of lumbar 5 or the first piece of the sacrum, the left common and external iliac vessels need to be mobilized. An attempt should be made to identify the ascending and/or ilio-lumbar veins. (See description for approach to degenerated discs.) If these vessels are lacerated or torn from their origins there will be troublesome bleeding. With difficulty they can be stopped by carefully placed atraumatic silk sutures. One one occasion, the abscess had partly eroded the posterior aspect of the right common iliac artery at its origin; dissection in this area completed it. The bleeding was controlled by passing tapes round the aorta and the two common iliac arteries, and the defect was visualized and repaired with fine atraumatic silk.

While excising L-5 body and the upper part of the sacrum care must be taken not to damage the lumbosacral nerve trunks, especially when chiselling and removing bone from the far side. It is difficult to wedge

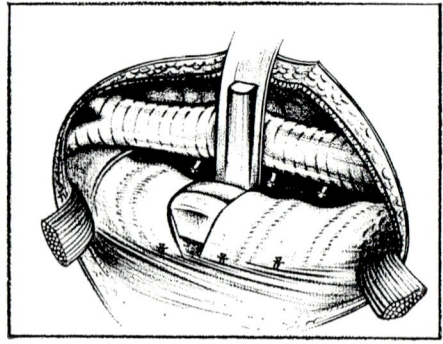

FIG. 37. Great vessels retracted, lumbar disease excised and bone grafts in position, part of psoas muscle turned up and turned down to give the exposure required.

in a large bone graft if part of the sacrum is removed, for the bony bed will diminish rapidly in size the further down the sacrum one goes. It will then have to be decided whether a posterior spinal fusion should be carried out at a later date, or if the anterior graft will suffice. At the end of the operation the psoas muscle, if divided, may be approximated with a few sutures or left as it is.

Interbody Fusion for Lumbar Disc Lesions

The following description is for the exposure of intervertebral discs between L3 and 4, L4 and 5, and L5 and S1 vertebrae. Usually only the lower two spaces need to be exposed (for removal of discs and interbody fusion) as it is not common to have a symptomatic degenerated disc between lumbar three and four vertebrae.

We prefer the extraperitoneal approach from the left side; extraperitoneal because the exposure is easier and there is little or no postoperative meteorism; from the left side because the left common iliac vessels are longer than the right and therefore can be retracted across to the right without undue tension.

In a few cases we have used a subumbilical midline incision and approached the spine transperitoneally for two reasons:
(1) Anticipated difficulties of dissection in the extraperitoneal area in patients who had had previous abdominal operations for unrelated conditions.
(2) For obese patients, the transperitoneal approach was used during the earlier part of our experience. However, we have been using the extraperitoneal approach without difficulty for patients with similar physique since that time.

If the aorta bifurcates at a high level, the lowest lumbar disc is best exposed between the common iliac vessels; if the bifurcation is low, the disc is approached from the left side of the left common iliac vessels.

Position: Previously, we used a supine position with a bridge in the low back to hyper-extend the lower lumbar vertebrae. Subsequently we have found it much easier to do the operation with the patient lying on

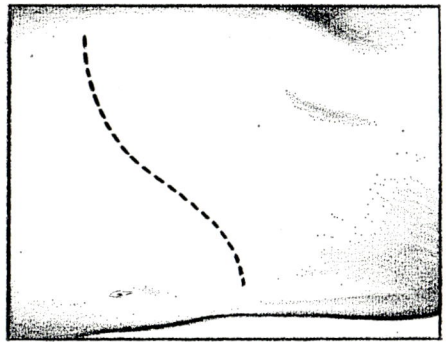

FIG. 38. S-shaped incision over left flank.

his right side; during dissection, the soft tissues fall away from the spine and little retraction is required. This is especially so when operating on obese individuals with pendulous abdomens. However, the advantage of the supine position is that an elevated bridge at the lumbosacral region will open up the disc space to accept well-fitting bone grafts, and when the bridge is lowered the grafts are absolutely tight. This disadvantage can be partly overcome by the use of vertebral spreaders.

A bridge or sandbag is used in the lumbar region to correct the scoliosis due to lying in the lateral position and is removed at the end of the operation to facilitate closure of the abdominal wound.

Incision: The incision starts in the midline midway between the symphysis pubis and the umbilicus and forms a lazy S to a point midway between the iliac crest and the lowest rib in the flank (Fig. 38). It may be shifted cranially to approach the disc between the third and fourth lumbar vertebrae.

Procedure: The skin incision is made with a scalpel; thereafter, an electric cautery is used to incise successively subcutaneous fat, superficial and deep fascia, external oblique, internal oblique and transversalis muscles, and fascia. All layers are divided in the line of the skin incision. The external oblique muscle may be split along its fibres but it will be found that the split does not correspond to the line of skin incision. Medially, the anterior and posterior rectus sheaths are divided with scissors up to the midline leaving the rectus muscle intact. Care must be taken to dissect the peritoneum off the posterior rectus sheath as sometimes here the peritoneum is thin and adherent, especially in multipara. Occasionally the semicircular fold of Douglas coincides with the line of incision at the posterior rectus sheath and thus the peritoneum can be stripped off directly without having to cut the sheath. It is best to start stripping peritoneum laterally as there is a good layer of extraperitoneal fat to work in and to develop the plane of dissection. Having found the plane, one can then work towards the rectus muscle, then laterally and backwards to expose the psoas muscle and sheath, the abdominal aorta

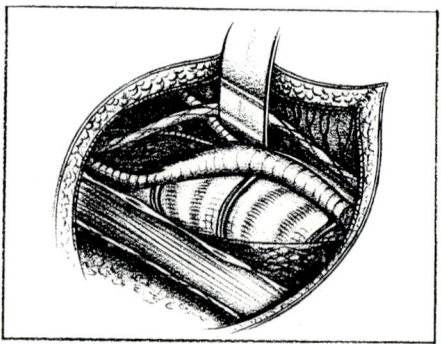

FIG. 39. Ureter behind retractor; the rest of the diagram shows the aorta and its branches, the last two lumbar discs, the psoas muscle with the overlying sympathetic chain and the genito-femoral nerve. For clarity, the great veins are not drawn in.

and the common iliac vessels, cranially for about a hand's breadth and caudally into the pelvis until a good length of the iliac vessels are exposed at about the level of the second piece of the sacrum. During dissection the ureter is identified and is displaced towards the right side together with the peritoneum (Fig. 39). If the peritoneal cavity is inadvertently opened it is closed with atraumatic catgut.

By means of Deaver retractors, the peritoneum is retracted medially and the psoas muscle laterally; this brings the great vessels into view. The iliac artery is freed from its sheath by means of scissors and stripping with the index finger. Some sympathetic fibres passing over the artery will be divided as a consequence.

Dissection is then carried proximally towards the bifurcation of the aorta. Occasionally para-aortic lymph glands hinder dissection, but they can be dissected off with patience. By this stage, the intervertebral disc between lumbar four and five vertebrae comes into view and by blunt dissection, pushing extraperitoneal connective tissue and the left sympathetic chain towards the left, more of it will be seen. Working caudally again along the line of the common iliac artery the common iliac vein will be seen on a deeper plane. The fifth set of lumbar vessels if present may be encountered lying on the body of lumbar five vertebra. These vessels are ligated and divided. They may not be present; instead, an ascending lumbar vein may need ligation and division. The common iliac vein and its continuation, the external iliac vein, is carefully freed caudally, thus leading to the ilio-lumbar vein running upwards, laterally and posterior to the medial border of the psoas muscle (Fig. 40). A good length of the ilio-lumbar vein is freed for ligation and division. This vein may be absent, may be single, double or triple; and if single, may be short and of wide bore or may bifurcate immediately. In the latter case, one branch of the Y may lie deep to the other and is not easily seen. Thus it may be damaged and cause troublesome bleeding. If the vein is short and of wide bore, it is safer to use a stitch ligature; otherwise during retraction of the common iliac vein, the ligature may slip.

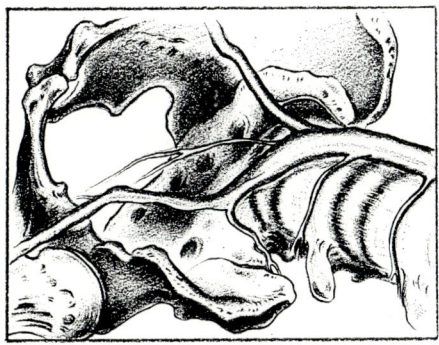 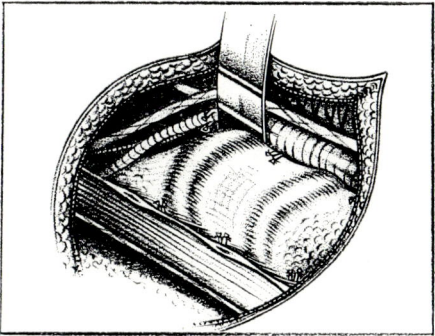

FIG. 40. FIG. 41.

FIG. 40. Drawing of an injection specimen showing the left common iliac vein tethered down by the ilio-lumbar vein.

FIG. 41. Ilio-lumbar and lumbar vessels ligated. Great vessels displaced towards the right exposing the fourth and fifth lumbar discs.

After dividing the ilio-lumbar vein, and cauterizing and dividing some occasional muscular arterial branches from the iliac artery, the common iliac vessels can be displaced towards the right side, exposing the lumbo-sacral disc. Using a slightly curved Morriston Davies' rib raspatory and a small piece of gauze, all the soft tissue is gradually stripped towards the right side. This exposes the whole of the lumbar four-five disc, lumbar five body, lumbosacral disc and the upper part of the sacrum (Fig. 41). During stripping small vessels will be encountered running into the anterior longitudinal ligament from the vena cava and they are diathermied and divided. This stage of the operation can be very tedious in some cases of spondylolisthesis because of dense fibrous adhesions between the spine and the big vessels. In such a case the left common iliac vessels are mobilized from the left and right alternately until they can be lifted off the spine. When the spine is approached in this manner, the midsacral artery and vein and the hypogastric plexus are not damaged.

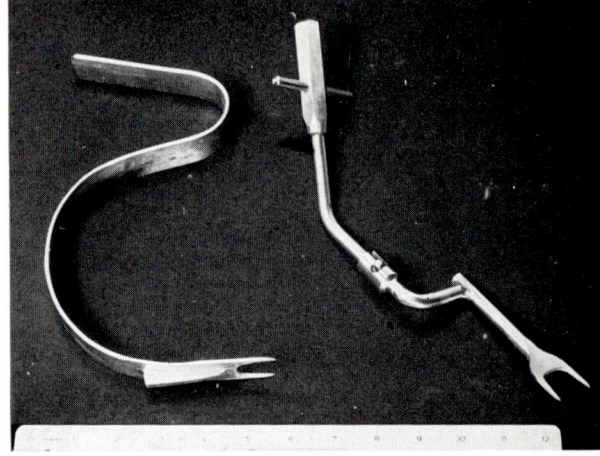

Fig. 42. Harmon's retractors.

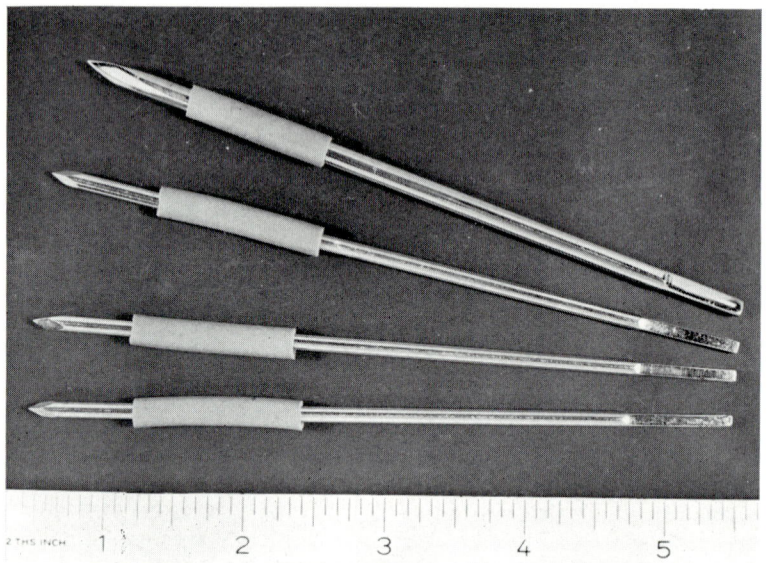

Fig. 43. Steinmann's pins with protective rubber tubing.

With a little difficulty in retraction one can dissect upwards to expose the disc between lumbar three and four vertebrae after ligating and dividing a further set or two of lumbar vessels. Self-retaining retractors are used to straddle the disc space: on the right side a Harmon's retractor is best (Fig. 42), but if this is not available Steinmann pins (Fig. 43) are effective. Harmon's retractor is too bulky to be used on the left side; there, a Deaver's retractor is better. The intervertebral discs are now well exposed. A discogram may be carried out and this will also confirm the level of the disc. If the level of the lesion is in doubt, we use the saline acceptance test. A normal disc should accept with great difficulty, one to 1·5 ml. of saline.

With a long-bladed scalpel, the anterior longitudinal ligament and annulus fibrosus is cut in the form of a rectangle almost across the whole width of the disc and removed; alternatively, it may be hinged towards one side or other and used for retraction (Fig. 44). The nucleus pulposus is removed with long-neck rongeurs designed by Hodgson (Fig. 21). A pituitary rongeur is useful to remove the remaining bits left in the deeper recesses of the disc space. Sometimes an opening may be found in the annulus posteriorly and it may be plugged with prolapsed nucleus. This can be drawn out of the spinal canal in its entirety.

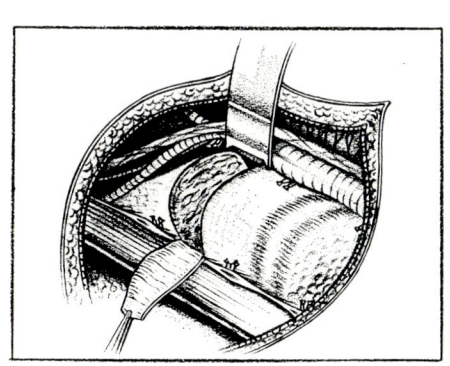
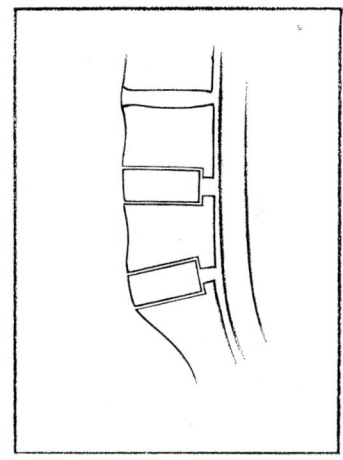

FIG. 44.   FIG. 45.

FIG. 44. Harmon's spiked retractors inserted on far side, annulus fibrosus hinged towards the left, nucleus pulposus removed revealing cartilage plate on upper surface of sacrum.

FIG. 45. Cartilage plate excised. Note rim of bone left posteriorly.

Having cleared out all the nucleus, one can then judge the depth of the cavity. With chisels the cartilage plate of the adjacent vertebral bodies is shaved off and removed. A narrow rim of bone is left at the back of the vertebral bodies to ensure that the bone grafts will not extrude into the spinal canal (Fig. 45). The size of the cavity is estimated; it is packed with gelfoam and a piece of gauze while the next disc is dealt with in the same manner. The retractors are removed and placed astride the next disc. In this way a minimum of traction is exerted on the big vessels.

Iliac grafts are then cut from the left crest, slightly larger than the cavity in the vertical plane and to a depth of at least two-thirds or more of the antero-posterior diameter of the vertebral bodies. Usually two grafts are required for each intervertebral space. They are impacted well in while the assistant provides hyperextension of the lumbar spine. If the anterior longitudinal ligament and the annulus fibrosus was used as a hinged flap, it may be sutured back to the annulus opposite the hinge. In fact this is not necessary and it does no harm to remove the flap after impacting the bone grafts (Fig. 46).

Before closing the abdominal wound in layers the divided ilio-lumbar vein and/or ascending lumbar vein is checked to ensure that the ligatures are not on the point of slipping. It is not necessary to leave a drain in the abdominal wound, but one may be left in the iliac wound for twenty-four to forty-eight hours. Blood loss averages 250 ml. and a transfusion is rarely required. Post-operatively, patients are allowed up and about as soon as possible.

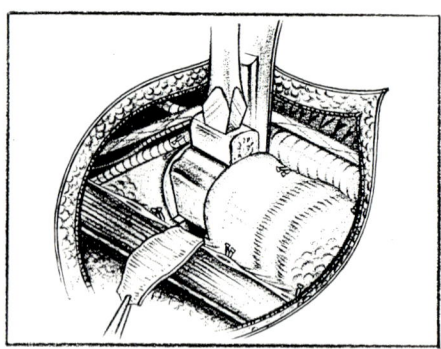

FIG. 46. Two blocks of autogenous iliac graft being impacted into disc space.

High Bifurcation of the Aorta

Having stripped the peritoneum off the big vessels, one can palpate the lumbosacral angle and note its relation to the bifurcation of the aorta. If this is high, at or above the upper half of lumbar body four, it is easier to approach the lumbosacral disc between the common iliac vessels.

A vertical incision is made in the extraperitoneal connective tissue over the disc in the mid-line. The midsacral vessels must be ligated and divided. By careful blunt dissection the disc is exposed as described previously (Fig. 47). This procedure causes a minimum of damage to the hypogastric plexus; in fact we have not encountered any case of loss of sexual prowess in the male. The rest of the procedure is similar to that already described.

Occasionally one may be able to reach the disc above by enlarging the incision upwards. Otherwise this disc is best approached from the left side of the aorta and left common iliac vessels. There is then little need to mobilize the left common iliac vessels as extensively as described previously.

Complications. (1) Deep vein thrombosis. (2) Osteomyelitis of the bone graft. (3) Paralytic ileus and retention of urine. (4) Warm left leg due to damaged lumbar sympathetics.

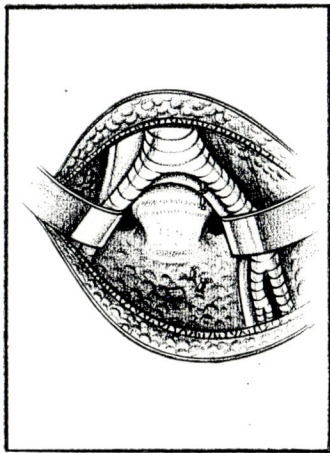

Fig. 47. Exposure of lumbo-sacral disc between the bifurcation of aorta; note ligated presacral vessels.

Perineal Approach to the Sacral Spine

This was carried out in two cases only. A transverse curvi-linear incision is made with its centre at the coccyx which is excised; the front of the sacrum is approached by pushing the rectum forwards. The abscess is opened and cleaned out; no grafting is necessary or possible.

Complications of Surgery for Tuberculosis of the Spine

These are listed below: some apply to operations other than for tuberculosis.

(1) Wound sepsis.
(2) Pleural effusion.
(3) Pulmonary embolism.
(4) Cystitis and bed sores in paraplegics.
(5) Post-operative ileus.
(6) Convulsions due to streptomycin on the exposed dura.
(7) Fistula between subarachnoid space and pleural cavity.
(8) Damaged ureter.
(9) Fractured grafts.
(10) Slipped grafts.
(11) Paraplegia.

The only common complication was paralytic ileus when the operation involved the dorsolumbar and lumbar region, but this was of a mild form. Pulmonary embolism is almost unknown among the Chinese in Hong Kong. Cases of incomplete paraplegia occasionally become complete post-operatively, but in time there was full recovery.

Discussion

The surgery involved in the exposure of the spine from the front is a major undertaking; hence we do not advocate this procedure where facilities for surgery, anaesthesia and nursing care are inadequate. The surgeon must have a thorough knowledge of normal and abnormal anatomy, and of surgical techniques such as the repair of major vessels. With experience, the surgeon will find that most of the procedures described are not much more difficult than many routine orthopaedic or general surgical procedures. Even frail patients tolerate the operation surprisingly well. The exceptions are the transoral and the split-sternum approaches; the transoral because one is working in a confined space and there are the ever-present dangers of damaging the vertebral vessels and of secondary infection; the split-sternum, because there is a great deal of anatomy to be dealt with on the way to the spine. This approach is even more difficult when there is a marked kyphosis and a pigeon chest so that one has to work in a deep hole; such cases are best tackled through the neck or through a standard thoracotomy incision.

The radical treatment of spinal tuberculosis, correction of kyphoses and the treatment of disc lesions is well established in our hands; but the treatment of fixed deformities in scoliosis, other than those due to hemivertebrae, is still in its early stages. However, we feel that this line of treatment is worth pursuing and that a better fixation device should be developed for closing a wedge and holding it closed.

The anterior approach to fractured spines is rarely indicated though we have used this route for stabilization of fresh, unstable dorsolumbar fractures. A case can probably be made out for the anterior fixation of cervical spine fractures, if these are unstable.

In spinal surgery we advocate the use of electric cautery wherever possible, as it shortens the operating time considerably. It is best to use a needle at the end of a pair of diathermy forceps; the needle can easily be replaced whenever the one in use is caked with burnt tissue.

References

BAILEY, R. W. and BADGLEY, C. E. (1960). Stabilization of the cervical spine by anterior fusion. *J. Bone Jt. Surg.*, **42A**, 565.
BURNS, B. H. (1933). An operation for spondylolisthesis. *Lancet* **i**, 1233.
CAUCHOIX, J. and BINET, J. P. (1957). Anterior surgical approaches to the spine. *Ann. Roy. Coll. Surg. Engl.*, **21**, 237.
CLOWARD, R. B. (1963). Lesions of the intervertebral disks and their treatment by interbody fusion methods: the painful disk. *Clin. Orthop.* **27**, 51.
DIGBY, K. H. (1941). *Surg. Gynec. Obstet.*, **73**, 84.
DOMMISSE, G. F. (1959). Lumbo-sacral inter-body spinal fusion. *J. Bone Jt. Surg.*, **41B**, 87.
FANG, H. S. Y. and ONG, G. B. (1962). Direct anterior approach to the upper cervical spine. *J. Bone Jt. Surg.*, **44A**, 8, 1588–1604.
FEY, B. (1925–27). *Arch. Urol.*, **5**, 169 (quoted by Monat).
GERAUD (1750). Observation sur un coup de feu à l'épine. *Mém. Acad. Roy. Chir.*, **2**, 515.
GJESSING, M. H. (1951). Osteoplastic anterior fusion of the lower lumbar spine in spondylolisthesis, localized spondylosis and tuberculous spondylitis. *Act. Orthop. Scand.*, **20**, 200–213.
GREY, T. G., ROGERS, L. C., and GORDON-TAYLOR, G. (1956). Modern operative surgery, Ed. 4 pp. 1678–1679, London, Cassell.
HARMON, P. H. (1961). Anterior extraperitoneal lumbar vertebral body fusion. *Clin. Orthop.* **18**, 169.

Hodgson, A. R. (1965). An approach to the cervical spine. (C3–7). *Clin. Orthop.*, **39,** 129–134.
Hodgson, A. R. (1965b). Correction of fixed spinal curves. *J. Bone Jt. Surg.*, **47A,** 6, 1221–1227.
Hodgson, A. R. and Stock, F. E. (1956). Anterior spinal fusion. A preliminary communication on the radical treatment of Pott's disease and Pott's paraplegia. *Brit. J. of Surg.*, **44,** 185, 266–275.
Hodgson, A. R., Stock, F. E., Fang, H. S. Y. and Ong, G. B. (1960). Anterior spinal fusion—the operative approach and pathological findings in 412 patients with Pott's disease of the spine. *Brit. J. of Surg.*, **48,** 208, 172–178.
Hodgson, A. R., Yau, A., Kwon, J. S. and Kim, D. (1964). A clinical study of 100 consecutive cases of Pott's paraplegia. *Clin. Orthop.* **36,** 128–149.
Iwahara, T. (1944). A new method of vertebral body fusion. *Surg.*, **8,** 271 (Japan).
Jaslow, A. (1946). Intercorporal bone graft in spinal fusion after disc removal. *Surg. Gynec. & Obstet.* **82.**
Kocher, T. (1911). Textbook of operative surgery. (Trans. from the fifth German Ed. by H. J. Stiles and C. B. Paul.) Ed. 3 Vol. 2; 434–435. London: Adam & Charles Black.
Maisonneuve (1852). Accident de l'Hotel des Princes. *Gazette des Hôpitaux,* 85.
Mercer, W. (1963). Spondylolisthesis, with a description of a new method of operative treatment and notes of ten cases. *Edin. Med. J.*, **43,** 545.
Monat, T. B. (1939). *Brit. J. Urol.*, **11,** 126.
Robinson, R. A., Walker, A. E., Ferlic, D. C. and Wieching, D. K. (1962). The results of anterior interbody fusion of the cervical spine. *J. Bone Jt. Surg.*, **44A,** 1569.
Rodolfi (1859). Palla di fucile penetrata nel cello e incunecta al lato destro della colonna vertebrale. Extrazione del proiettile. *Gaurigione Grazz. Med. Ital.* (Lombardia), **4,** 404.
Sacks, S. (1960). Cervical spine fusion by the anterior approach. *Mediese Bydraes,* **6,** 493.
Southwick, W. O. and Robinson, R. A. (1957). Surgical approaches to the vertebral bodies in the cervical and lumbar regions. *J. Bone Jt. Surg.*, **39A,** 631–644.
Thomson, St. Clair, and Negus, V. E. (1947). Diseases of the nose and throat. A textbook for students and practitioners. Ed. 5. 489–509. Cassell: London.
Wilson, C. P. (1951). The approach to the nasopharnyx. *Proc. Roy. Soc. Med.* Section of Laryngology, **44,** 9–14 (quoted by Grey-Turner, Rogers and Gordon-Taylor).
Yau, A. and Hodgson, A. R. (1968). Penetration of the lung by the paravertebral abscess in tuberculosis of the spine. *J. Bone Jt. Surg.*, **50A,** 243.

Chapter 10

AN OPERATIVE TREATMENT FOR CONGENITAL DISLOCATION AND SUBLUXATION OF THE HIP IN THE OLDER CHILD

ROBERT B. SALTER

The purpose of this chapter in the present edition of Recent Advances in Orthopaedics is not to discuss all of the many operative methods of treatment for congenital dislocation of the hip at various ages; such material, which could hardly be considered recent, is ably presented in other publications and need not be repeated here. Rather, the purpose of this chapter is to present one surgeon's experience with one operative method of treatment—innominate osteotomy—for congenital dislocation and congenital subluxation of the hip in the older child.

This operative method will be discussed in relation to its design, principle, indications, prerequisites, contra-indications, preoperative management, operative technique, post-operative management, results and complications as well as common errors and pitfalls.

General Considerations

By careful *clinical* examination, congenital dislocation of the hip can usually be diagnosed on the first day of life at which time the hip is *dislocatable* but not necessarily permanently dislocated. Early diagnosis is still the most important aspect of congenital dislocation of the hip; nevertheless, despite continuing emphasis on early diagnosis, a disturbingly large number of congenital dislocations remain undiagnosed until after the child has started to walk—particularly if the dislocation is bilateral. Furthermore, even with early diagnosis and early treatment, some children fail to respond and have a residual subluxation of the hip when they have reached the age of walking.

The dysplasia of the acetabulum, which from clinical and experimental observations is considered to be secondary to the displacement of the hip, is minimal at birth but progresses in severity as long as an abnormal relationship exists between the femoral head and the acetabulum. The potential for normal development of the hip joint after reduction is maximal at birth and gradually diminishes thereafter; this potential for normal development remains relatively adequate during the first year or year and a half of life. After about eighteen months of age however, the dysplasia is sufficiently severe and its reversibility sufficiently limited that normal development of the acetabulum and femoral head after non-operative treatment is no longer assured in a sufficiently high percentage of children. For this group of patients, over the age of eighteen months, as well as for those in whom earlier non-operative treatment has failed to produce a satisfactory joint, innominate osteotomy has proved to be most helpful.

For the purposes of the present discussion the term 'older child' refers to a child over the age of eighteen months; furthermore, the discussion refers only to the 'typical' type of congenital dislocation and excludes the atypical or teratologic type of dislocation such as that associated with arthrogryposis and spina bifida.

An Explanation of the Instability Following Reduction in the Older Child

In children between the ages of eighteen months and six years, initial *reduction* of a congenital *dislocation* can usually be obtained by a period of traction followed by either closed or open reduction. Reduction of a congenital *subluxation*, however, occurs with simple abduction and flexion of the hip. The reduced hip is stable in the position of abduction, flexion and varying degrees of rotation; however, the reduction is unstable in that the hip either re-dislocates or re-subluxates when the lower limb is brought back into the functional position of walking. The main problem in treatment therefore, is not the reduction but the *instability of reduction*.

Clinical observations in children and experimental observations in animals have led the author to believe that in the older child the most significant aspect of acetabular dysplasia is an abnormal direction in which the acetabulum faces (*acetabular mal-direction*); the acetabulum, instead of facing downward, faces more anteriorly and more laterally than normal. This phenomenon explains why the reduced hip is stable in a position of abduction and flexion, why it re-dislocates or re-subluxates laterally in the position of adduction and why it re-dislocates or re-subluxates anteriorly in the position of extension. This phenomenon also explains why, in the presence of femoral anteversion, the combination of external rotation and extension results in anterior re-dislocation or re-subluxation. Thus, operative treatment in the older child should include correction of the acetabular mal-direction.

A second factor contributing to the instability of reduction in congenital *dislocation* is the elongation of the joint capsule which is somewhat analogous to a hernial sac. Thus, any operative treatment for a *dislocation* in the older child should also include resection of redundant capsule and careful capsular repair (capsulorrhaphy). In a *subluxation*, the capsule is not unduly stretched and therefore does not require capsulorrhaphy.

A third factor contributing to the instability of reduction in the older child is contracture of muscles about the hip—particularly the adductors and the iliopsoas. These muscle contractures limit movement in the reduced hip and contribute to the instability of reduction when the hip is placed in the functional position of walking. Thus, operative treatment in the older child should also include lengthening or release of these tight muscles.

Thus, three factors—acetabular mal-direction, capsular elongation and contracture of the adductors and iliopsoas muscles—would seem to be most significant in explaining the instability of the reduced hip in the older child; therefore, all three factors must be dealt with during the treatment of a *dislocation* whereas in the treatment of a *subluxation*, since capsular elongation is not a significant factor only the acetabular mal-direction and muscle contractures must be corrected.

The Design of Innominate Osteotomy

The aim of innominate osteotomy in the treatment of congenital dislocation and subluxation of the hip in the older child is to correct the associated acetabular mal-direction and thereby to render the *reduced* hip stable in the functional position of weightbearing. Studies in the

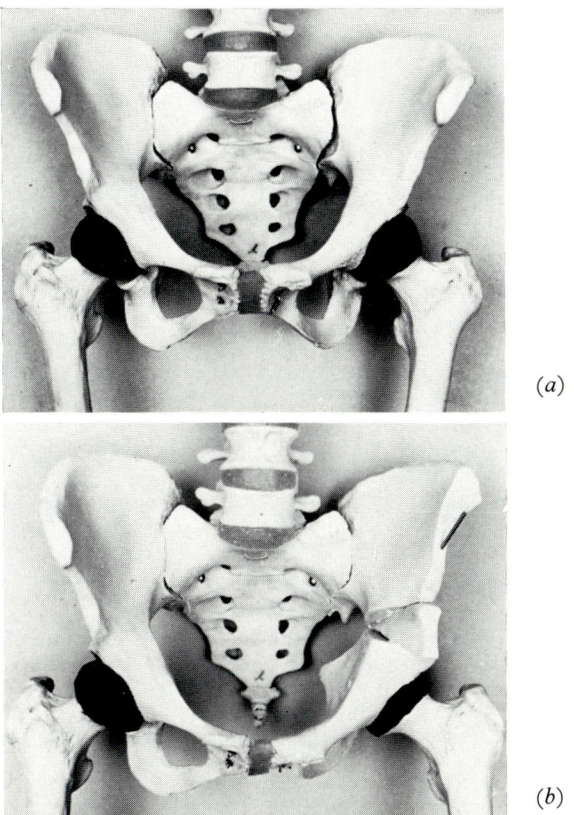

FIG. 1. The design of innominate osteotomy shown in a model of a normal pelvis. (a) Note that in the functional position of weight-bearing, the femoral heads are poorly covered anteriorly and laterally even by the normal acetabulum. (b) Following complete division of the innominate bone and *rotation* of the distal fragment through the symphysis pubis, the acetabulum has been re-directed in such a way that it covers the femoral head more adequately with the hip in the functional position of weightbearing. The triangular bone graft in the open wedge osteotomy maintains the new position of the distal fragment.

Department of Anatomy and in the postmortem room revealed that if the innominate bone was divided completely just above the acetabulum, the distal half of the innominate bone containing the entire acetabulum, could be re-directed by *rotating* this portion through the symphysis pubis; furthermore, neither the *capacity* nor the *contour* of the acetabulum would be altered. The new position of the open wedge osteotomy could be maintained by means of a triangular shaped bone graft taken from the

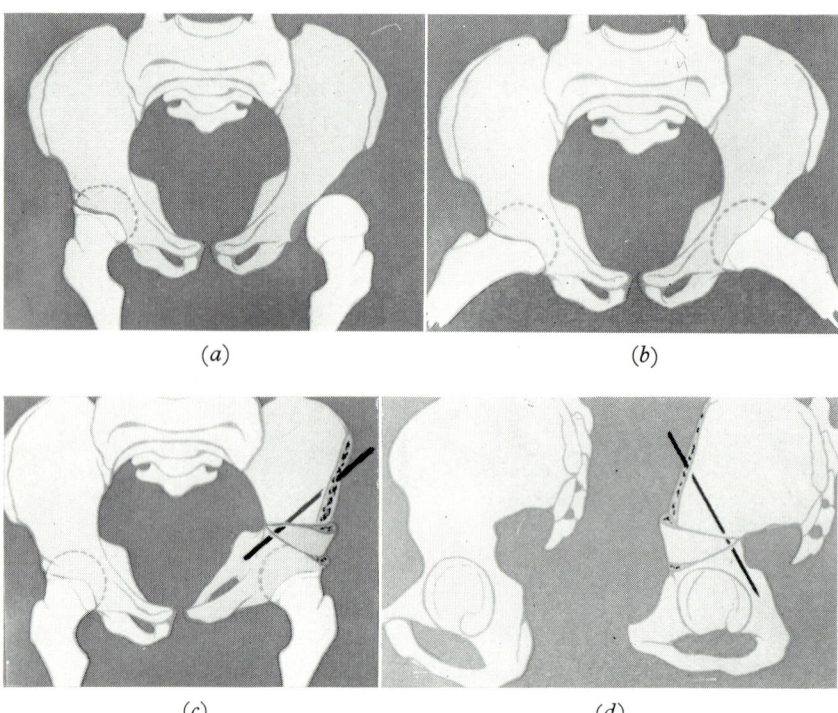

FIG. 2. The principle of innominate osteotomy. (*a*) The congenitally unstable hip is dislocated in the adducted and extended position. Note the abnormal direction of the acetabulum. (*b*) The reduced hip is stable in the position of abduction and flexion. (*c*) Following re-direction of the acetabulum by innominate osteotomy, the reduced hip is stable in the functional position of weightbearing. Note that the osteotomy site is kept closed posteriorly and that the Kirschner wire passes medial to the acetabulum. (*d*) In the lateral projection the osteotomy site is seen to be open anterolaterally and closed postero-medially. The Kirschner wire passes posteriorly to the acetabulum.

proximal portion of the innominate bone. The osteotomy site could be secured by means of a heavy Kirschner wire which traverses the proximal fragment, the graft and the distal fragment (Fig. 1).

The principle of innominate osteotomy. The principle of innominate osteotomy is *re-direction of the entire acetabulum* in such a way that the reduced dislocation or subluxation, which previously was stable in the position of abduction and flexion, is made stable in the functional position of weightbearing (Fig. 2). This procedure permits early weightbearing which, in a stable joint, is the best stimulus for subsequent development of the various components of the joint.

Examination of radiographs before and after innominate osteotomy provides evidence that a 'sloping acetabular roof' actually indicates acetabular mal-direction and furthermore, that the acetabular maldirection can be corrected by *rotation* of the distal fragment of the innominate bone (Fig. 3).

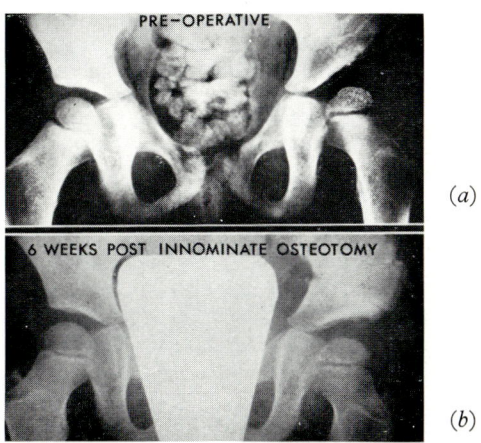

FIG. 3. Pre- and post-operative radiographs of the hips of a four-year-old girl. (*a*) Residual acetabular dysplasia and subluxation of the left hip following one year of non-operative treatment. Note the appearance of a 'sloping acetabular roof'. The day following this radiograph an innominate osteotomy was performed. (*b*) The same patient, six weeks after innominate osteotomy and immediately after removal of the Kirschner wire. Note the triangular shaped bone graft. In the postoperative film the acetabulum appears comparable to that on the normal side. The only change that had taken place between these two radiographs was re-direction of the acetabulum by means of an innominate osteotomy. Therefore, the correct interpretation of the preoperative radiograph is acetabular maldirection rather than a 'sloping acetabular roof'.

Indications for innominate osteotomy. The indications for innominate osteotomy are clearly defined. For a *complete dislocation* the upper age limit is approximately six years, since in children beyond this age it is difficult to obtain a *reduction* of the hip with impunity. For a *subluxation* however, there is no such limit since reduction is obtained by simple abduction and flexion of the hip. The indications are as follows:

(1) *Congenital Dislocation*. Primary Operation (no previous treatment). Ages $1\frac{1}{2}$ years to approximately 6 years.
(2) *Congenital Subluxation*. Primary Operation (no previous treatment). Ages $1\frac{1}{2}$ years to adult life.
(3) *Residual Dislocation or Subluxation*. Secondary Operation (failure of previous treatment). Ages $1\frac{1}{2}$ years to adult life.

Prerequisites for innominate osteotomy. The feasibility and advisability of applying the *principle* of innominate osteotomy to the problem of a given child's hip joint depends on certain definite prerequisites which must be met. Indeed, the absence of any one of these prerequisites represents a definite contra-indication for innominate osteotomy. The essential prerequisites for innominate osteotomy are as follows:

(1) *Ability to bring the head of the femur opposite the acetabulum.* In a dislocation, this requires a period of preoperative traction.
(2) *Release of contracture of adductors and iliopsoas muscle.* This is just as important for a subluxation as for a dislocation.
(3) *Complete and concentric reduction of the femoral head in the depth of the true acetabulum.* In a dislocation this requires a careful open reduction.
(4) *Reasonable congruity of the hip joint surfaces.*
(5) *A good range of hip joint motion.*
(6) *The correct age of the patient—as mentioned under indications.*

The contra-indications for innominate osteotomy. The principle of innominate osteotomy should not be applied for any hip which does not have all the prerequisites listed above. Thus, the *contra-indications* for innominate osteotomy can be enumerated as follows:

(1) *Inability to bring the head of the femur opposite the acetabulum.*
(2) *Residual tightness of the adductors and iliopsoas muscle—even after release.*
(3) *Incomplete reduction of the femoral head in the true acetabulum.* Innominate osteotomy above a *false* acetabulum is *not* in keeping with the principle of innominate osteotomy and cannot be expected to improve the situation. The same is true for a hip that appears to be subluxated but in which the femoral head is actually articulating with an acetabulum that has gradually "wandered" upward and laterally.
(4) *Incongruity of the hip joint surfaces.*
(5) *Marked limitation of hip joint motion.*
(6) *Dislocation in a child over the age of six years.* The upper age limit for a *unilateral* dislocation can be a little higher but for a *bilateral* dislocation it should be a little lower.

Application of the Principle of Innominate Osteotomy

For the purpose of demonstration, the preoperative management, operative technique and post-operative management are depicted and described in relation to a three-year-old girl with unilateral congenital dislocation of the hip (Fig. 4).

PRE-OPERATIVE MANAGEMENT

Preliminary continuous traction is important in the treatment of congenital *dislocation* of the hip at any age but particularly so in children over the age of eighteen months. In children under the age of three

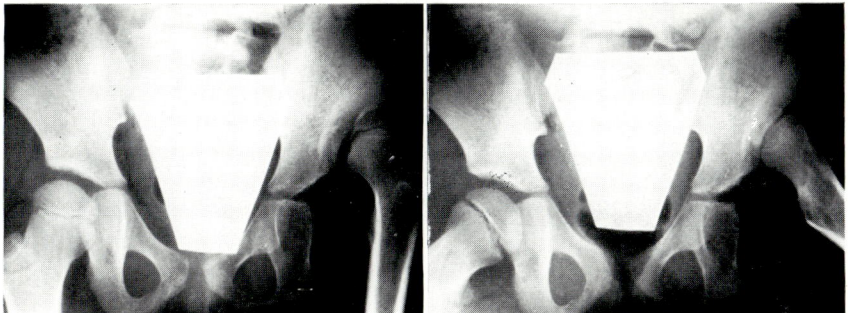

Fig. 4. Radiographs of the hips of the three-year-old girl whose treatment is to be described. Note the complete congenital dislocation of the left hip; the femoral head is high and is articulating with a false acetabulum.

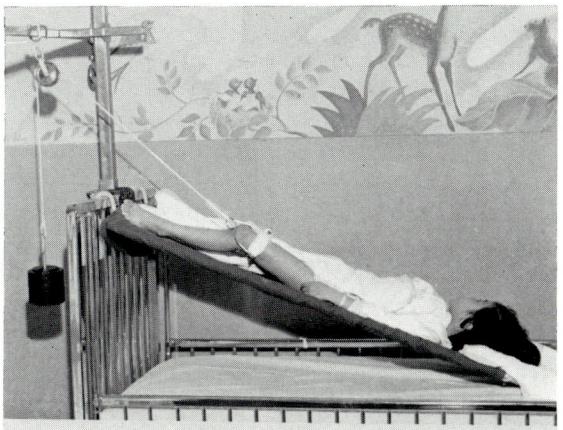

Fig. 5. Preoperative skeletal traction for the child whose radiographs are shown in Fig. 4.

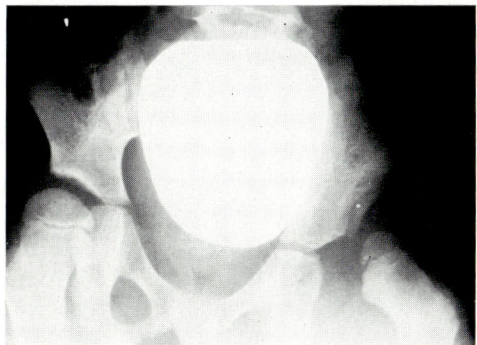

Fig. 6. Radiograph of the hips of the same child as shown in Fig. 4 after three weeks of skeletal traction. The femoral head has been gradually brought down to a position opposite the acetabulum.

years, *tape traction* for two weeks is usually sufficient to bring the femoral head opposite the acetabulum. In children three years of age or older, *skeletal traction* is usually necessary and may have to be continued for longer than two weeks (Fig. 5). In the three-year-old child under consideration, the femoral head was brought down to a position opposite the acetabulum after three weeks of skeletal traction (Fig. 6).

OPERATIVE TECHNIQUE OF COMBINED OPEN REDUCTION AND INNOMINATE OSTEOTOMY

The various stages of the combined operation are best illustrated by a series of photographs taken during the procedure. For this child's left hip the operation included open reduction, release of the adductors and iliopsoas muscle, innominate osteotomy and capsulorrhaphy (Figs. 7–49).

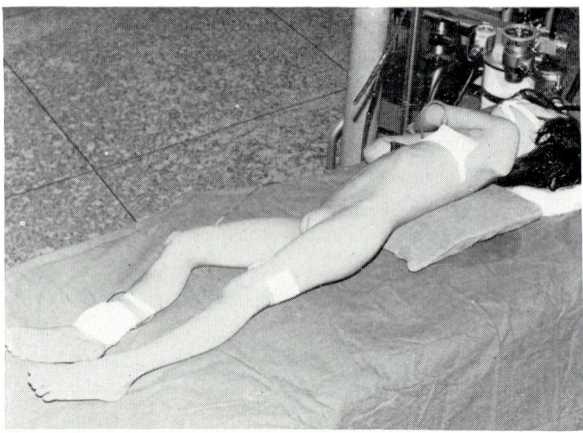

FIG. 7. Position of child on the operating room table. The child is placed partly on her side with a sand bag behind the chest (not behind the hip). For the purpose of skin preparation and draping the child must be completely on the side. An intravenous infusion is started before the operation and cross-matched blood is available. In young children a cut down at the ankle is the most dependable form of infusion. Blood loss is measured throughout the operation and blood is administered only if the loss exceeds 10% of the child's estimated blood volume.

POST-OPERATIVE MANAGEMENT

The child remains in the single hip spica cast for six weeks, after which the cast is removed in the operating room. The intradermal wire suture is removed and a radiograph is taken (Fig. 50). The Kirschner wire is then removed through a small skin incision. General anaesthesia is usually preferable for removal of the Kirschner wire—particularly in young children. At this time a bilateral long leg abduction cast is applied to maintain the hips in abduction and internal rotation and at the same time to allow flexion and extension (Fig. 51). The abduction cast is maintained for four weeks following which a further radiograph is taken.

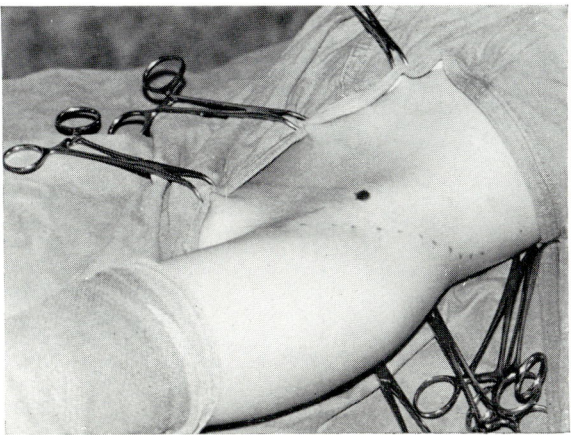

Fig. 8. Following the skin preparation, the hip is draped to the mid-line anteriorly and posteriorly and beyond the costal margin. The lower limb is draped separately so that it may be moved freely during the operation. The dot is over the anterior superior spine and the dotted line indicates the site and extent of the incision.

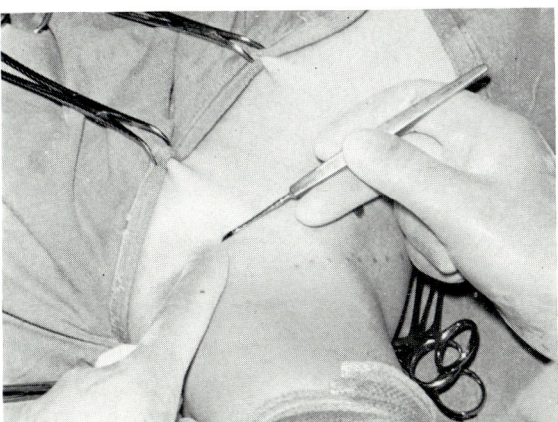

Fig. 9. Subcutaneous adductor tenotomy is performed to release any residual contracture so that maximum abduction may be obtained.

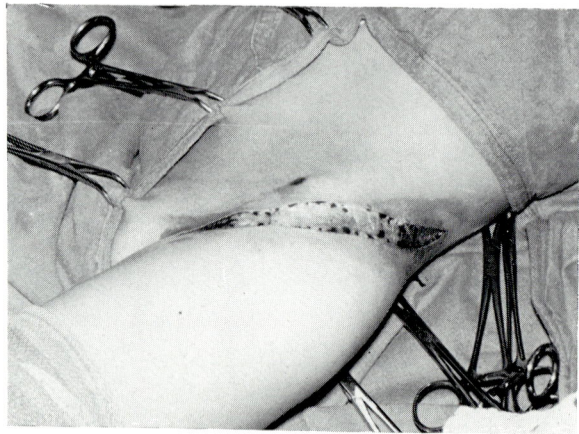

Fig. 10. The oblique skin incision which begins just below the mid point of the inguinal ligament and passes laterally below the anterior superior spine to a point beyond the middle of the iliac crest.

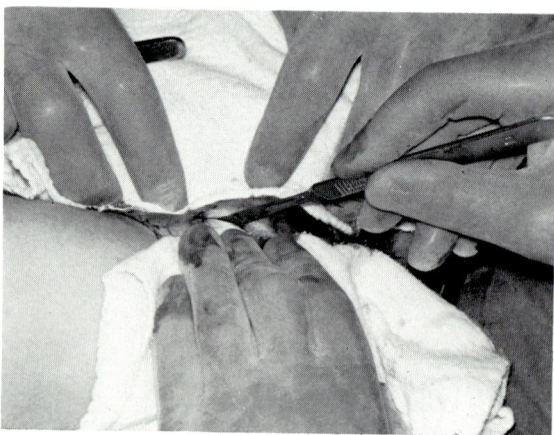

Fig. 11. Pressure is applied to the wound edges with large sponges to minimize bleeding and the iliac crest is exposed. The cartilaginous iliac apophysis is incised from the anterior superior spine to the mid point of the liac crest.

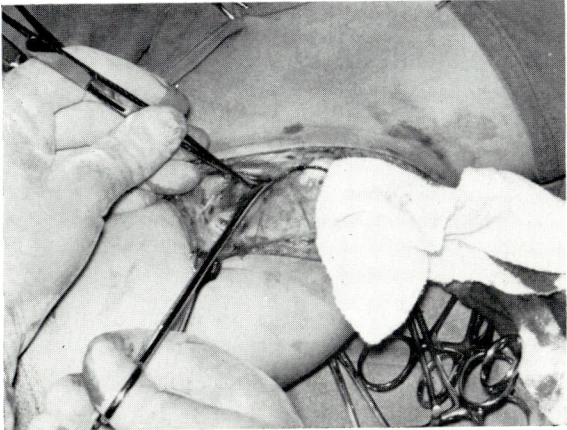

FIG. 12. The deep fascia is incised between the sartorius and the tensor fascia femoris muscles. The interval is opened by blunt dissection to expose the rectus femoris muscle which is then dissected free from the underlying joint capsule. The reflected head of the rectus femoris is divided at this time.

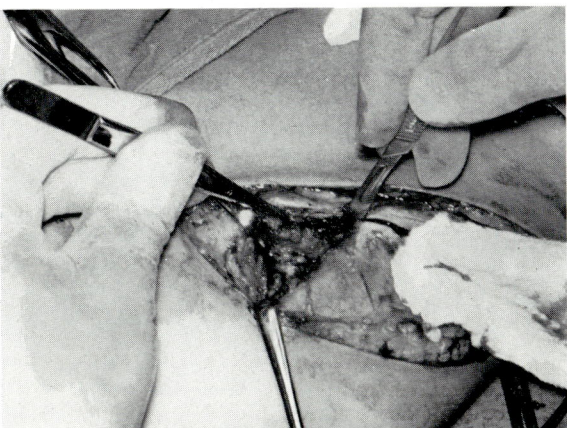

FIG. 13. The incision in the iliac apophysis is then extended downward to the anterior inferior spine.

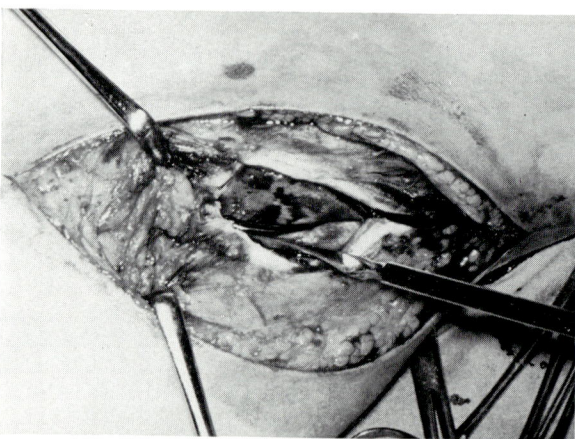

Fig. 14. The periosteum is elevated in a continuous sheet from the outer aspect of the ilium with a long handled periosteal elevator to expose the outer side of the sciatic notch. Wide exposure facilitates this part of the operation.

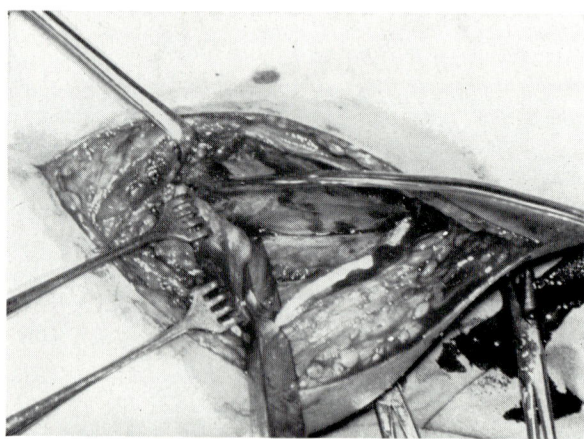

Fig. 15. The periosteum should always be elevated from the site of the false acetabulum (shown at the tip of the suction tube) and distally to the level of the cartilaginous portion of the true acetabulum. The elevator is in the sciatic notch. The periosteum is elevated from the bone behind the sciatic notch. It is important to stay *within* the periosteum in order to avoid injury to the superior gluteal artery and the sciatic nerve.

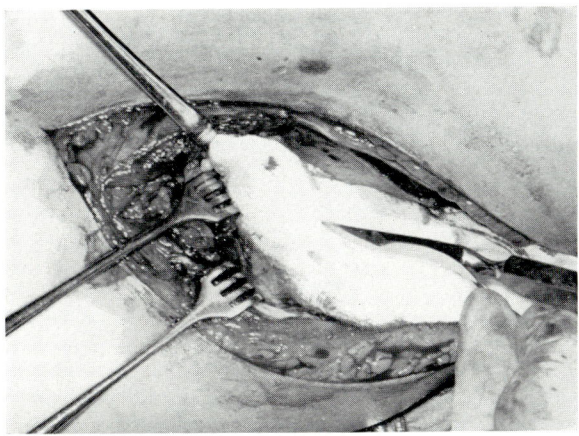

Fig. 16. The dissected space is packed with a large sponge, not only to dilate the interval between the periosteum and the sciatic notch but also to control any oozing from the separated tissues.

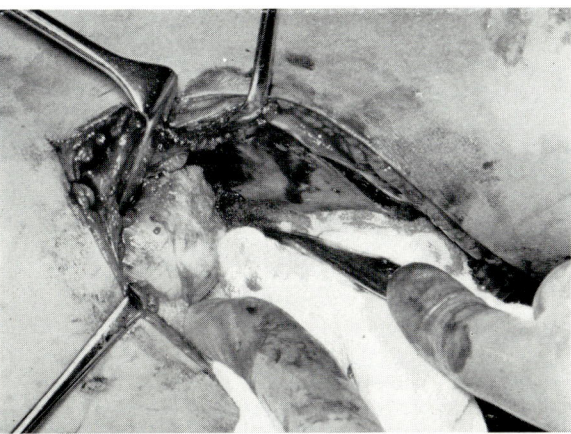

Fig. 17. The fibrous capsule of the hip joint is then exposed superiorly and anteriorly by blunt dissection. The dissection is carried medially right down to the inner edge of the acetabulum.

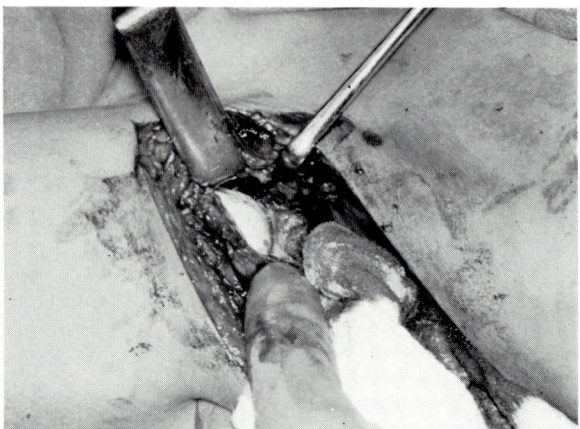

FIG. 18. The capsule of the hip joint is then opened about 1 cm. distal to the edge of the acetabulum and parallel to it.

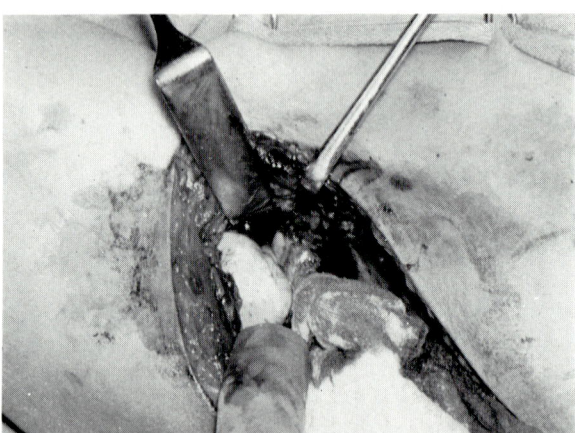

FIG. 19. The capsular incision extends medially right down to the *depths* of the acetabulum to open the joint widely and to make room for a *complete* reduction of the femoral head. The capsular incision is then extended upward over the femoral head. The ligamentum teres is excised only if it is hypertrophied. At this point the femoral head can be reduced into the acetabulum. The reduction is stable with the hip in flexion, abduction and internal rotation but the hip re-dislocates when it is extended, when it is adducted and when it is externally rotated. The fibro-cartilaginous labrum (limbus) is *never* excised. The acetabulum maldirection can be appreciated at this time.

OPERATIVE TREATMENT FOR CONGENITAL HIP DISORDERS 339

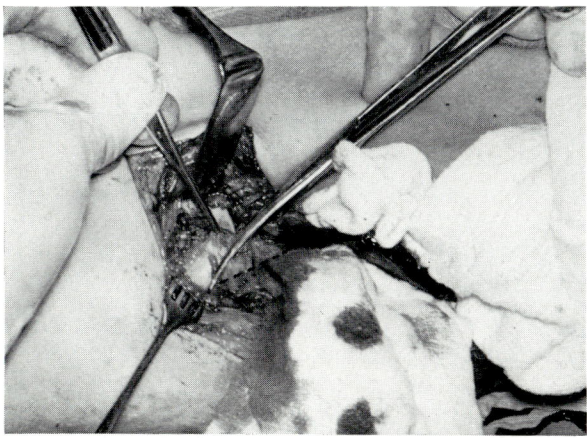

Fig. 20. With the femoral head reduced beyond the labrum, an incision is made with scissors in the distal flap of the capsule at right angles to the first incision, thereby forming a 'T'. The dotted line indicates the site of the next cut in the capsule.

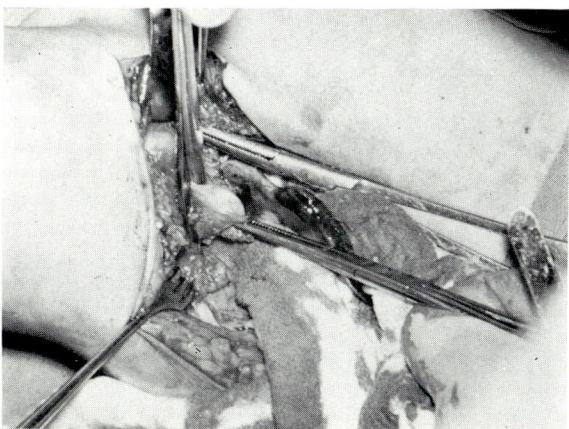

Fig. 21. The T-shaped incision in the capsule leaves a redundant proximal portion of the lateral flap. This triangular part of the flap is then excised along the dotted line shown in Fig. 20.

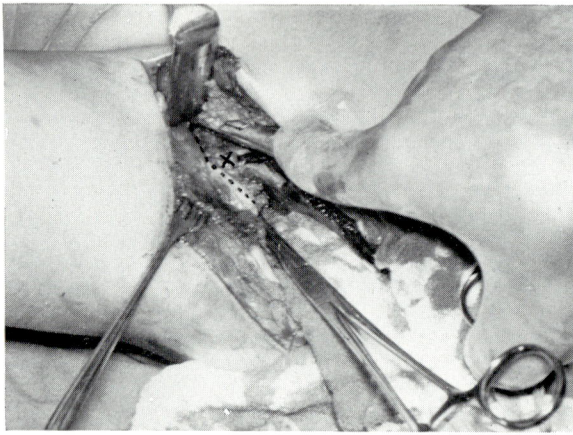

Fig. 22. The distal half of the lateral flap can then be shifted medially beyond the anterior inferior spine (X) when the hip is in the stable position of flexion, abduction and internal rotation. The cut edges of the resected area of the capsule then come together accurately as shown along the dotted line. These edges will be sutured *after* the innominate osteotomy has been completed. In the meantime, the femoral head is allowed to re-dislocate.

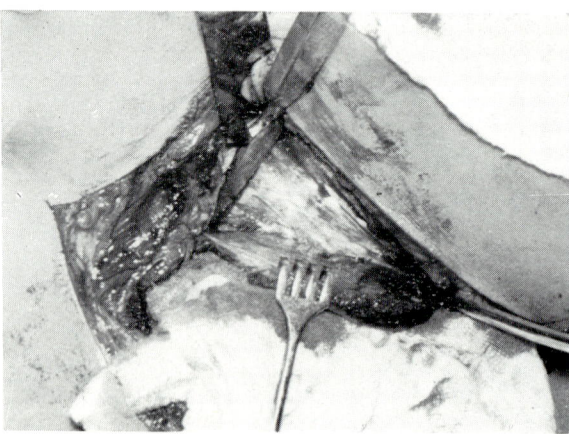

Fig. 23. The periosteum is then elevated from the inner aspect of the ilium with a long handled periosteal elevator (the rake retractor is on the inner side of the iliac crest). The sciatic notch is then exposed subperiosteally from the inner side (the elevator is in the notch). This space is then packed, not only to dilate the interval between the sciatic notch and the periosteum but also to control any oozing from the separated tissues.

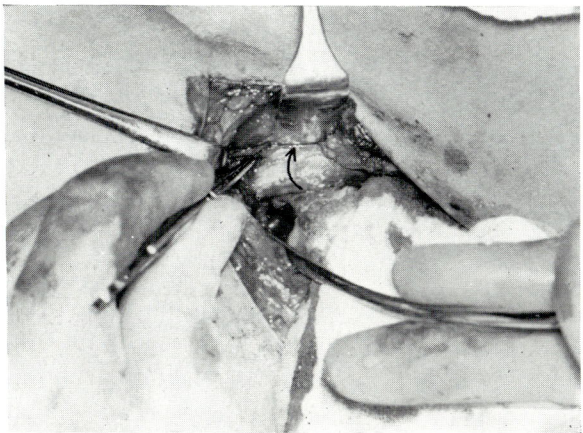

Fig. 24. The tendinous part of the iliopsoas muscle, which is always tight, is then exposed on its deep surface at the level of the pelvic brim and rolled over so that the tendinous portion can be separated from the muscular portion.

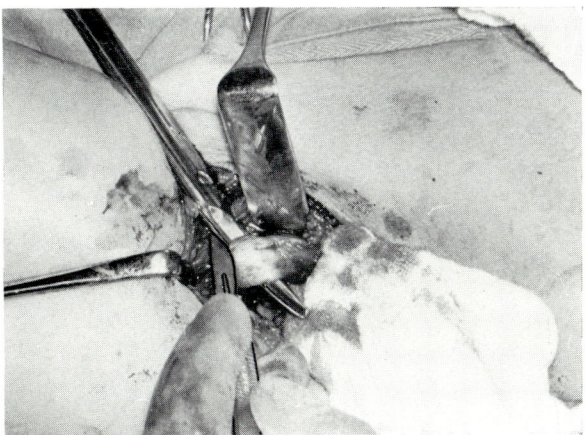

Fig. 25. The scissors pass between the tendinous portion of the iliopsoas muscle and the muscular portion. The tendinous portion of the iliopsoas muscle is then cut with a scalpel while the scissors protect the muscular portion. The cut edges of the tendinous portion then retract, the muscular portion stretches and the contracture is thereby released without losing the continuity of the muscle.

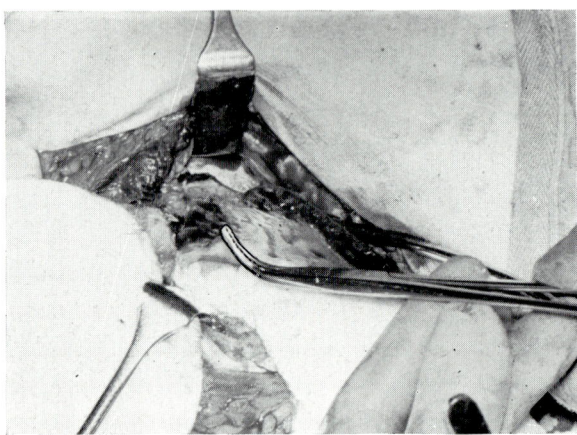

Fig. 26. The right angled forcep (Negus forcep) which is used to grasp the end of the Gigli saw.

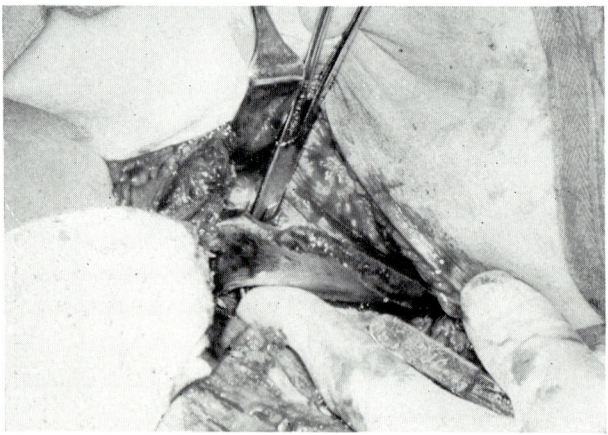

Fig. 27. The right angled forcep is passed into the sciatic notch subperiosteally from the inner side and guided through the notch to the outer side with the index finger of the opposite hand.

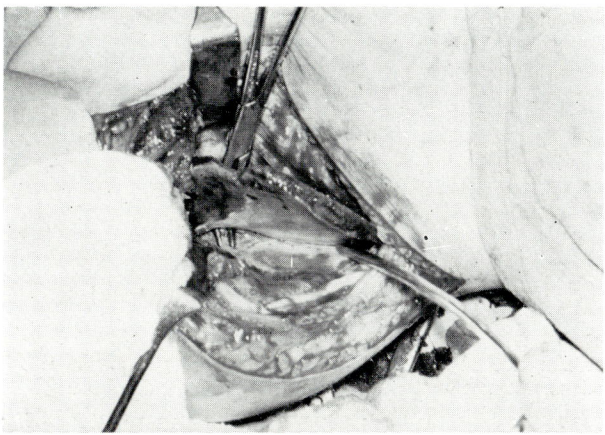

FIG. 28. A wide exposure and good haemostasis facilitates this part of the operation. The open ends of the Negus forcep can be seen ready to grasp the end of the Gigli saw.

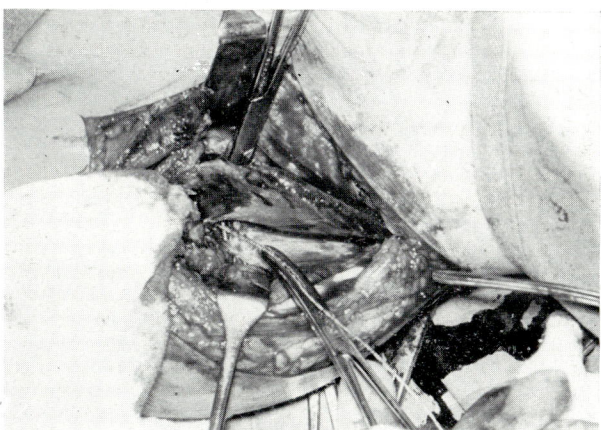

FIG 29. A loop at one end of the Gigli saw is passed over one blade of the Negus forcep.

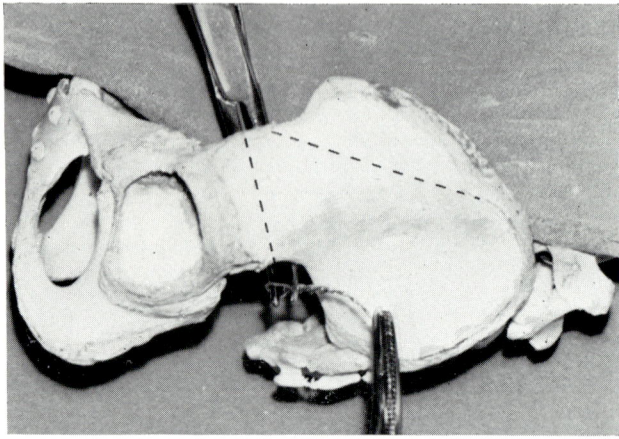

FIG. 30. The dotted line indicates the site of the innominate osteotomy from the sciatic notch to the anterior inferior spine in this dissected pelvis. The loop at one end of the Gigli saw has been passed over one blade of the Negus forcep. The second dotted line indicates the site of removal of the bone graft.

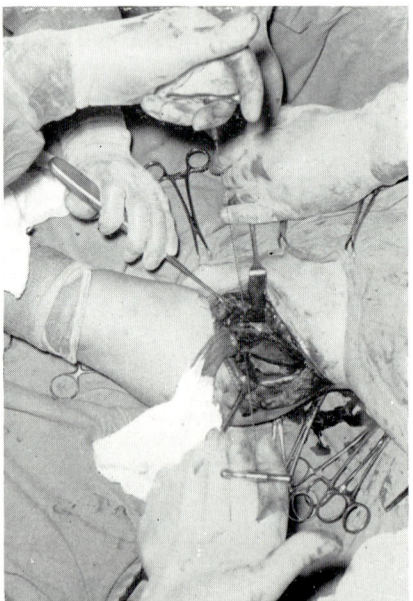

FIG. 31. The skin margins are retracted widely and the surgeon's hands, holding the ends of the Gigli saw, are kept far apart with continuous tension on each end of the saw. If the hands are kept close together or if the tension on the Gigli saw is released with either hand, the saw will tend to bind in the bone.

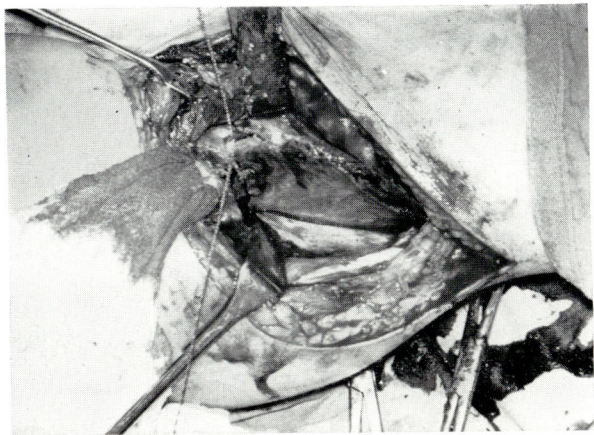

Fig. 32. The Gigli saw is seen emerging from the osteotomy site anteriorly at the anterior inferior spine. The saw cut is made at right angles to the sides of the ilium. After completion of the osteotomy, the distal fragment tends to displace posteriorly and this must always be overcome.

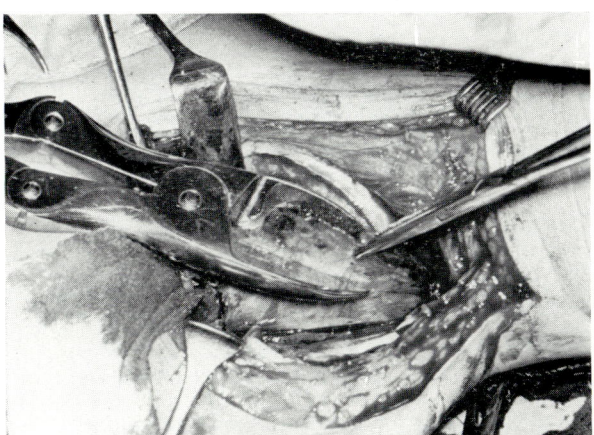

Fig. 33. The triangular shaped bone graft is then removed from the iliac crest with large straight double action bone cutters. The base of the triangle represents the distance from the anterior superior spine to the anterior inferior spine. The portion to be removed is held firmly with a forcep.

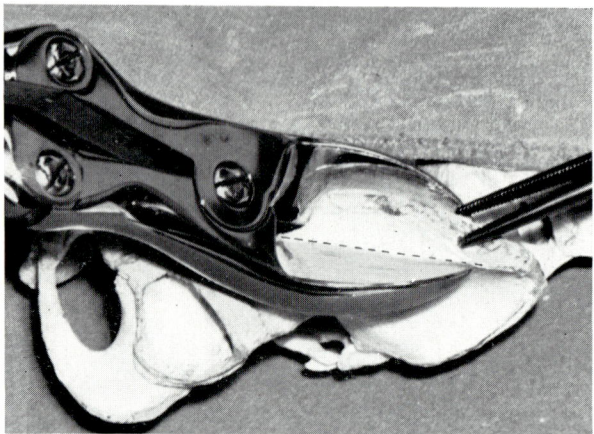

Fig. 34. A comparable view to Fig. 33, in the dissected pelvis.

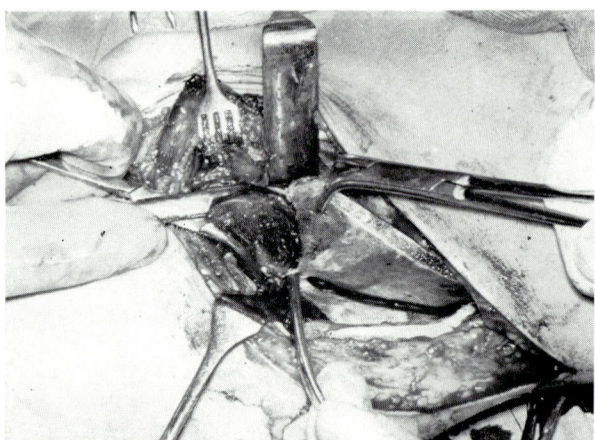

Fig. 35. One towel clip grasps the proximal fragment but only to steady it. There should *not* be any upward pull on the proximal fragment. A second towel clip, which is placed well posteriorly, grasps the distal fragment, which is then *rotated* downward and forward in line with the ilium. This rotation occurs at the symphysis pubis. The distal fragment should never be allowed to remain posterior to the proximal fragment. The osteotomy is opened anteriorly and kept closed posteriorly. The osteotomy site should never be spread apart with instruments—such as laminectomy spreaders or self-retaining retractors—because such a maneouvre actually moves the proximal fragment upward and the distal fragment downward, lowering the hip without obtaining any re-direction of the acetabulum.

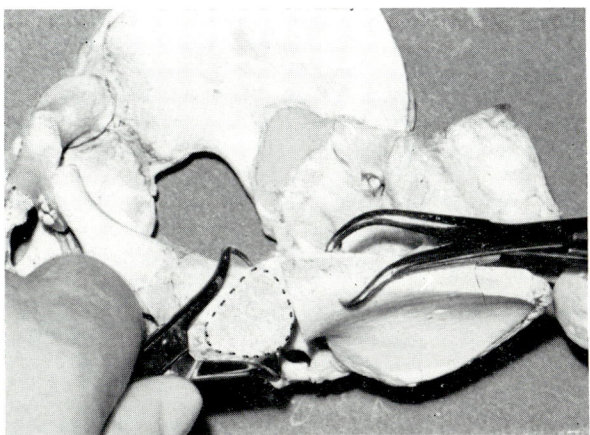

Fig. 36. A comparable view to Fig. 35, in the dissected pelvis. The dotted line marks the cut edge of the distal fragment.

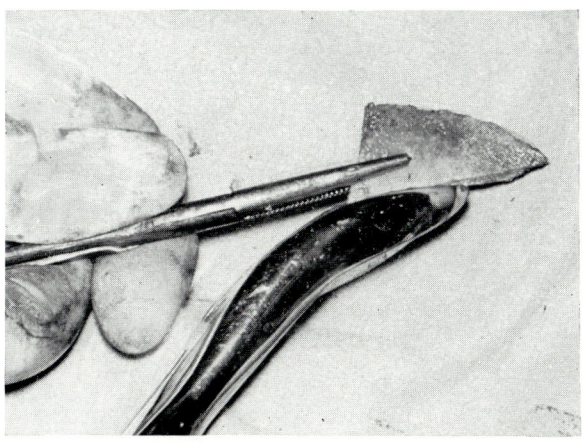

Fig. 37. The bone graft is then shaped with bone cutters to fit the open osteotomy site. Since the base of the triangular graft represents the distance between the anterior superior spine and the anterior inferior spine, the graft is always about the same size relative to the size of the patient.

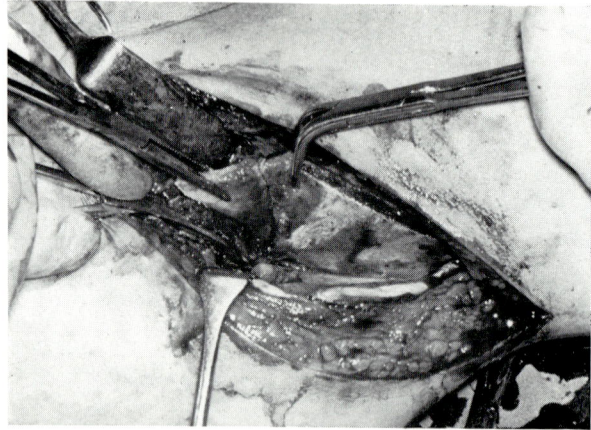

Fig. 38. While the osteotomy site is kept open anteriorly with the distal fragment *rotated*, the bone graft is inserted. The osteotomy site should be kept closed posteriorly and the distal fragment should be kept slightly anterior to the proximal fragment.

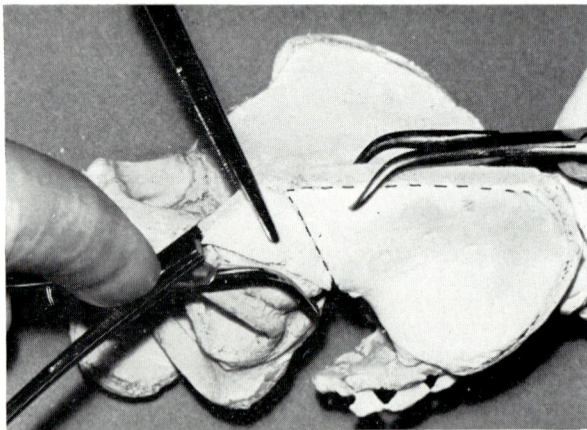

Fig. 39. A comparable view to Fig. 38, in the dissected pelvis. The dotted lines mark the cut edges in the proximal fragment of the innominate bone.

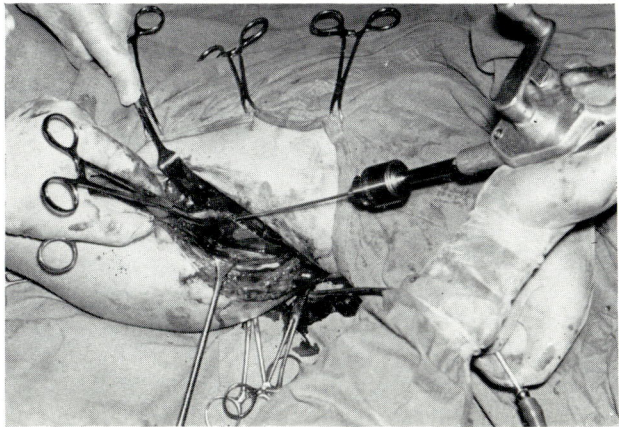

FIG. 40. A heavy Kirschner wire is drilled through the proximal fragment, across the graft and well into the distal fragment, posterior and medial to the acetabulum. The osteotomy site must be held firmly in the corrected position at this time. The wire should never be passed into the joint nor even left pointing in the direction of the joint. With a second Kirschner wire of equal length to the first, the length of wire in the distal fragment can be ascertained.

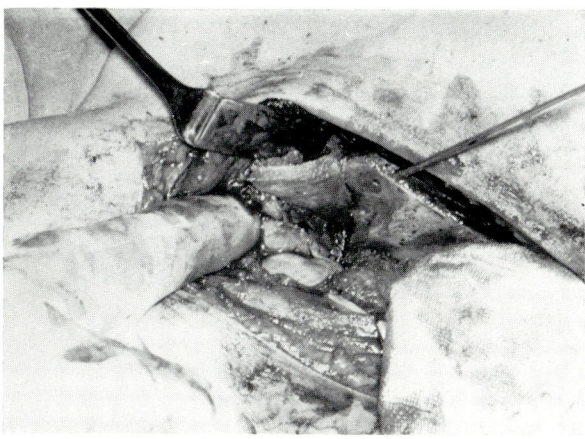

FIG. 41. A finger is inserted into the acetabulum to be certain that the Kirschner wire has not entered the joint. At this point, a second Kirschner wire was inserted to ensure stability of the osteotomy site. (When the innominate osteotomy is being performed for a *subluxation*—in which case the capsule is not opened—the hip should be moved passively at this stage to be certain that the Kirschner wire has not entered the joint.)

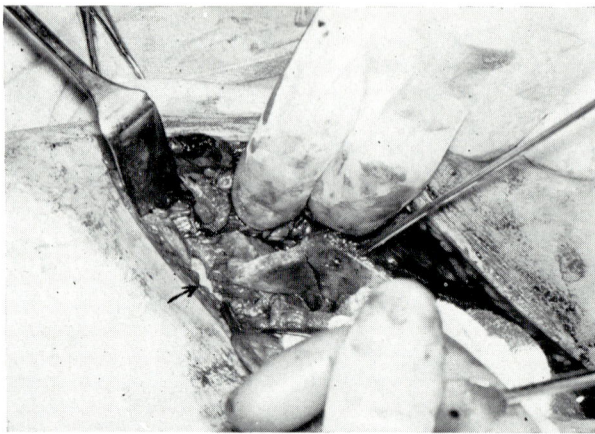

Fig. 42. Since the acetabulum has been re-directed and is therefore more like a normal acetabulum, the reduction, which should be done at this time, is more difficult than before; it is comparable to the reduction of a traumatic dislocation in a normal hip. By the same token, the reduction is now stable in the range of motion used for walking. In this photograph the femoral head is seen to be well covered anteriorly and laterally by the reduced acetabulum. (The arrow points to the femoral head.)

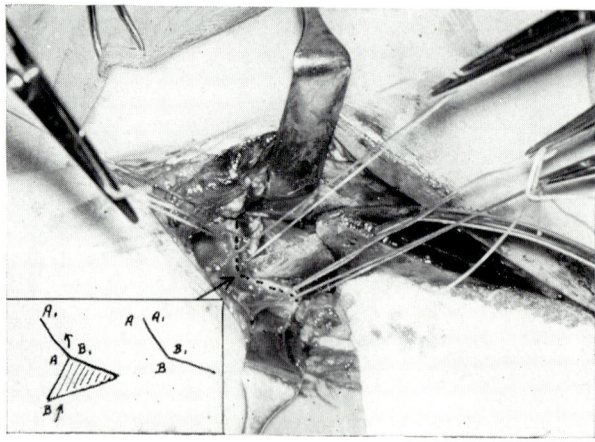

Fig. 43. The distal half of the lateral flap is moved medially *beyond* the anterior inferior spine following which the cut edges of the resected area of the capsule come together accurately. Multiple sutures are used to repair the capsule as shown along the dotted line (the arrow points to the anterior superior spine). This form of capsulorrhaphy is important in that it keeps the hip internally rotated and increases the stability of the reduction. The line drawings indicate the medial advancement of the distal portion of the lateral flap (A to A_1 and B to B_1).

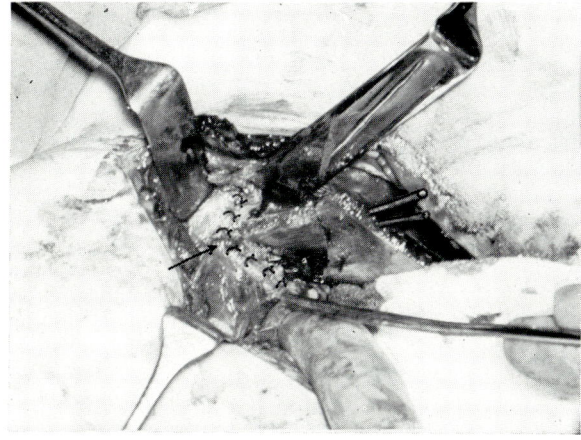

Fig. 44. The capsulorrhaphy has been completed; the sutures and the two Kirschner wires have been inked in so that they may be seen in this photograph. At this stage the reduction should be completely stable in the range of motion used for walking. During the remainder of the operation an assistant holds the lower limb with the hip in flexion, abduction and internal rotation to keep tension off the suture line in the capsule.

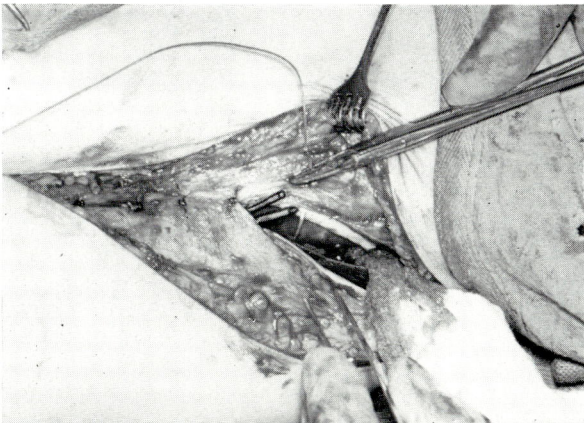

Fig. 45. The periosteum and muscles are replaced by suturing the cut surfaces of the iliac apophysis. The Kirschner wires which are outlined with ink, and are seen just to the left of the suture needle, have been cut so that they protrude through the suture line.

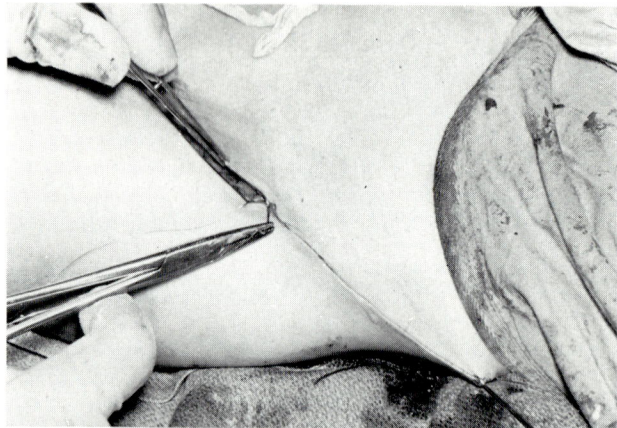

Fig. 46. The proximal flap of skin and subcutaneous fat is then brought over the cut ends of the Kirschner wires, and the skin is closed with continuous intradermal wire suture.

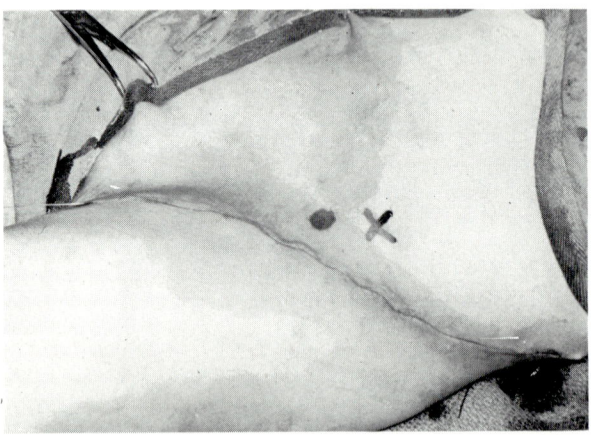

Fig. 47. The dot marks the preoperative site of the anterior superior spine; the X marks the site of the palpable buried ends of the Kirschner wires. A thick dressing is applied while the lower limb is held in a position of abduction, flexion and internal rotation. An anteroposterior radiograph is taken while the child is still under anaesthetic and before the hip spica cast is applied.

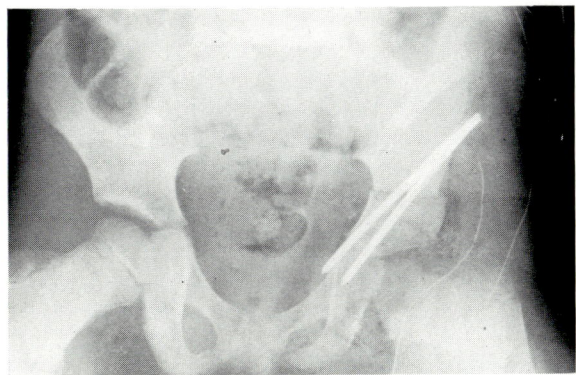

Fig. 48. The radiograph of this child's hip taken in the operating room. Note in comparison with the preoperative radiograph (Fig. 4), the improved acetabular index and the complete reduction of the femoral head which is well covered by the re-directed acetabulum. The osteotomy site is closed posteromedially and the Kirschner wires pass medial and posterior to the acetabulum. The alteration in the contour of the obturator foramen indicates that the distal half of the innominate bone has been *rotated* through the symphysis pubis.

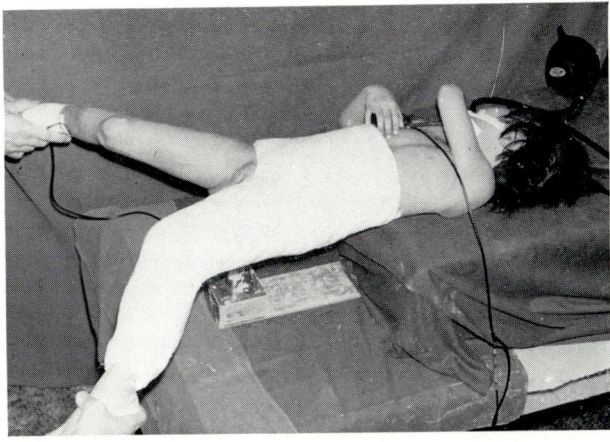

Fig. 49. A single hip spica cast is applied with the hip in moderate flexion (about 30°), slight abduction and slight internal rotation. (Occasionally femoral retroversion is present rather than femoral anteversion; in the presence of femoral retroversion, it is necessary to immobilize the hip in slight external rotation.)

The child is then allowed to walk with the assistance of a physiotherapist or a nurse; the child soon learns to use crutches and within a few weeks is allowed to walk unaided.

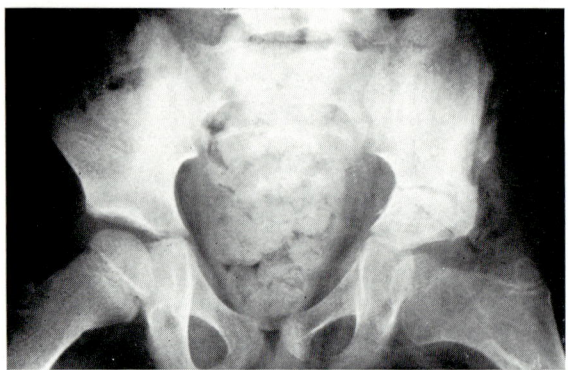

FIG. 50. Radiograph of the same three-year-old child six weeks after open reduction and innominate osteotomy. The Kirschner wires have just been removed. Note that the osteotomy has united and that new bone formation has begun in the site of graft removal from the iliac crest. At this stage, an abduction plaster cast was applied.

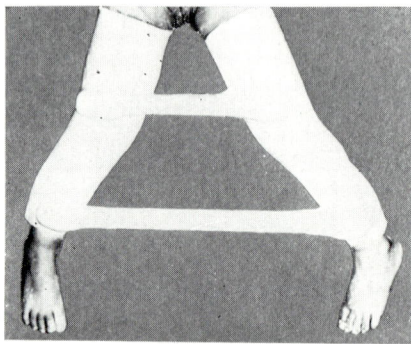

FIG. 51. Bilateral long leg abduction cast which is applied six weeks after operation to protect the capsular repair for a further four weeks.

Bilateral dislocation. With bilateral dislocation the second hip is usually operated upon two weeks after the first. It is important to leave the child in the hip spica cast however, to protect the first hip during the operation on the second hip. Part of the hip spica is cut away to obtain exposure of the second hip but a proximal portion of the cast is left intact to maintain the optimum position of the first hip.

Subluxation. The technique of innominate osteotomy is the same for subluxation as for dislocation with three exceptions: (1) the capsule is not opened; (2) opening of the osteotomy site is facilitated by externally rotating the hip, flexing the knee, placing the heel on the opposite knee and then passively extending the hip (the intact capsule then pulls the distal fragment downward and forward); (3) the child is allowed to start walking in six weeks when the hip spica is removed rather than in ten weeks.

Results of Innominate Osteotomy

The following results represent the first five years of the author's personal experience with innominate osteotomy in the treatment of congenital dislocation and subluxation of the hip. The one hundred and thirty-four operations were either performed by, or supervised by the author. At the time of this study (1966) the shortest follow-up period was four years and the longest was eight years. The anatomical results were based on the Severin classification and the patients were divided into three clinical groups on the basis of the indications for operation (Table I).

TABLE I
Clinical Groups (Based on the Indication)

1. Congenital Dislocation: Primary Operation (No previous treatment) Ages $1\frac{1}{2}$ to 8 years	74 Hips
2. Congenital Subluxation: Primary Operation (No previous treatment) Ages $1\frac{1}{2}$ to 15 years	16 Hips
3. Residual Dislocation or Subluxation: Secondary Operation (Failure of previous treatment) Ages $1\frac{1}{2}$ to 15 years	44 Hips

As would be expected, the results are much better when innominate osteotomy is performed as the *primary* treatment of a previously untreated hip than when it is performed as *secondary* treatment following the failure of previous treatment—either closed or open. Many of the patients in the secondary treatment group, in addition to having a residual dislocation or subluxation had such complicating problems as avascular necrosis of the femoral head, pressure necrosis of articular cartilage, dense fibrous adhesions between the capsule and the femoral head, and severe femoral anteversion.

The anatomical results in the three clinical groups of patients are shown in Tables II, III and IV.

Complications

Most of the complications listed below occurred during the first year of experience with innominate osteotomy.

(1) *Superficial wound infection*—3 in 134 operations—no residual problem.
(2) *Deep wound infection*—1 in 134 operations—this child had a deep infection following a previous operation also.

TABLE II
Congenital Dislocation of the Hip
Children over the age of 1½ years   74 Dislocations   No previous treatment
ANATOMICAL RESULTS OF PRIMARY OPERATION
(Combined open reduction and innominate osteotomy)
Based on Severin Classification
Operations - 1958 to 1962

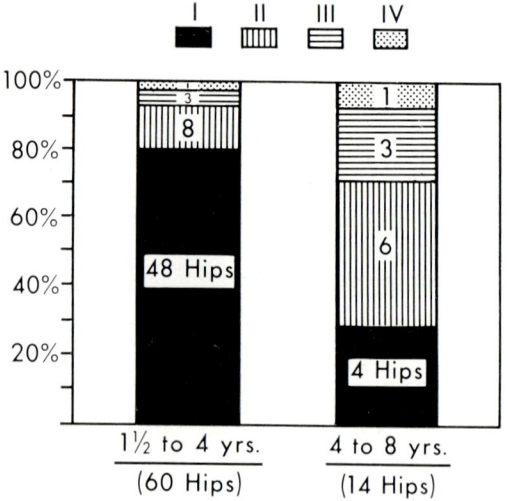

Ages 1½ to 4 years - Excellent + Good - 93%
Ages 4 to 8 Years - Excellent + Good - 72%

(3) *Slipping of the graft requiring revision*—4 in 134 operations. All of these occurred in the early stages before Kirschner wire fixation of the graft was used.

(4) *Redislocation or resubluxation:*
   (a) Early redislocation requiring closed reduction—3 in 134 operations.
   (b) Late redislocation requiring open reduction—3 in 134 operations.
   (c) Late resubluxation requiring capsulorrhaphy—6 in 134 operations.

These complications have not occurred since we have been using the above described method of capsulorrhaphy (resection of redundant capsule and advancement of the distal portion of the lateral flap).

(5) *Avascular necrosis of the femoral head*—12 in 134 operations (9%). There was no instance of avascular necrosis when innominate osteotomy was performed alone (without open reduction and capsulorrhaphy).

OPERATIVE TREATMENT FOR CONGENITAL HIP DISORDERS 357

TABLE III
Congenital Subluxation of the Hip
Children aged 1½ to 15 years   16 Subluxations   No previous treatment
ANATOMICAL RESULTS OF PRIMARY OPERATION
(Innominate osteotomy alone)
Based on Severin Classification
Operations - 1958 to 1962

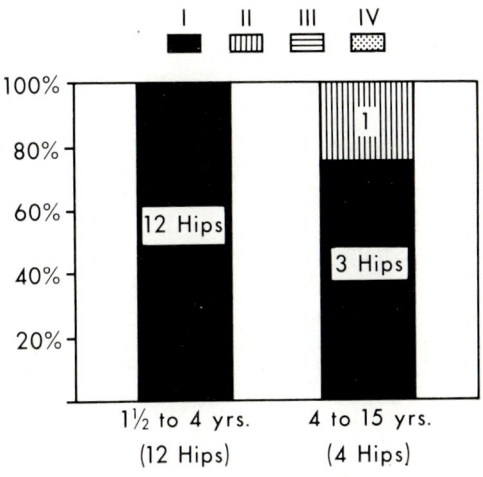

TABLE IV
Residual Dislocation or Subluxation of the Hip
(Following Failure of Previous Treatment)
Children aged 1½ to 15 years   44 Hips
ANATOMICAL RESULTS OF SECONDARY OPERATION
(Innominate Osteotomy ± open reduction)
Based on improvement in grade of result (Severin Classification)
Operations 1958 to 1962

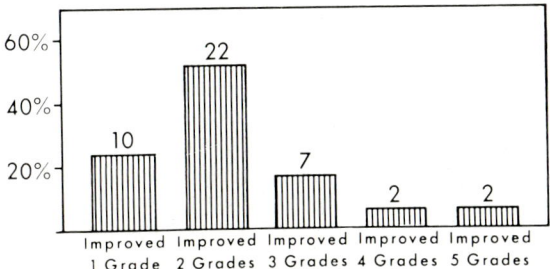

Improved 2 or more grades - 77%
Made worse - one hip (deep infection)
3 hips required femoral osteotomy in addition

There were no deaths and no injuries to the sciatic nerve. Four of the patients who had an innominate osteotomy in their teens for residual subluxation have delivered normal babies without difficulty. The first child of one of these patients weighed ten pounds.

Common Errors and Pitfalls

Many surgeons throughout the world have followed the original article on innominate osteotomy (1961) faithfully and have achieved satisfactory results. As with many new operative procedures, however, so also with innominate osteotomy, some surgeons have modified the originally described operative technique—either wittingly or unwittingly—while others have not adhered to the indications, prerequisites and contra-indications. Under such circumstances, as might be expected, the results have been less than optimal. The author is grateful to those surgeons who have communicated their problems since such communications make it possible to warn others of the more common errors and pitfalls in both judgement and operative technique that can lead to unsatisfactory results.

These errors and pitfalls are discussed in relation to the following aspects of the operative treatment for congenital dislocation and subluxation of the hip in the older child: (1) clinical judgement in selection of patients; (2) pre-operative management; (3) the operative technique of open reduction and capsulorrhaphy; (4) the operative technique of innominate osteotomy; and (5) the post-operative management.

(1) *Clinical judgement in selection of patients.*
   (a) Failure to adhere to the indications for innominate osteotomy.
   (b) Failure to observe the prerequisites for innominate osteotomy.
   (c) Failure to adhere to the contra-indications for innominate osteotomy.

(2) *Pre-operative management.*
   (a) Failure to use continuous traction until the femoral head is opposite the acetabulum.
   (b) The use of "well leg traction" with bilateral dislocation, particularly when used on the second hip after operation on the first hip.

(3) *Operative technique of open reduction and capsulorrhaphy.*
   (a) Failure to perform a subcutaneous adductor tenotomy for residual adduction contracture.
   (b) Inadequate operative exposure of the anatomical structures.
   (c) Failure to obtain a complete and concentric reduction of the femoral head in the *true* acetabulum.
   (d) Mistaking a well developed false acetabulum for a true acetabulum.
   (e) Failure to release the tendinous portion of the iliopsoas muscle. This is probably the commonest error of operative technique.
   (f) Failure to perform an adequate capsular repair (capsulorrhaphy).

(4) *Operative technique of innominate osteotomy.*
   (a) Inadequate operative exposure of the sciatic notch.
   (b) Failure to stay within the periosteum—particularly in the region of the sciatic notch (potential danger to the superior gluteal artery).
   (c) Use of an osteotome or power saw to divide the innominate bone (potential danger to the superior gluteal artery and the sciatic nerve).
   (d) Opening the osteotomy site with a mechanical spreader (the proximal fragment may be forced upward rather than the distal fragment being *rotated* downward and forward).
   (e) Leaving the osteotomy site open posteriorly (the hip joint is lowered without re-directing the acetabulum).
   (f) Allowing the distal fragment to displace posteriorly and medially (decreases the amount of re-direction of the acetabulum).
   (g) Failure to *rotate* the distal fragment (inadequate correction of the acetabular maldirection).
   (h) Use of thin Kirschner wires (which may bend or break).
   (i) Inadequate penetration of the Kirschner wires into the distal fragment (subsequent loss of correction).
   (j) Insertion of a Kirschner wire into the joint (damage to the joint surface and interference with a concentric reduction).
   (k) Insertion of Kirschner wires from below rather than from above (potential danger to intraperitoneal and retroperitoneal structures).

(5) *Post-operative management.*
   (a) Immobilization of the hip in other than the most stable position. In the presence of anteversion the hip should be immobilized in slight internal rotation whereas in the presence of retroversion the post-operative position should be one of slight external rotation.
   (b) Immobilization of the hip in a forced or extreme position (may lead to avascular necrosis of the femoral head or pressure necrosis of the articular cartilage).
   (c) Immobilization of the hip in a hip spica cast for much longer or much shorter than six weeks.
   (d) Unsupervised walking during the first few weeks after weight-bearing is allowed.

AVOIDANCE OF ERRORS AND PITFALLS

The above mentioned errors and pitfalls can be avoided by adhering strictly to the indications, prerequisites and contra-indications as well as to the described details of pre-operative management, operative technique and post-operative management. It is respectfully suggested that the operation of innominate osteotomy be performed in the anatomy laboratory or in the postmortem room before it is performed *for* a living patient.

The Advantages of Innominate Osteotomy

The following advantages of innominate osteotomy which are quoted from the original article (1961) seem to be valid. They are as follows:

(1) Correction of the abnormal direction in which the entire acetabulum faces produces immediate stability of reduction in the functional position of weightbearing without altering the congruity of the acetabulum or decreasing its capacity.

(2) After innominate osteotomy, the area of articular cartilage of the femoral head and acetabulum in contact in the functional position of weightbearing, is considerably increased because the femoral head is better covered by the acetabulum. As a result, pressure of weightbearing is distributed over a larger area of articular cartilage; it is suggested that this may be an important factor in helping to prevent degenerative changes in the articular cartilage with subsequent function of the joint.

(3) Both reduction and stability are provided by a single operative procedure; femoral osteotomy is obviated unless the femoral anteversion is extreme.

(4) The stability of reduction permits early resumption of function of the hip, thereby avoiding the undesirable effects, as well as the hardships, of prolonged immobilization.

(5) Early weightbearing on a completely reduced and completely stable hip seems likely to provide the best possible stimulus for subsequent normal development of both the femoral head and the acetabulum.

Since the development of innominate osteotomy in 1957, the results in the author's experience, have continued to be encouraging. Early recognition and early gentle treatment, however, are still the most important aspects of congenital dislocation and subluxation of the hip; it is to be hoped that eventually all these children may be effectively treated by non-operative means during the most favourable first few months of life.

References

SALTER, R. B. (1961). Innominate osteotomy in the treatment of congenital dislocation and subluxation of the hip. *J. Bone Jt. Surg.*, **43B**, 518.

SALTER, R. B. (1966). Role of innominate osteotomy in the treatment of congenital dislocation and subluxation of the hip in the older child. *J. Bone Jt. Surg.*, **48A**, 1413.

SALTER, R. B. (1967). Movie Film. "The Principle and Technique of Innominate Osteotomy" (Available for loan from the Film Library of the American Academy of Orthopaedic Surgeons, 29 East Madison Street, Chicago, Illinois 60602, U.S.A.)

Chapter 11

THE CONCEPT OF ARREST OF OSTEOARTHRITIS IN THE HIP AND KNEE

ARTHUR J. HELFET

"If a man will begin with certainties, he shall end in doubt; but if he will be content to begin with doubts, he shall end in certainties."
Advancement of Learning, IV-8
FRANCIS BACON

We may be on the threshold of change in our understanding of primary osteoarthritis and with it a change in our approach to management of this condition. The term 'primary osteoarthritis' is in itself inaccurate and misleading, and the alternative of 'osteoarthrosis' only slightly better. The prevailing view which was expressed by Harrison

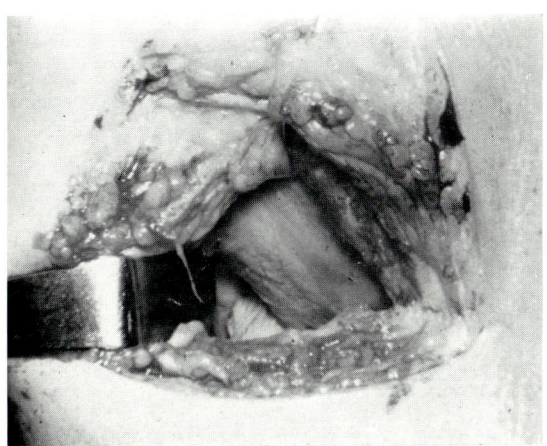

FIG. 1. Patterns of erosion on the medial femoral condyle etched by a deranged meniscus in a middle-aged patient.

et al. in 1953 is that the primary lesion is one of patchy degeneration of articular cartilage, mainly in non weight-bearing areas. There are grounds for doubt whether it is primarily a disorder of cartilage, or whether it is always, or indeed usually, a primary disorder. In the knee, for instance, the initial patterns of erosion are etched by a deranged meniscus, not in an area of weight-bearing but of the articular cartilage opposing the derangement of the meniscus (Fig. 1). And these erosive lesions of articular cartilage are profoundly affected in degree by the aging process in the meniscus.

In the past the degenerative process was recognized, but it was not understood and the outlook appeared hopeless. A primary condition without known etiology provides no basis for an active approach to treatment. So palliation of symptoms and attempts to preserve function were the optimum of standard practice. This usually meant aspirin, physical therapy including injections of either lactic acid or hydrocortisone, with or without splinting, until the condition became intolerable. In other words, the joint was made to last as long as possible before radical surgery (arthrodesis, débridement and drilling, or arthroplasty) was advised. Consequently, surgical experience was limited to the severely damaged joint and this in itself delayed understanding of the changing conditions involved.

The significance of the reparative changes in the hip joint and juxta-articular bone after intertrochanteric osteotomy for osteoarthritis was realized only recently, and crystallized in the term 'Arrest of Osteo-arthritis' by Karl Nissen in his presidential address to the Orthopaedic Section of the Royal Society of Medicine.

In reviewing the results of displacement osteotomy he pointed out that the disease in every respect had been arrested and moreover, that besides the relief of symptoms and restoration of function, X-rays revealed actual reversal of the degenerative process. It is therefore reasonable to affirm that the degenerative process may at least be arrested, and the consequent assumption that the earlier the operation is carried out the better the result, is borne out in clinical practice. This approach has led us to re-examine the whole osteoarthritic process. Taking the knee and hip joints (which lend themselves to precise clinical examination and simple access) we have been able to trace the sequence of changes in the development of osteoarthritis and to compare the results of treatment by soft tissue operation in the knee with those of osteotomy in the hip.

Osteoarthritis of the Knee

The entity to be considered as the osteoarthritic knee is recognized by limitation of at least the extremes of movement, notably the synchrony of extension with external rotation of the tibia on the femur, and the synchrony of flexion with internal rotation (Fig. 2). It is incorrect and confusing to label the painful menopausal knee arthritic if its range of movement is complete.

In osteoarthritis limitation of movement is always associated with pain and most of the pain is due to abnormal tensions produced during attempts at normal movement which cannot be achieved.

The pattern of movement of the knee is not that of a hinge joint but part of a spiral of a helix. When weight-bearing, the tibia rotates laterally as the knee joint straightens. It rotates medially when the knee bends. The synchrony of these movements is controlled by the obliquity of the thigh muscles and guided by a figure-of-eight rotator mechanism composed of the cruciate ligaments and menisci.

If this synchrony is prevented forcibly as by the weight of the falling body, the rotator mechanism is injured. Most cartilage tears are caused by nothing more than this disruption of the rotator mechanism of the knee, and are signalled in every instance by inability to rotate the tibia to its full extent and therefore to extend or flex the knee completely. In addition each particular variety of meniscus rupture produces its own complex of symptoms, signs and sequelae, so that an accurate diagnosis of site as well as extent can usually be made.

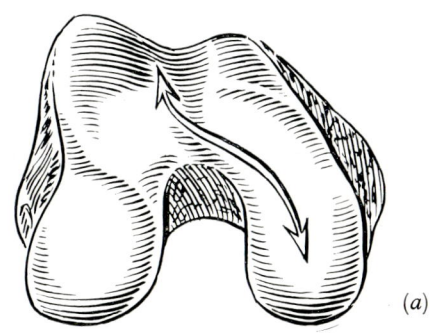

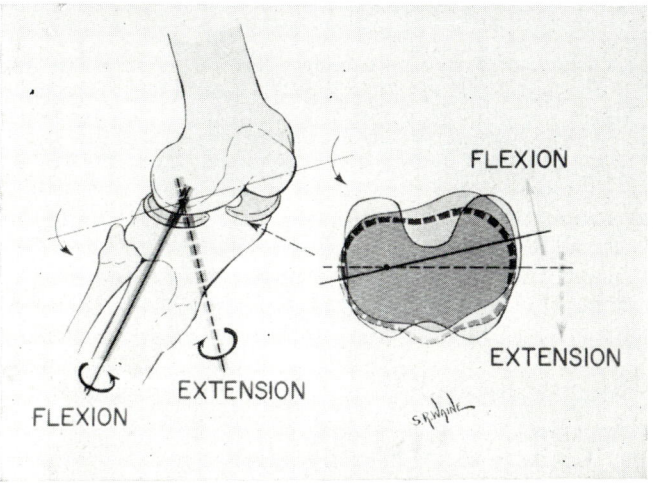

FIG. 2.
(*a*) The articular surface of the bicondylar lower end of the femur. The lateral tuberosity of the tibia rotates on the round lateral femoral condyle while the medial tuberosity of the tibia follows the sinuous track on the medial condyle. (From 'Internal Derangements of the Knee'. A. J. Helfet, Pitman Medical.)
(*b*) Diagrammatic representation of the helicoid movement of the knee joint.

As accurate and reliable physical signs were demonstrated the whole concept developed, leading to the *inescapable conviction that most osteoarthritis of the knee in middle age and over is due to minor derangements of the menisci*; moreover the pain and the distribution can usually be cured by simple operation.

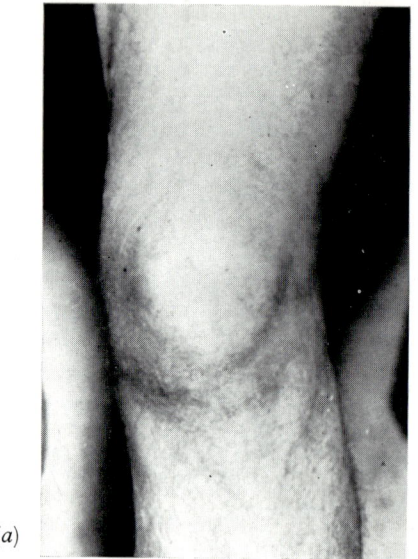 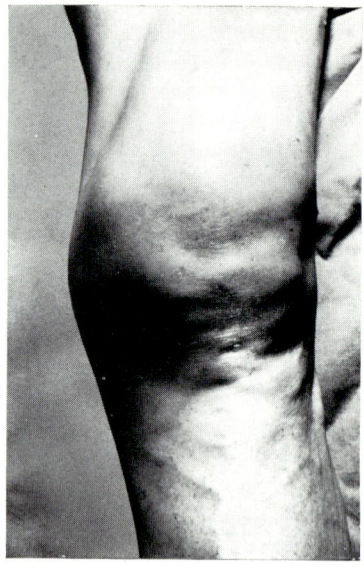

FIG. 3.

(a) Locked knee of a young footballer. The protrusion of the medial femoral condyle and the blocked rotation of the tibial tubercle are evident.

(b) The classical osteoarthritic knee with medially rotated tibial tubercle, prominent medial femoral condyle, prominent patella and wasted thigh.

The physical signs of the displaced meniscus in the young footballer (Fig. 3a) are all demonstrable in the osteoarthritic knee (Fig. 3b)—limitation of external rotation of the tibia on the femur and therefore lack of full extension; limitation of internal rotation and therefore lack of full flexion; pain and finger-point tenderness of the joint line over the

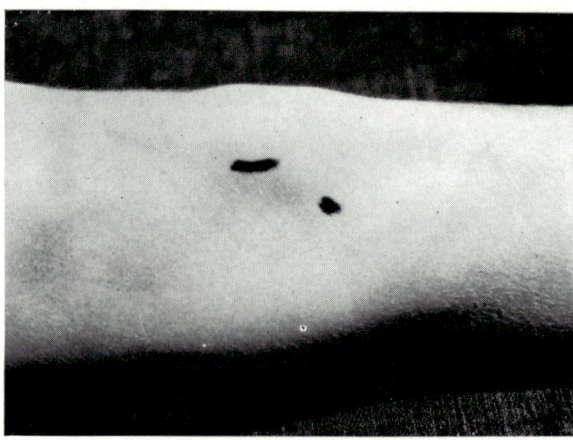

FIG. 4. Knee marked to show areas of tenderness from the anterior horn of the medial meniscus and the medial border of the patella.

deranged part of the meniscus; protrusion of the medial femoral condyle; and wasting of the quadriceps. When lateral rotation of the tibia is blocked, the patellar ligament prevents full excursion of the patella and when the quadriceps contracts the medial border of the patella is forced to impinge against the medial trochlear groove. Consequently after a time, a new physical sign develops, namely tenderness of the medial articular surface of the patella without tenderness of the lateral border (Fig. 4).

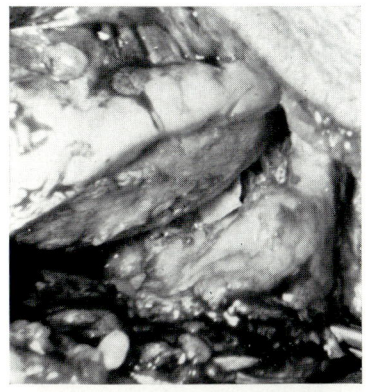

(a) Operation photograph showing marked osteoarthritic changes and with a fragment of meniscus blocking the back of the joint.

(a)

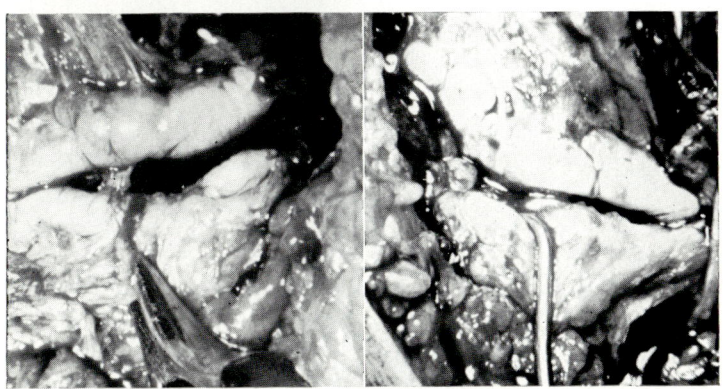

(b) (c)

FIG. 5.

(b) With the knee straight the internal derangement results in lack of congruity or rotational alignment of the femur and tibia.

(c) After removal of the medial meniscus the joint surfaces are now congruent, with the result that even with this degree of osteoarthritis the patient subsequently had comfortable function.

The fixed deformity in the osteoarthritic knee is always flexion and internal rotation of the tibia on the femur; consequently the patella is also fixed more medially and distally than normal in relation to the medial femoral condyle.

Operation is designed to restore a normal pattern of movement and especially full extension and external rotation of the tibia on the femur.

Usually all that is needed is simple meniscectomy, and limited débridement of the medial facet of the patella and of any osteophytes on the edge of the medial femoral condyle if these obstruct movement (Fig. 5); normally only the medial meniscus need be removed but occasionally both menisci. If the tibia can now be fully extended and externally rotated, no more need be done—except of course adequate rehabilitation.

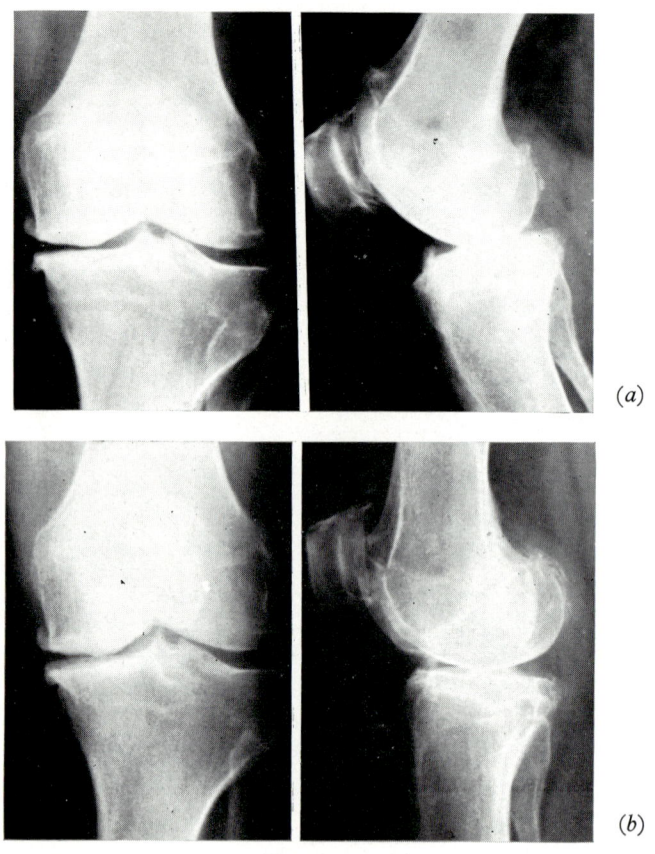

FIG. 6.
(a) A.P. and lateral X-ray in an osteoarthritic knee.
(b) Four years after operation showing the improved appearance.

More extensive operation, the so called 'house-cleaning', is unnecessary and, indeed, causes excessive injury to the knee joint.

To recover comfort in walking, to increase the range, and to enable the patient to negotiate stairs, he must recover and maintain the necessary muscle tone and power—and if muscular control is preserved the patients remain comfortable.

Recovery of movement in the normal pattern, even if not complete, has a pronounced effect in relieving osteoarthritic pain and in permitting normal walking and activity. It is interesting that it is not necessary to touch the articular cartilage, because recovery of comfort is striking despite the persistence of articular ulcers and erosions. The important thing is that the knee must be able to move in its normal pattern without tension, and once the patient can fully extend the knee, comfort and function are recovered. Eventually resolution of juxta-articular sclerosis and restoration of bone trabeculation is seen on X-ray (Fig. 6). It must be concluded that Nissen's criteria for the 'arrest' of arthritis have been borne out; the formerly degenerating joint is, in fact, regenerating.

Osteoarthritis of the Hip

Without treatment, the osteoarthritic hip invariably degenerates. The joint space narrows, the joint margins become sclerosed and cystic changes appear in adjacent bone (Fig. 7). As the range of movement

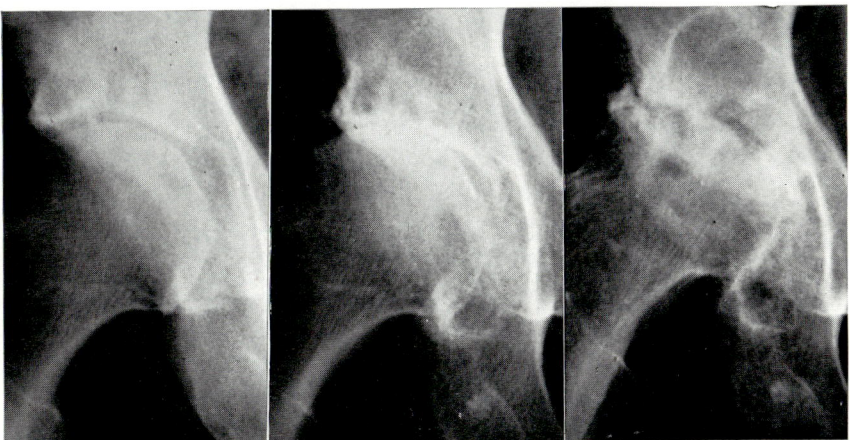

FIG. 7. The progression of radiological changes in osteoarthritis over a period of seven years. (From 'A System of Orthopaedics and Fractures' by A. Graham Apley. Butterworths, London.)

decreases, pain on movement increases. The hip becomes deformed; the deformity is one of increasing flexion and external rotation with, in addition, either abduction or adduction (Fig. 8). Finally ache or bone pain develops which lasts into the night and prevents sleep.

Intertrochanteric displacement osteotomy has a striking effect (see D'Aubigné, Fig. 2, page 382). Displacement of the shaft is essential to relieve tension and to compensate for deformity; but it is neither necessary nor reasonable to attempt abduction or adduction by a precise number of degrees as advised by Pauwels. To plan the specific rotation of the 'impingement point' on the ball-shaped head of the femur from measurements on a flat X-ray is an extraordinary mechanical feat even if its purpose were adequately justified. Before operation pain on walking is due to the tension produced by the attempt to bring the foot forward normally—a movement which is obstructed by the fixed deformity. This compares with pain in the obstructed knee.

Similarly the surgical objective is to recover a pattern of movement which allows the limb to come forward without tension despite the existing deformity. All that is needed besides medial displacement, is rotation at the osteotomy site so that the leg and foot point forwards. This works well whatever the initial deformity.

Realignment compensates for the fixed flexion, external rotation, and ab/or adduction deformity; the limb can now move forward without tension even though the hip is still deformed. The realignment does not in itself produce an improved range of movement but the altered arc of movement provides relief from repeated tension and results in slow recovery of range which gradually increases as the joint surfaces remould.

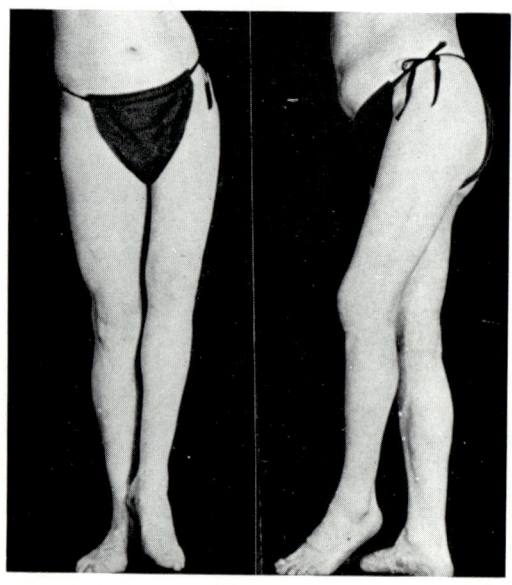

FIG. 8. Characteristic deformity in osteoarthritis of the hip. (From 'A System of Orthopaedics and Fractures' by A. Graham Apley. Butterworths, London.)

After operation early movement of the hip and knee, using light traction and a knee sling, is encouraged, and the patient is allowed to walk on crutches within two or three weeks. Full weight-bearing is permitted when the osteotomy has consolidated three or four months later. By this time active non weight-bearing exercises have usually resulted in a greater range of movement than before operation.

There is evidence that in osteoarthritis of the hip the earlier osteotomy is performed the more beneficial the effect. Consequently in bilateral osteoarthritis it may be a mistake to operate on the worse hip first. Within a year the patient considers this his better hip and as the other deteriorates further, he usually asks for osteotomy of that hip. It might be wiser to advise operation on the less affected hip first, so that the arrest of the early osteoarthritis is that much more complete. Further, the use of compression devices allows the second (more advanced) hip to be operated on soon after the first.

Trueta, Goran Bauer and others have shown that in osteoarthritis, a state of excessive hyperemia of the head of the femur exists. Nissen postulates that the osteotomy cuts off the excessive blood supply, thus reducing pain, and that as a result of metabolic changes the joint is remoulded.

Osteotomy of the Tibia

The success of osteotomy in the relief of disability from osteoarthritis of the hip led Wardle, Helal, Apley and Coventry among others to advocate osteotomy of the upper end of the tibia for osteoarthritis of the

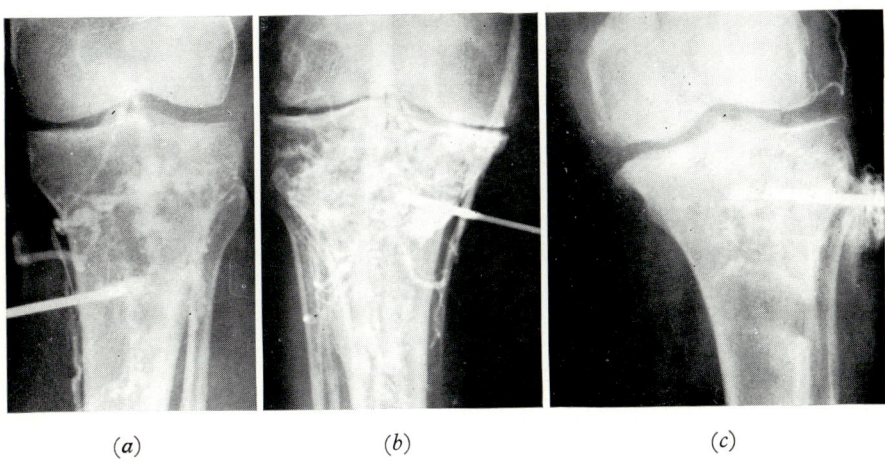

(a)　　　　　　　　　(b)　　　　　　　　　(c)

FIG. 9. (Reproduced by courtesy of B. Helal.)
(a) Intra-osseous venogram of a normal knee.
(b) Of an osteoarthritic knee—note the venous congestion in the sub-chondral zone.
(c) Is a similar knee in which, after inserting an acrylic plug, the venous pattern has returned to normal.

knee. Pain has been relieved, but the results are qualified by the finding that in a number of patients intra-articular operations on the knee itself have to be carried out at a later stage. Wardle, Helal and Apley by manometric studies of the medullary circulation found that in osteoarthritis a state of venous congestion exists and they believe that by dividing the bone this venous congestion is relieved. Moreover, in the healing of an osteotomy, a layer of new bone forms across the medullary canal; this blocks the venous flow and so decompresses the upper segment. This has led Helal, working with Apley, to insert a barrier of acrylic cement across the bone in lieu of an osteotomy (Fig. 9).

In the author's series osteotomy of the upper end of tibia has been used only for correction of deformity—that is, for gross valgus or varus deformities. For plain osteoarthritis a simple correction of the internal derangement of the knee to restore a normal pattern of movement without tension especially in extension, has been quite satisfactory.

The earlier the operation the quicker and better the result. And improvement is maintained; hence Nissen's concept of early arrest of osteoarthritis has validity.

Non-referred Pain in the Knee with Osteoarthritis of the Hip

Pain felt in the knee may be referred from the hip joint and is recognized as a symptom of osteoarthritis of the hip. This referred pain is muscular in origin and is felt in front or on the sides of the knee depending on the muscle group which is contracted. A patient with flexion and abduction or adduction deformity may feel pain in front or on the sides of the knee. As extension contracture, if it ever occurs, is a rarity, pain is not felt behind the knee. It should be noted too that it is difficult with fixed flexion of the hip to walk with a straight knee. The trunk tends to overbalance forward. The fixed deformities of osteoarthritis of the hip are *always* flexion, *either* adduction or abduction, and *usually* external rotation as demonstrated.

Surprisingly often, with long-established osteoarthritis of the hip, careful examination of the knee reveals fixed limitation of extension, and external rotation of the tibia on the femur, prominence of the medial femoral condyle, and tenderness of the medial meniscus and medial border of the patella. Fixed adduction contracture of the hip may also be associated with laxity of the medial ligaments of the knee.

It is apparent that pain in the knee need not necessarily be referred from the hip and the question arises whether the changes in the knee are independent of the hip and part of a generalized osteoarthritis or whether they are secondary to and the consequence of fixed deformity of the hip. The latter is almost certainly the case for the pattern of disorder in the knee depends on the particular deformity of the hip.

For example, fixed external rotation and flexion of the hip eventually leads to flexion and internal rotation contracture of the tibia on the femur with consequent internal derangement of the knee of the typical pattern.

In normal walking, sinuous and synchronous adaptations of movement take place between hip and knee. During flexion, the hip rotates outwards while the tibia rotates inwards, and vice versa during extension. Walking with a fixed flexion-external rotation deformity of the hip demands compensation by flexion of the knee and, in order to point the foot forward, limited external rotation of the tibia during extension. In time, these factors effect permanent fixed limitation of extension and external rotation of the tibia with retraction of the aging, harder medial meniscus. This is shown in Fig. 3(b) by the limitation of external rotation of the tibia and the prominent medial femoral condyle. These signs persist both while walking and at rest. When present, they represent or portend the typical patterns of erosion of the medial femoral condyle and medial border of the patella, and are a frequent cause of pain—pain which may be relieved by simple meniscectomy and when necessary, débridement of the medial border of the patella. These changes are consequent too, on the normal aging of menisci, which as has been noted, in the young are shiny, smooth and elastic, and with age, become harder, contracted and fibrous and retract from the edges of the joint. This hard retracted meniscus causes deep patterns of erosion on the femoral condyle and secondarily on the trochlear groove and patella. To recapitulate, so-called osteoarthritis develops which is relieved only by separate operation.

Adduction deformity adds a valgus strain to the knee and causes medial ligaments and sometimes cruciates to stretch, so producing instability of the knee. The medial meniscus may be and usually is retracted as seen in the patient depicted in Fig. 3. For many years her left hip had been arthritic, flexed, adducted and externally rotated. The X-ray of the knee taken with valgus stress, showed the degree of medial capsule laxity, while the limited external rotation of the tibia and protrusion of the medial femoral condyle denotes a retracted meniscus. These changes plus laxity of the cruciate ligaments were confirmed at operation. All were secondary to the fixed deformity of the hip and pain felt in the knee was local in origin and not referred.

To stabilize this knee, it was necessary to remove the meniscus and in addition to do an extra-articular tendon transplant of the semitendinosus into a groove in the medial femoral condyle, plus medial transfer of the tibial tubercle. An advanced example of change secondary to the arthritis of the hip joint, it stresses the importance of examination of the knee joint itself when pain is present with osteoarthritis of the hip.

Discussion

What is the common factor in restoration of function and alleviation of pain by osteotomy at the hip or by soft tissue operation at the knee? Change in the abnormal arterial or venous circulation must play a part, but only a part; it may not even be the prime factor. I suggest that the important feature is the *relief of tension on the soft tissues of the joint—during movement.*

Limitation of rotation (and therefore of the extremes of extension and flexion) is constant in osteoarthritis of the knee; and limitation of rotation accompanied by flexion and abduction or adduction is the pattern of contracture in osteoarthritis of the hip. Attempts to walk therefore come up immediately against these limiting factors. Neither the hip nor the knee can achieve full extension and the synchronous movement of rotation also is blocked.

When the thigh moves forward, both the hip and the knee flex and the accommodating adaptation of sinuous movement of these joints is well demonstrated; the tibia rotates inwards on the femur which rotates outwards in the acetabulum. Then, when the hip extends and the knee straightens, the tibia rotates outwards while the femur rotates inwards.

In the early stages of osteoarthritis pain is felt only at the extremes of movement. Once there is fixed contracture pain is more pronounced and is felt earlier. Displacement derotation osteotomy at the hip immediately reduces the soft tissue tension due to movement against these fixed deformities. In a different fashion, correction of derangement of the knee by soft-tissue operation leads to a normal tensionless pattern of movement.

The temporary relief of pain which sometimes follows muscle division for arthritis of the hip has the same explanation. But to maintain comfort and function, it is essential to recover and maintain tone and power of the muscles acting on the joint. This is not easily achieved after extensive muscle division, which is the probable explanation for the return of pain and dysfunction after this operation.

The use of intra-articular injections of hydro-cortisone, a common, though perhaps ill-considered practice, must be mentioned only to be discounted. We have no evidence that cortisone does or can play any part in

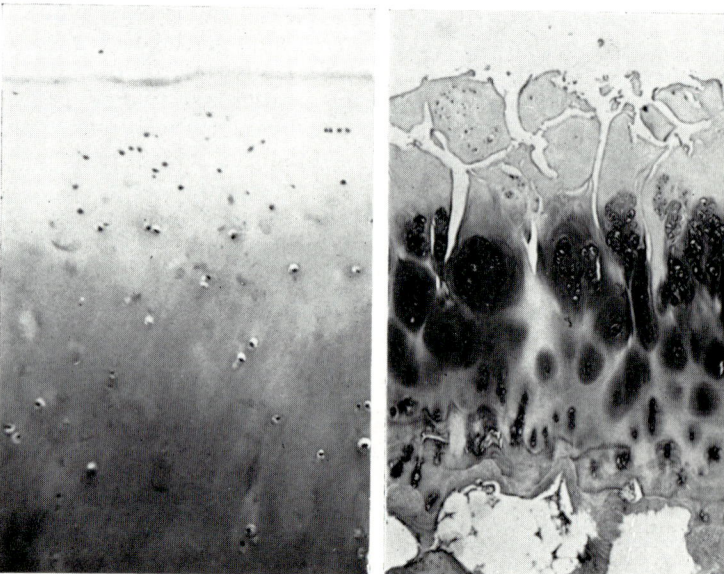

Fig. 10. Human articular cartilage stained to demonstrate collagen and mucopolysaccharides.
(a) Normal, showng the lamina splendens; normal distribution of chondrocytes; a collagen layer free of mucopolysaccharides which are evenly distributed in the deeper layers.
(b) Osteoarthritic (different scale), showing disruption of surface with obvious mucopolysaccharide leak; the chondrocytes clump and show a high rate of polysaccharide production.

the arrest of osteoarthritis. And indeed it is probably harmful for after a series of these injections, the articular cartilage at operation may resemble that found in neuropathic joints and often is yellow and malacic. One injection in a recently injured joint may be soothing, but the temptation to repeat this should be resisted.

Miller and Kasahara have demonstrated small myelinated nerve fibres of unknown function spread on the undersurface of joint cartilage. Rosenberg et al. have shown by biochemical staining the differences between normal, traumatized and osteoarthritic articular cartilage (Fig. 10). The 'skin' is broken and it appears that the mucopolysaccharides of the matrix are washed out into the joint. Cartilage cells clump and

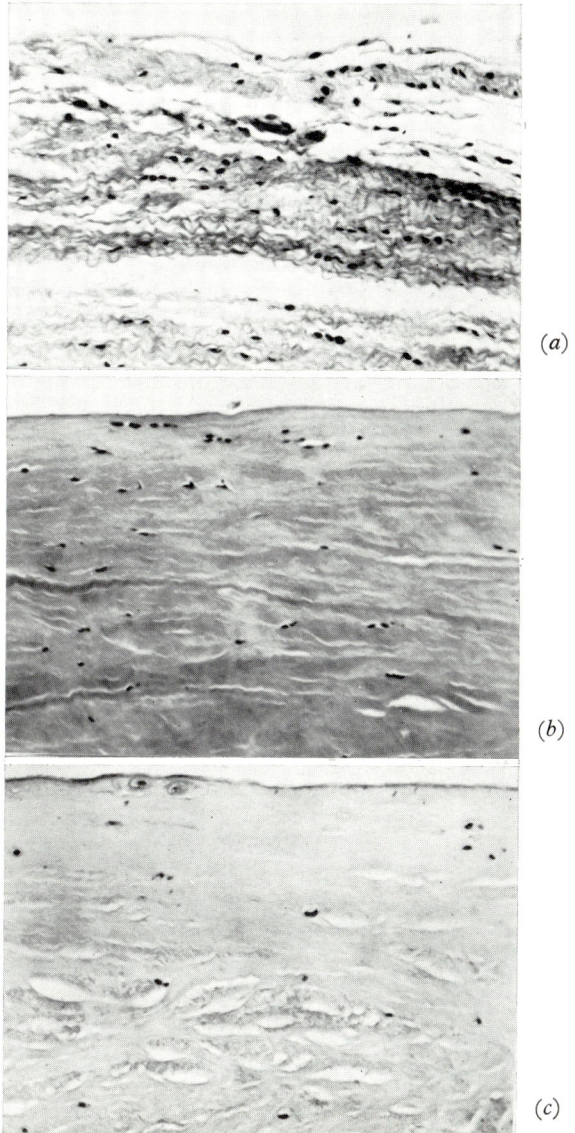

Fig. 11. Microscopic appearance of menisci at ages of (a) 8 years, (b) 24 years and (c) 77 years. The youngest meniscus shows patterned layers of collagen and numerous ovoid-nucleated cells. Gradually, with increasing age the collagen is replaced by fibrous tissue; the cells diminish in number and their nuclei become round and cartilaginous. Finally, in the 77-year-old, the collagen is completely replaced by fibrous tissue, with the glass-like appearance of chondrification; the cells are very few in number and are cartilaginous.

only around these areas is the presence and perhaps the formation of mucopolysaccharides demonstrated. No local repair is demonstrable except when the cartilage is completely eroded down to the underlying bone.

In the meantime, the aging meniscus or the meniscus in the osteoarthritic is changed from the shining, compressible, pliable structure which, in the normal young knee, is cellular and composed of avascular collagenous tissue. As it ages and degenerates the meniscus becomes less cellular, more fibrous and invaded by blood vessels and inflammatory cells (Fig. 11). This fibrosis, with hardening, contraction and change in shape of the meniscus may well be the predisposing factor in the derangement of the joint. The meniscus tends to contract and therefore to retract; and minimal trauma by a twist or stumble disrupts one end (usually the anterior horn) from its attachment to the anterior tibial spine. It may be considered a 'pathological' derangement comparable to pathological fracture of the neck of the femur in the aged osteoporotic. Change in the shape of the content of the helical joint causes the block to movement and initiates the patterns and sequelae of typical 'osteoarthritis'.

It is extraordinary that the patient with a knee on which it is painful to bear weight and which aches sufficiently to prevent sleep, after simple surgery (removal sometimes of only a meniscus sufficient to allow the knee to extend fully on the table) has usually lost these symptoms within 24 hours. Ten days later he can walk and take weight comfortably because the removal of an obstruction to movement has relieved all pain in spite of the fact that the erosion and ulcers in the articular surface are unaltered.

Lent Johnson has shown that the articular ends of bones do not have a constant or stable bone pattern but are subject to a continuous process of resorption and laying down of new bone, so that the relation and proportion between bone and articular cartilage is always changing. He has shown that in the course of time the actual shape may alter. Change or improvement in the circulation of the head of the femur or the upper end of the tibia after operation is probably important in remodelling these bone ends to a more suitable shape for their new and tensionless patterns of movement. In other words while the relief of pain is due to relief of tension, the improved architecture is the result of improved circulation.

Summary

It has been argued that (1) it is reasonable to incriminate abnormal local tensions *during movement* as an important cause of arthritic pain and disability; (2) the degenerative process of osteoarthritis can be arrested; and (3) the earlier arrest is effected the better and quicker function and comfort recover.

Pain and dysfunction at the knee may be relieved by intra-articular operation to correct the internal derangement; at the hip by intertrochanteric derotation-displacement osteotomy which compensates for any fixed deformity. Review after these operations demonstrates not only arrest of the arthritic process but also that in many instances sclerosis, cyst formation and abnormal patterns of trabeculation in juxta-articular bone tend to resolve. It is postulated that both these procedures prevent abnormal local tensions during movement.

Changes in the circulation to the bone ends are probably instrumental in restoring bone structure and joint contours suitable to the new patterns of movement.

References

BAUER, G. (1967). Pattern of distribution of SR-85 in osteoarthritis of the knee. Paper read at the Orthopaedic Research Society, San Francisco.

COVENTRY, M. B. (1965). Osteotomy of the upper portion of the tibia for degenerative arthritis of the knee. *J. Bone Jt. Surg.*, **47A**, 984–990.

HARRISON, M. H. M., SCHAJOWICZ, F. and TRUETA, J. (1953). Osteoarthritis of the hip: a study of the nature and evolution of the disease. *J. Bone Jt. Surg.*, **35B**, 598–626.

HELAL, B. (1965). The pain in primary osteoarthritis of the knee. *Post. med. J.*, **41**, 172–181.

JOHNSON, L. E. (1959). Kinetics of osteoarthritis, laboratory investigation. **8**, No. 6, 1223–1241.

MILLER, M. R. and KASAHARA, M. (1963). Observations on the innervation of human long bones. *Anat. Rec.*, **145**, 13–23.

NISSEN, K. I. (1963). The arrest of early primary osteoarthritis of the hip by osteotomy. *Proc. roy. Soc. Med.*, **56**, 1051–1060.

PAUWELS, F. (1951). Des affections de la hanche d'origine mecanigne et de leur traitement par l'osteotomie d'adduction. *Rev. Chir. Orthopaed.*, **37**, 22–30.

ROSENBERG, L. Personal communication.

WARDLE, E. N. (1962). Osteotomy of the tibia and fibula. *Surg. Gynec. Obstet.*, **115**, 61–64.

Chapter 12

ARTHROPLASTY IN THE TREATMENT OF DEGENERATIVE OSTEOARTHRITIS OF THE HIP

R. MERLE d'AUBIGNÉ

Reconstruction of the hip joint is obviously one of the great challenges offered to the orthopaedic surgeon. Anatomical and physiological conditions make its realization more attainable than in other weight-bearing joints. The high incidence of disabling hip lesions, whether traumatic, inflammatory or degenerative, is a great stimulus to research.

The problem is a difficult one: no complete or final solution has yet been reached. But great advances have been made in the last thirty years and it is not unreasonable to hope that within a few years it will be possible to offer patients with progressive disabling hip disorders restoration of nearly normal hip function, with complete security.

Before 1935, attempts to restore mobility of the hip were made in three directions.

(1) **Resection of the femoral head and neck,** generally gave mobility and in some cases, surprisingly enough, also relative stability. It was advocated in England by Girdlestone, as the 'pseudarthrosis operation'. In Germany Hackenbroch tried to obtain greater stability by associating a valgus osteotomy either at the same time or at a second operation. Milch was the United States advocate of this procedure.

(2) **Reconstruction of the joint** using a more ambitious and elaborate procedure was tried by Putti in Italy and by Royal Whitman in the U.S.A. Putti, after a limited resection, reshaped the head and the acetabulum, and interposed a hood made of fascia lata. I remember visiting Putti in Bologna, in 1932, and realizing for the first time, that, with good technique, really mobile hips could be obtained.

Whitman, using a more extensive resection, maintained the neck stump in the acetabulum (with or without fascial interposition) by lowering the greater trochanter. This technique was advised and used by Mathieu in France, and we employed it in a few cases before the last war.

These reconstruction operations produced greater stability than resection, but mobility and painlessness were seldom obtained together.

Smith-Petersen concentrated all his efforts on inserting an inert and rigid interposition material able, of course, to prevent adhesions between bony surfaces, but also to induce the healing process to form spherical and smooth surfaces covered by fibro-cartilage. The first 'cups' he used, made of glass or plastic material broke: in his final technique he used a vitallium mold, and left it in place as a permanent interposition material. His whole technique, meticulous and atraumatic, has survived and a great number of patients have enjoyed, thanks to it, great improvement of their condition. I used it for more than 500 patients and still do, for some well chosen cases of hip lesions.

(3) **Replacement of part or the whole of the joint.** As Smith-Petersen's operation did not solve the problem of extensive destruction or necrosis of the head, other surgeons worked on a different line: instead of interposition they inserted a prosthesis as a substitute for the femoral head.

These attempts were made first in the U.S.A. by Austin Moore and others, using a metallic prosthesis; and in France by Judet who used an acrylic prosthesis. The immediate results were good and Judet had many followers. But, after a few years, most of the good results deteriorated and the acrylic prosthesis was abandoned in favour of the metallic types: Moore's, Thompson's, and others. With the use of metal, the extensive bone absorption due to fragmentation of the methacrylate no longer occurred.

But in osteoarthritis the results of the prosthesis remained inferior to those of the cup. For this reason, different authors have developed techniques of arthroplasty in which both joint components are replaced; after excision of the joint a double articulated prosthesis is inserted. This has been the work of Charnley and of McKee, both in England. We have followed them along this path and the results obtained appear to be really promising.

But the first question is: what, at the present time, is the place of arthroplasty in the treatment of degenerative osteoarthritis?

To answer this question we must consider three factors:

the physiological conditions of the hip; the pathological conditions of osteoarthritis; and the clinical result obtained:

(a) by operations other than arthroplasty, and (b) by the different types of arthroplasty.

Physiological Conditions of the Hip

Some conditions are favourable for surgical reconstruction: spherical bone surfaces maintain themselves in permanent and complete contact without the aid of ligaments; provided the femoral head is congruent with the acetabulum it is kept in place by the peri-articular muscles. Good muscle tone is, therefore, essential for stability: not only to maintain the bone surfaces in contact, but also to keep the pelvis horizontal when the patient stands on one leg: as the line of gravity of the body falls medially, the tendency to adduction of the hip must be counter-balanced, at each step, by strong contraction of the abductors. To allow walking without a limp, a mobile hip must have a stable femoral head, and good leverage action of the abductors.

Pathological Conditions of Osteoarthritis

The degenerative process may affect either the passive or the active parts of the joint or both.

Passive parts: the articular cartilage is always affected: but we know that it can regenerate. Sometimes the shape of the bone extremities is practically normal with spherical surfaces, normal direction of the neck, and little or no abnormal bone production. In such cases a conservative procedure, such as osteotomy, may be successful.

Often, however, the bony part of the mechanism is greatly abnormal, this being either the cause of the degenerative process (congenital dysplasia), or its result (bone absorption in the weight bearing part, bone production elsewhere or both). Normal mobility cannot then be restored by an extra-articular procedure.

Active parts: the necessary integrity of the peri-articular muscles is frequently lacking in osteoarthritis. Weakness is often caused by mechanical disturbances, congenital or acquired, of the bone extremities. But before the disability is so severe that arthroplasty is considered, years have elapsed with pain and limitation of motion, and muscle atrophy or even muscle degeneration may have taken place.

The evaluation of muscle power before operation is difficult and uncertain, as pain inhibits the muscular contraction. For this reason it is very hazardous to promise a normal gait after an arthroplasty. But it is remarkable how many patients recover good and strong muscular action provided the normal leverage is re-established and weight-bearing has become completely painless.

Clinical Results

Whatever the physiological and pathological conditions, the only safe basis for appreciation of the different methods of treatment is the clinical results.

It has been our constant effort for the last twenty years to collect the necessary information. As the results can only be established by comparison between the pre-operative and the post-operative functional state, records have been kept, as objectively as possible using, since 1945, the same scale of evaluation, shown here (Table I).

This grading of hip function could very probably be improved, as it has been by different authors. But having used it for 20 years in more than 5000 hip patients, including nearly 2000 cases of osteoarthritis, I can say that using three numbers, it provides a fairly accurate evaluation of hip function.

Evaluation of the improvement brought about by operation is particularly difficult in osteoarthritis where pain is the most important feature. It has been shown in Sweden that after any treatment, operative or not, the patient will acknowledge improvement in 70 per cent of cases. The opinion of the patient is only of value when the percentage rises higher than this. But objective observations of the gait, the duration of walking time, the use of a cane, and of particular movements, if carefully measured and noted, are of great value.

The following section describes how the methods used at the Hôpital Cochin have changed over the last 20 years. They must be compared between themselves, and with arthroplasty.

TABLE I

Grading of Functional Value of the Hip

	Painlessness	Mobility	Ability to walk
0	Pain intense and permanent	Ankylosis with bad position of the hip	Unable to walk
1	Pain severe at night	No movement with pain or slight deformity	Only with crutches
2	Pain severe when walking, preventing any activity	Flexion under 40°	Only with two sticks
3	Pain tolerable with limited activity	Maximum flexion between 40° and 60°	With one stick, less than one hour, very difficult without stick
4	Pain mild when walking, disappearing with rest	Maximum flexion between 60° and 80°, can reach his foot	A long time with a stick—a little without stick but with limp
5	Very mild and inconstant pain, permitting normal activity	Maximum flexion between 80° and 90°, abduction at least 15°	Without stick but with slight limp
6	No pain	Maximum flexion more than 90°, abduction to 30°	Normal

Tenomyotomy (Voss's operation)

This was used in only 20 cases, when the age or the general condition of the patient precluded a major operation. Pain was abolished or diminished in a little more than half the cases. In most cases the pain recurred after some weeks or months. Moreover, when the abductors were cut, the limp in some patients was seriously aggravated. This operation has been abandoned in our department.

Osteotomy

This has been restricted in our series to hips with relatively good mobility. In the early stage, when abduction still exists and particularly in congenital dysplasia with coxa valga and a shallow acetabulum, varus osteotomy with correction of the anteversion gives very satisfactory results. As a rule arthroplasty is out of the question in these cases.

In more advanced cases, where arthroplasty might be considered, 250 of our cases were treated by the so-called *McMurray's osteotomy*, with transfer of the shaft medially and superiorly, with or without lateral angulation. The cases selected for osteotomy were those who still had a fair range of flexion, and where the radiographs showed *relatively congruent articular surfaces.*

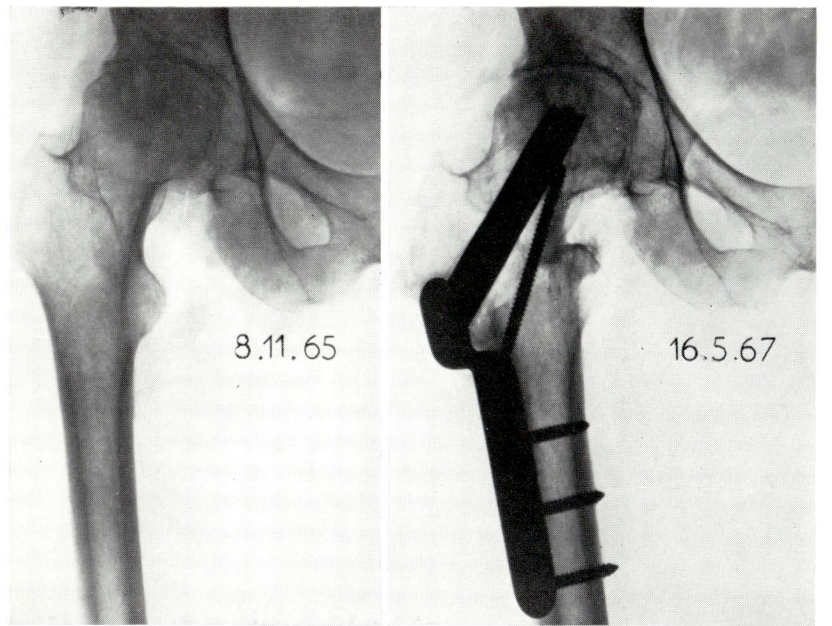

(a)   (b)

FIG. 1. Female, age 58 years.
(a) Severe osteoarthritis with preserved mobility and parallel joint space.
(b) Two years after displacement osteotomy; painless, walks without a cane.

TABLE II

Results of Displacement Intertrochanteric Osteotomy.

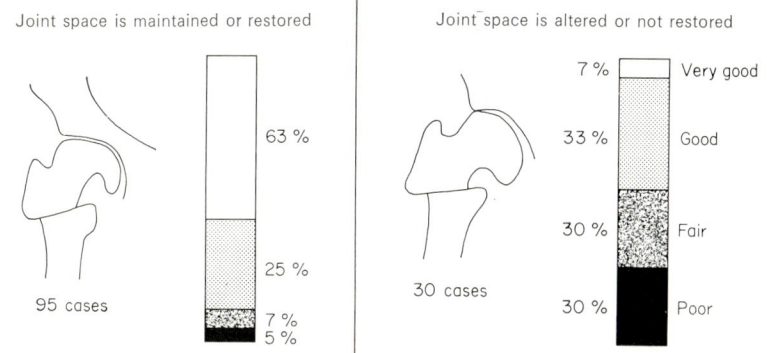

When parallelism of joint space is present before operation or can be restored by exact varus or valgus displacement, together with medial shaft displacement, results are regularly good. When joint space is not parallel, results are very irregular.

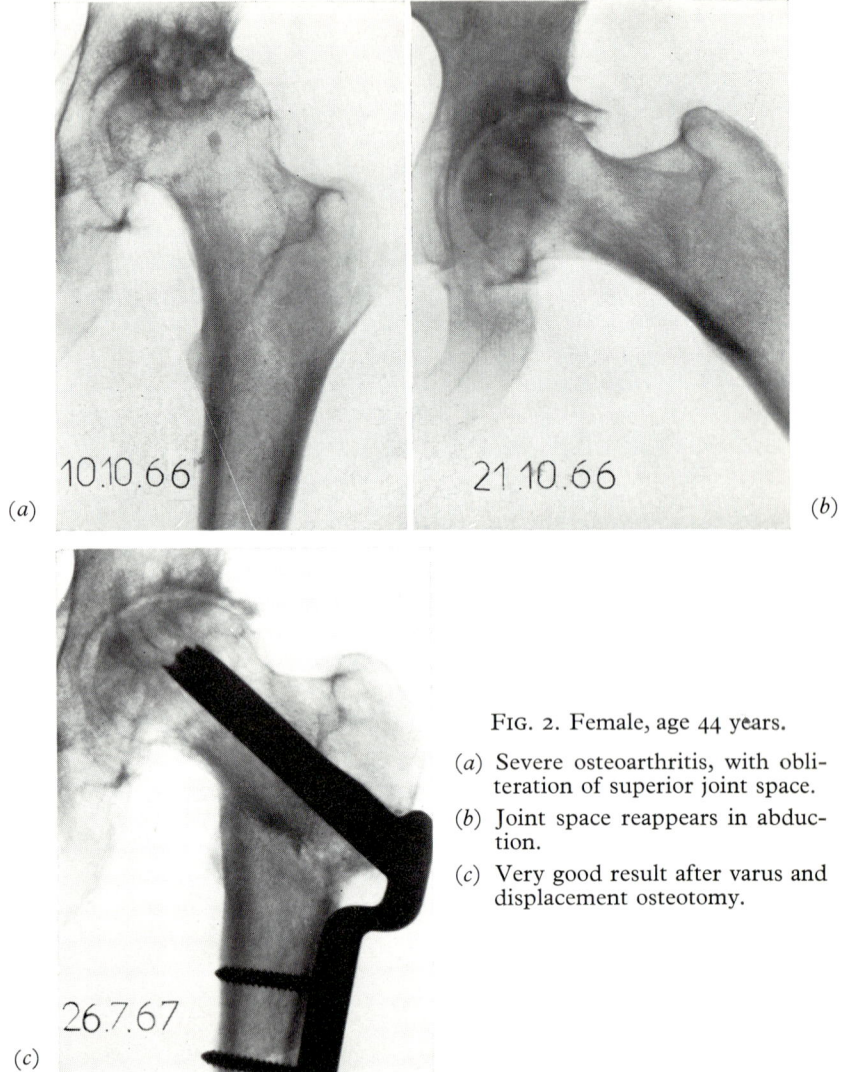

Fig. 2. Female, age 44 years.
(a) Severe osteoarthritis, with obliteration of superior joint space.
(b) Joint space reappears in abduction.
(c) Very good result after varus and displacement osteotomy.

All our osteotomies are fixed by a solid blade plate and the patients are allowed out of bed after a few days. One hundred and fifty results, followed up for one to six years, have been reviewed recently by our friend J. Kerboul.

Osteotomy gives a high percentage of excellent and good results clinically (no pain, normal gait) and radiologically (re-appearance of a good articular space) when parallelism of the weight-bearing surfaces is either preserved—by simple displacement without angulation—so restored, by producing the precisely correct amount of varus or valgur angulation. In our series, these conditions were observed in the X-rays

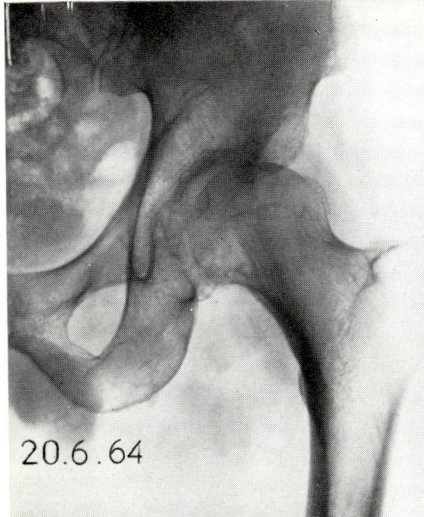
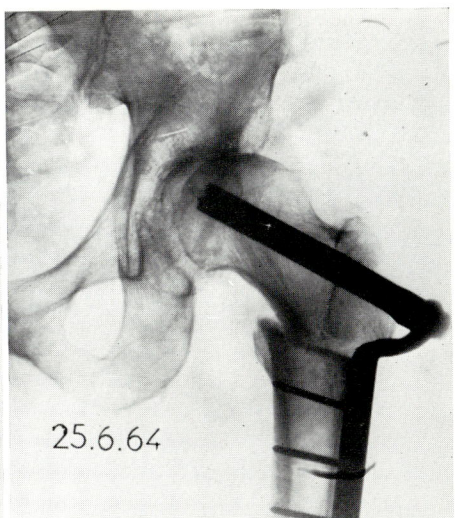
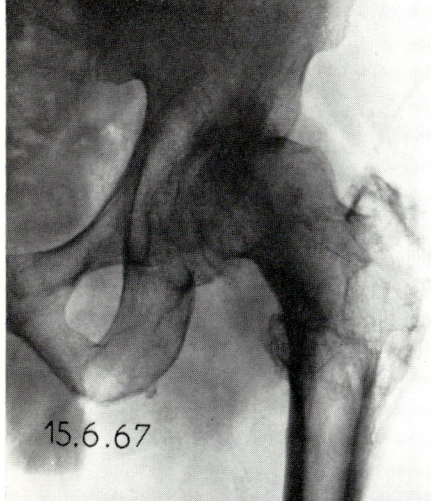

FIG. 3. Male, age 52 years.

(a) Very painful osteoarthritis with preserved mobility. Non-parallel joint space.

(b) After osteotomy: unmodified joint space.

(c) Three years later, improved, but still painful.

of 95 cases: functional results were excellent or good in 88·5 per cent of cases, with only five failures.

When the post-operative X-rays show persistent incongruity only 40 per cent of the results are classified as good.

It is our opinion that osteotomy should not be considered in a great number of advanced osteoarthritic hips, namely:

all cases where parallelism of the articular surfaces is destroyed and impossible to restore; all cases where limitation of joint movement of one or, more often, both hips, make restoration of mobility necessary. In our series, patients with great limitation of mobility and with marked adduction or flexion deformity, were not treated by osteotomy. Intra-articular procedures were used: resection, arthrodesis or arthroplasty.

Resection

Complete resection (30 cases) gave relief of pain after one year or more in all cases except one, but useful mobility in only 16 cases (one out of two). Only five patients (young and with good muscles) regained a relatively good gait after two or three years, but all the others had to use a cane at all times. Moreover, in many cases the mobility is very limited. An associated osteotomy did not improve the results. Consequently, we believe that resection is an operation of the past, except for high painful congenital dislocation, where pain is regularly relieved without alteration of the gait and, as a last resort, for failed arthroplasties.

Arthrodesis

Arthrodesis provides the surgeon with his most satisfied patients: before the advent of total hip replacement no other operation could claim such a high proportion of completely painless patients, able to walk and stand for as long as they like. When obtained in the right position, when the opposite hip and the vertebral column are sound, and when the homolateral knee has preserved a complete range of motion, bony ankylosis is surprisingly well tolerated, especially by patients who were pre-operatively used to limited mobility.

But the picture has its dark side: first, bony ankylosis is permanent

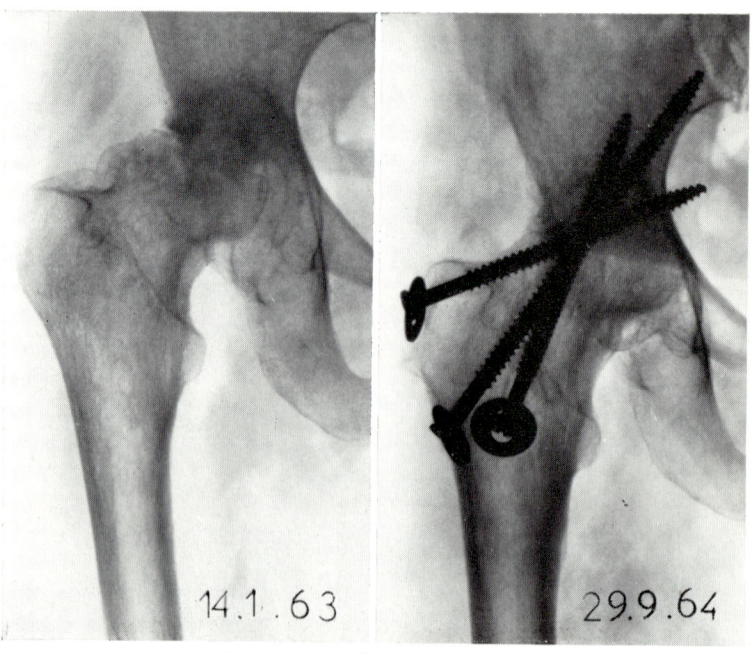

FIG. 4. Female, age 66 years.
(a) Severe pain but flexion up to 90°.
(b) Two years after operation. No pain in the hip, but some low back pain.

and may lead to considerable trouble if the opposite hip is affected by progressive stiffness, especially in relatively young women. Ankylosis in slight flexion makes sitting easy, but may cause lumbar pain; and in extension the limb is rather cumbersome.

And, above all, absence of bony union is not exceptional in sclerotic osteoarthritic hips: some pain may persist, a cane may be necessary: the patient will then resent as a failure the loss of his pre-operative mobility.

Consequently neither resection, osteotomy nor arthrodesis is able to solve all the problems of advanced cases of osteoarthritis: bilateral hips with great limitation of mobility and/or deformity, require arthroplasty. Even in unilateral cases arthroplasty has many indications, and will have more if its results become more regular, more complete and more lasting.

'Prosthesis' Arthroplasty

In 1953, reviewing 153 cases of Judet's acrylic arthroplasties, we drew attention to the frequent deterioration after the first year, and to the important bone absorption around the prosthesis in these cases. We presented these results to the American Orthopaedic Association in

TABLE III

Results of Arthroplasty using Moore's prosthesis.

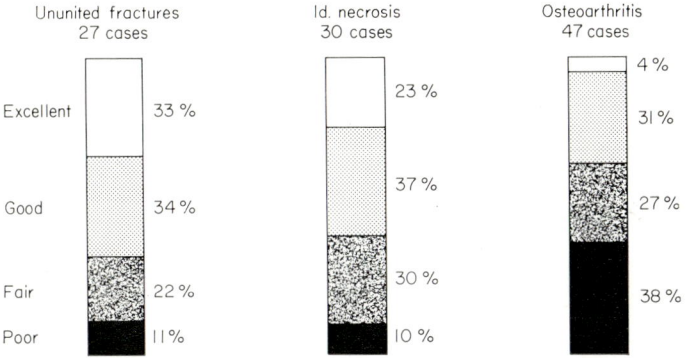

In ununited fractures or necrosis, where the cartilage of the acetabulum is preserved, results are good in 70 per cent of the cases. In osteoarthritis, when acetabulum is altered, results are good only in 30 per cent

1954 and proposed the use (instead of the purely cephalic Judet's prosthesis), of a metallic one more solidly fixed to the superior end and shaft of the femur. As soon as Austin Moore's vitallium prosthesis was available we used it concurrently with our own device. With these we avoided the late deterioration due to massive bone absorption. But the results, in osteoarthritis, were not substantially better than those observed after acrylic arthroplasty. Reviewing 47 cases we found 35 per cent good, 27 per cent fair, 38 per cent poor.

This brought us back to cup arthroplasty. But before describing our experience with cups, let us say that the results of prosthesis, whether acrylic or metallic, were very different and, as a matter of fact, remain today quite good *in traumatic cases*, where the prosthesis replacing the ununited or necrotic head was introduced into a sound acetabulum, with its normal cartilage, and where normal length of the neck is restored. This means that a prosthetic head firmly fixed on the femur and moving in a sound acetabulum gives a practically normal hip 9 times out of 10.

Cup Arthroplasty

Since 1948 about 400 cup arthroplasties for osteoarthritis have been done by me or my collaborators. At first the technique used was that which we had learned from Smith-Petersen: an anterior approach with wide exposure of the anterior part of the iliac bone; and extensive bone excision on both sides to allow great mobility of the cup. From 1950 on, we have always used the lateral approach with section of gluteus medius and minimus, and tried, by preserving the neck lever, to obtain stability as well as mobility.

Two hundred and fifty-three cases were reviewed in 1964, with a follow up of two years or more.

Pain was completely or nearly completely relieved in 52 per cent and substantially relieved in another 20 per cent.

Mobility was improved as a rule, but not always, and never completely restored if it was limited before the operation. But deformity rarely recurs.

Walking ability: only 20 per cent of these patients walk without a cane; 46 per cent walk well with a cane. It is fair to observe that before operation all these patients either did not walk or used one or two canes.

Most of the patients are satisfied.

But, considering the time spent in hospital, the extensive operative procedure, and the prolonged and expensive rehabilitation, we consider that in the unilateral cases only 64 per cent of the results are satisfactory, and in the bilateral cases 68 per cent. Among the 62 patients with poor results (21 operated on both sides) 23 have stiffness and pain, 23 have sufficient mobility but are painful, and 13 (most bilateral) do not complain of pain but of lack of mobility.

Like many surgeons, we were not satisfied with these results. I firmly believe that this inadequacy is not due to technique. Of course, some of these operations have been performed by young surgeons, but always helped by me or one of my experienced associates.

It is clear that failures are mostly related to persistent pain, and it is interesting to note that pain sometimes disappears when movement is lost or even reduced. A possible hypothesis is that the pain is due to friction of the cup on one or both altered bone extremities.

In favour of this hypothesis are the excellent results obtained by cup arthroplasty in old fractures of the acetabulum. Out of 33 cases of such cases treated by cups in our department and reviewed after two years, 24 are classified as excellent or good. They have a practically normal hip, can walk as far as they like, and went back to sport: one of them is a well-known alpinist. Of course this is not osteoarthritis but trauma, with sound periarticular parts. As the cup is fixed in the acetabulum the good result is probably due to the normal head with good cartilage moving in a prosthetic acetabulum.

This observation is in line with that of the regularly good results of head prosthesis in a sound acetabulum. It suggests that foreign bodies are painless in the hip as long as they are firmly fixed in one bone and move on the other covered with normal cartilage.

TABLE IV

Comparison of Results of Cup Arthroplasty.

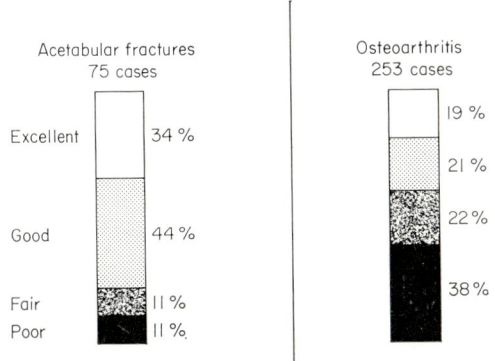

In old acetabular fractures with sound femoral head—good results. Results are good in less than half cases in osteoarthritis

Artificial Hip Joint

With this in mind, we were extremely interested in the attempts made in England by Charnley and by McKee, using complete artificial hip joints.

Their approach to the problem is slightly different. McKee, having confidence in the good tolerance of vitallium implants, tries to protect the acetabulum against the wear imposed by the prosthetic head. Charnley's idea was clearly expressed by the title of his first publication: 'low-friction arthroplasty'. His prosthesis was designed after very serious experimental work with engineers. Teflon was chosen for the acetabulum as having the lowest coefficient of friction, with the metallic head.

At our first visit to Manchester we saw beautiful results. But John Charnley was having trouble with late intolerance to Teflon, and was experimenting with other materials. At the present time, he seems quite satisfied with high density polythene. We are going to start a series with Charnley's prosthesis.

But in the meantime we have in the last three years used McKee's prosthesis in 223 cases. Before giving the clinical results, I would like to discuss the problems facing the surgeon who inserts an artificial joint.

Three main bio-mechanical problems are to be considered in artificial joints: friction—wearing—fixation.

FRICTION

We have already recalled the good results obtained by substitution of an inert prosthesis for one of the articular surfaces of the hip. In these cases, where normal cartilage works on a vitallium one, we know from the human experience of C. Hirsch and N. Rydell, that the coefficient of friction is between 0·021 and 0·004. This is twice as much as the friction of cartilage on cartilage: 0·005 to 0·010 (Barnett) and about the same as that of a metallic skate on ice.

It is difficult to obtain such low friction in mechanics, apart from ball-bearings: industrial rollings with steel on bronze have a coefficient of 0·07 when lubricated by oil, ten times as much as cartilage, but of 0·52 when lubricated with saline: 100 times more than cartilage. The coefficient of friction should diminish when the pressure increases as is the case with normal cartilage; this is perhaps possible with steel on plastic, but not with metal to metal. Moreover, it is impossible to adjust one spherical surface to another with enough accuracy to allow only a very thin, monomolecular film of liquid to come between the surfaces. For these reasons, a relatively soft plastic acetabulum would be preferable to a metallic one.

But, however important the coefficient of friction may be, in view of the absence of proper lubrication in these artificial joints, the *wearing* of the prosthesis probably has more influence on the late results.

WEAR

Wearing of the surface may cause loosening which is always a bad mechanical condition. But, above all, the fine particles produced may cause a foreign body reaction in the neighbouring tissues, even with an apparently inert material. This happened with Teflon, and late aseptic abscesses were observed in many cases. But it has been shown that even small metallic particles may have properties entirely different from massive pieces.

FIXATION

Solid fixation of the prosthesis to the bone seems absolutely necessary. Many of the complications observed after insertion of a prosthesis appear to be caused by progressive mobility of the implant. A cement of methylmethacrylate is used by Charnley and by McKee and we have followed them. But it is questionable whether this is the best answer: methacrylate is an unstable, hard and rather fragile material. Its carcinogenic action in man is very improbable, but the selective discovery of a cement as well tolerated and with better mechanical properties should be one of the aims of research.

In the research unit of our department of the Hôpital Cochin, a device has been made to study the wear of different materials. This machine reproduces grossly the mechanical conditions of walking with limited and alternating rotational movement and intermittent pressure. The wear of the material is measured very accurately—the particles produced by wearing are examined microscopically, chemically, and also injected into animals.

Our experiments have shown very important differences between several plastic materials and metal. Of the plastics two appear preferable to metal: high density polythene, used by Charnley, and celoron. This last material showed practically no wear in the experiments: its tolerance is, at present, being tested in animals.

As the tolerance of plastic materials under wearing conditions was still doubtful after the experience of Judet with acrylic and of Charnley with

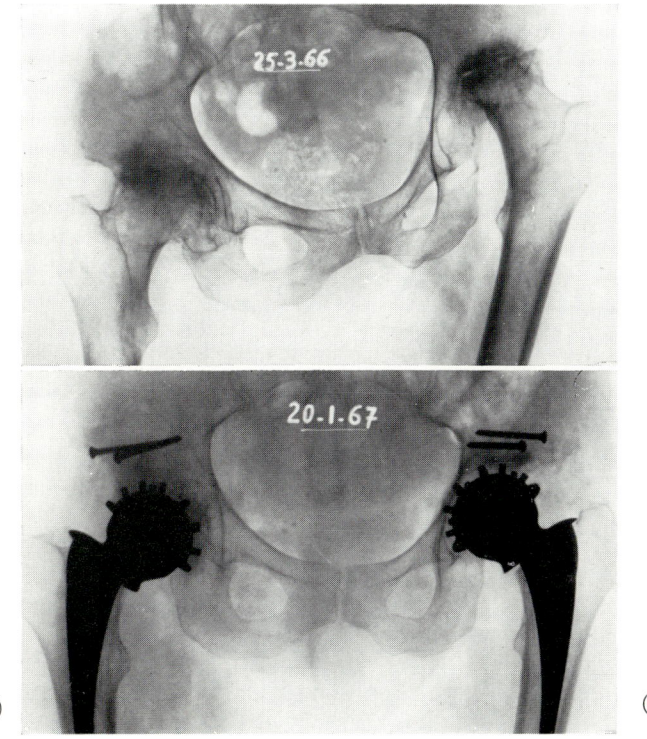

FIG. 5. Female, age 69 years.
(a) Very severe bilateral osteo-arthritis with adduction contracture and 10° range of flexion on both sides.
(b) One year after McKee's arthroplasty—painless—90° flexion—walks without a cane but with a slight limp.

Teflon, while tolerance of vitallium appeared highly probable, even in fine particles, our clinical experience has been with McKee's all-metal artificial joint.

Two hundred and twenty-three arthroplasties have been performed on 180 patients with a prosthesis similar to McKee's, but made in France.

Both portions are fixed with acrylic cement. Our technique differs from McKee's in that we use the postero-lateral approach instead of his antero-lateral. In most cases we cut the gluteus medius and minimus:

but when possible we believe that Austin Moore's posterior approach, leaving the abductors intact, is preferable. When a larger approach is necessary it may be preferable to cut the trochanter rather than the muscles, especially when shortening of the neck is to be expected: lowering of the great trochanter as advised by Charnley is then preferable.

The cup is placed in the same orientation as the normal acetabulum, and not as horizontally as McKee's; with the postero-lateral approach dislocation is not to be feared. The cup is fixed by pouring the methacrylate in a nearly liquid state into the acetabulum and into holes made around it.

The limb is maintained in suspension for one week, but the hip is actively mobilized from the second day. The patient is allowed to walk after a week if the abductors are intact, and after three weeks if they have been cut.

The early results from six months to two years after operation are available in 121 cases, of which one patient died from cardiac failure. Sixty-nine of these patients were operated for osteoarthritis (14 had bilateral operations). Eighty-three hips can be evaluated at the present time.

Up to now *we have had no infection.*

The immediate post-operative period is characterized by painlessness, and by free active movement in practically all cases.

Rehabilitation is quicker than with other types of arthroplasty. About half of our patients walk without a cane at the end of the third month.

Pain is relieved in practically all cases. Out of the 83 available cases 58 are completely free from pain, 13 have slight intermittent pain.

Mobility is very regularly restored. We have used this operation mostly in patients with very severe limitation of joint motion.

The results with regard to gait are also very satisfactory; 47 patients walk without a cane, 30 without limp, 31 use a cane, four use two canes.

The functional results are altogether much better and more quickly obtained than with any other sort of arthroplasty.

The problem is to know how long they will last. Our experience is rather short. But McKee has many patients with a follow-up of six or seven years with persisting good results.

Six of his early patients, when explored surgically for recurrence of pain, were found with their prosthesis loose.

The same loosening happened to two of our patients: in one of these the loose femoral prosthesis was removed and fixed again, with a very good result; in the other, refixing the loose acetabular part gave no improvement.

Some loosening of any foreign body introduced into bone with alternating stresses imposed on it, is to be expected. But we know that limited looseness can be tolerated and painless. It is suspected radiologically in nine of our patients, seven of whom are symptomless.

Nevertheless, certain thoughts must be present in one's mind before deciding upon this operation:

(1) If by chance operation is complicated by infection, how will the patient withstand removal of the prosthesis? Fortunately we have not

had this experience, but we know that removal is very laborious and often necessitates extensive bone destruction of the femur and ilium.

(2) If after some years the prosthesis becomes loose and painful, will the patient be fit to undergo another operation?

This second operation may be an extensive resection with subsequent instability. Is his present condition worth the risk?

These considerations have persuaded us to use total replacement only in cases where no other good alternative operation can be considered: bilateral osteoarthritis with great limitation of movement in patients around 70 is the best example.

But it can be considered in younger patients with bilateral ankylosis when a mobilizing operation *must* be done: as compared with resection, a total prosthesis will give a better functional result, and resection will be possible in case of failure.

TABLE V

Results with Various Operations for Osteoarthritis from 1960 to 1966 at the Hôpital Cochin, Paris.

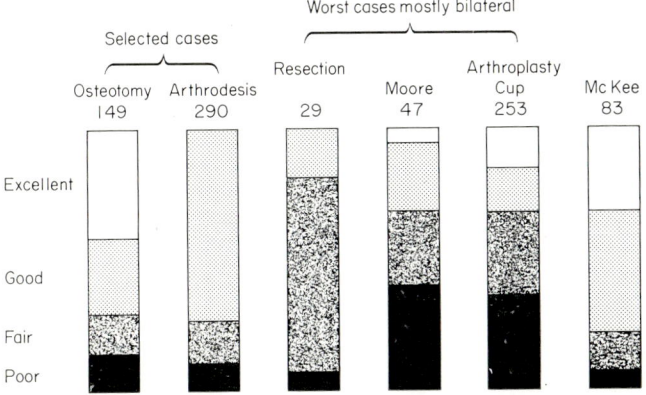

Osteotomy and arthrodesis give a great proportion of excellent or good results but are only possible in selected cases (parallelism of joint space and preserved mobility for osteotomy; unilaterality and stiffness for arthrodesis). In the really bad, advanced bilateral cases, McKee's arthroplasty results are largely superior to those of prosthesis and even of cup.

Conclusion

It is reasonable to hope that, as the years go by, improvements in technique and material, and a longer follow-up, will, in a growing number of cases, provide an efficient and regularly successful treatment for the most serious cases of osteoarthritis of the hip.

For the time being, arthroplasty has in our opinion and in our practice, a limited but definite place.

At an early stage of the disease, with mobility to 90° of flexion and without deformity, it is indicated only in cases where the degenerative process is due to a definitive or progressive lesion of one of the parts of the joint: a head prosthesis for aseptic necrosis of the head in old people with a sound acetabulum; a cup for old fractures of the acetabulum with a sound head, at any age.

At a more advanced stage of the disease, with good flexion but with slight external rotation or adduction deformity, osteotomy is still preferable to arthroplasty in all cases where a relatively *congruent joint space* can be preserved or restored.

In advanced cases, with a range of flexion of less than 50° and with marked adduction deformity, and in cases where the joint space is incongruent, osteotomy should be rejected on account of its many failures:

(*a*) In younger patients, strictly unilateral cases are preferably treated by *arthrodesis*. If the opposite hip is affected but still mobile and relatively painless, we use a *cup*.

(*b*) In patients over 60 we use the total prosthesis.

In the most serious bilateral cases, the indications for total prosthesis can be slightly enlarged especially when both hips are stiff and painful, when the patient is confined to bed or to a chair. Before total arthroplasty, we used in these cases to perform a complete resection on one side, then, if the mobility obtained was sufficient, an arthrodesis on the other: with this combination the patient was able to walk with one cane. Now we use a total prosthesis instead of resection even around the age of 50, as arthroplasty has a better chance of securing painlessness, mobility and stability; if early or late complications occur, resection will always be possible. For the opposite hip arthrodesis is preferred under 65 years, but in the aged, bilateral total arthroplasty is probably better.

With these limitations and with great precautions to minimize the danger of infection, we believe that in its present state total hip replacement is applicable to a considerable number of patients.

But, we must work for improvement of material and technique, and follow-up the results very carefully. If the early promise of this method is confirmed, it may, in a few years, change the picture of the treatment of osteoarthritis.

INDEX

INDEX

A

Acetabulum, dysplasia, in congenital dislocation of hip, 21, 326
  mal-direction, 326
Alkaptonuria, pattern of inheritance, 3
Allopurinol in gout, 46
Amish sect, 8
Amputation, silastic pads, 103
  traumatic, reattachment, 49–78
Anencephaly, incidence, 25
Ankle, equinus deformity, correction, 271
Anticoagulants after reattachment of severed limbs, 58
Anturan in gout, 46
Aorta, high bifurcation, management in treatment of lumbar disc lesions, 320
Arm, severed, reattachment, 65, 68, 72
Arteries, spasm, in reattached fingers, 65
Arthritis, gouty, mechanism, 37
  septic, simulation by pseudogout, 45
Arthrodesis in osteoarthritis of hip, 384
Arthroplasty in degenerative osteoarthritis of hip, 377–92
  'prosthesis', in osteoarthritis of hip, 385
Articular bone ends, transplantation, 219–63
    clinical data, 229
    errors and complications, 254–62
    experimental results, 225
    indications, 229
    lower limb, 238
    methods, 229
    patient reaction, 233
    upper limb, 234
Autoimmune disease, 5
Autosomes, 1, 2
  aberrations, 13

B

Benemid in gout, 46
Blood vessels, anastomosis after traumatic severance, 53, 57

Blood transfusion, after reattachment of severed limbs, 58
  vessels, management in reattachment of severed limbs, 52
Bolt bone graft, 117
Bone, anorganic, grafting, 186
  articular ends, transplantation, 219–63
    clinical data, 228
    errors and complications, 254–62
    experimental results, 225
    indications, 229
    lower limb, 438
    methods, 229
    patient reaction, 233
    upper limb, 234
  blood supply, 122
  cancellous, fixation, 81
    grafts, proliferative changes, 133
    remodelling, effect on osteogenesis, 148
    revascularization, 139
    use in grafts, 117
  cellular biology, 121
  compression as aid in orthopaedic surgery, 79–89
    bilateral, 87
    by screws, 81
    by tension band, 82
  cortical, contribution to osteogenesis in graft, 141
    fixation, 81
    grafts, cellular changes, 132
        proliferative changes, 132
    remodelling, effect on osteogenesis, 147
    revascularization, 138
    use in grafts, 117
  decalcified, use in grafting, 176, 184
  deproteinized, for grafting, 178, 184
  freeze-dried, remodelling, 172
    influence of irradiation on, 173
  freezing, 169, 213
  grafts, *see also* Bone, heterografts; Bone, homografts
    anatomical factors, 116
    autografts, fate, 115–53
    cancellous chips, 137

Bone grafts, cellular changes, 132
   clinical uses, 116
   cortical chips, 137
      shavings, 137
   degenerative changes, 132
   effect of steroids on, 146
   experimental study methods, 130–32
   foreign, fate, 153
   fragmentation, 137
   frozen, 213
   functions, 116
   growth control, 150
   host, effect on osteogenesis, 146
   infection, 146
   irradiation, effect on repair process, 146
   mitosis, 138
   necrosis, 136
   osteogenesis, 140
   preserved, comparison with autografts, 159
   proliferative changes, 132
   rejection, 165
   remodelling, 147
      rate, 166
   revascularization, 138
   site, contribution to osteogenesis, 145
      of donor bone, 161
   storage, 155
   transplantation immunity caused by, 163
  growth control, 129
  heterografts, anorganic bone, 186
   decalcified bone, 184
   deproteinized bone, 184
   fate, 180–88
   freeze-dried, 181
   frozen, 181
   Kiel bone, 185
   os purum, 184
   Oswestry bone, 186
   preserved, 181
   rejection mechanism, 180
  heterotransplantation, principles, 180
  homografts, freeze-dried, fate, 172
    influence of irradiation on remodelling, 173
   fresh, clinical use, 154
      fate, 162–7
   frozen, comparison with fresh bone, 160
   inflammatory response around, 165

Bone, homografts, limitations, 188
   osteogenesis, impaired, 166
   preserved, boiled and autoclaved, 175
   clinical results with frozen bone, 171
   clinical results with irradiated bone, 171
   clinical results with merthiolate-preserved bone, 174
   clinical use, 155
   comparison of remodelling in freeze-dried and frozen bone, 172
   decalcified, 176
   deproteinized, 178
   fate, 167–80
   sterilization, 169
  rejection, 165
  remodelling, rate, 166
  revascularization, impaired, 165
  transplantation immunity caused by, 163
  long, transplantation, 118, 119
  marrow, 122
   contribution to osteogenesis in grafts, 142
   supply, 122
  mitosis after grafting, 138
  preservation, 155
   at low temperature, 217
   by freezing, 169
   sterilization, 169
  remodelling, 128
   of grafts, 147
  repair, 125–8
  resorption, 128
  revascularization after grafting, 138
  transplants, pedicle, 120
  treatment in reattachment of amputated limbs, 52
Boplant, 181

C

Cadaveric tissue, collection, 215
  preservation, 216
Calcaneo-varus deformity, correction, 283
Calcaneus deformity, correction, 283
Calcification, cartilage, diagnostic significance, 41
Calcium, negative balance, and bone grafts, 146

Calcium pyrophosphate dihydrate crystals in gout, 38
Callosities, plantar, silicone treatment, 100
Cambium layer, 121
Capsule, suture in articular bone end transplant, 230
Capsulorrhaphy, 326, 358
Carpal bones, silastic replacements, 103
Cartilage, articular, in osteoarthritis, 372
  protection with silicone, 100
  calcification, diagnostic significance, 41
  growth-plate, transplantation, 118
Cerclage, tension, in repair of fractures, 84
Cerebral palsy. See Palsy, cerebral
Cervical disc lesion, interbody fusion, 296
Charnley compression device, 79
Chondrocalcinosis, 37–48
  diagnostic significance, 41
Chondro-ectodermal dysplasia, 8
Chondroitin sulphate B, 15
Chromosomes, 1
  aberrations, 5
  classification, 2
  deletion, 6
  disorders, clinical forms, 13
  mosaics, 6
  sex, 1
    aberrations, 13
  translocation, 6
  trisomy, 5, 13
Colchicine in treatment of gout, 45
Compression as aid in orthopaedic surgery, 79–89
  bilateral, 87
  by screws, 81
  by tension band, 82
  by tension plate, 85
Condyle, femoral, protrusion in displacement of meniscus, 365
Cortisone, effect on bone grafts, 146

D

Diabetic ulcers, silastic underlay, 110
Diaphyseal aclasis, pattern of inheritance, 3
Digits, transplantation, 119
Down's syndrome, 5, 13
Duchenne's muscular dystrophy, see Muscular dystrophy, Duchenne's
Dupuytren's contracture, 26
  association with epilepsy, 26–28
Dwarfism, diastrophic, 15

E

EDTA for bone decalcification, 177
Elbow joint, chondrocalcinosis, 44
  silastic prosthesis, 104
Ellis–Van Creveld syndrome, see Chondro-ectodermal dysplasia
Endosteum, 122
  contribution to osteogenesis in bone graft, 141
Epilepsy, association with Dupuytren's disease, 26–28
Epiosteum, 121
Equino-varus deformity, correction, 284
Equinus deformity, correction, 271
Ethebenecid in gout, 46
Extremities, severed, reattachment, 49–78
  postoperative management, 58
  refrigeration, 61

F

Fascia, treatment in reattachment of severed limbs, 55
Femur, articular transplant, 238, 241
  head, avascular necrosis, after reduction of hip, 356
  resection, in osteoarthritis, 377
  hyperemia, in osteoarthritis, 369
  neck, resection, in osteoarthritis, 377
Fibula, articular transplant, 248
  use for grafts, 118
Fingers, paralytic deformities, correction, 273
  severed, reattachment, 56, 73
    tendon repair, 64
  transplantation, 119
Foot deformities due to cerebral palsy, correction, 271
  in spina bifida, correction, 283

G

Gargoylism, 15
Gastrocnemius, contracture, treatment, 271

Genes, 1
  alternatives, 4
  disorders, 14
  major, 1
  multiple, inheritance, 5
Genetic and environmental factors in disease, distinction between, 9
  counselling, 29
  disorders, age of onset, 9
  factors in orthopaedics, 1–35
Gout, 37–48
  treatment, surgical, 47
  with drugs, 45
Gudushauri's fixation apparatus, 231

H
Hallux, silastic filler, 107
  valgus, correction, 271
Hand, amputation, traumatic, re-attachment, 49
  burned, silicone bath, 97
  severed, reattachment, 65, 70, 76
  silastic prosthesis, 103, 105
Harmon's retractors, 318
Haversian systems, 122
Heparitin sulphate, 15
Heredity, physical basis, 1
Hip, adduction tenotomy, 269
  arthroplasty, 377–92
    cup, 386
    'prosthesis', 385
    results, 379
  artificial joint, 387–91
  deformities in spine bifida, correction, 279
  dislocation, bilateral, management, 354
    congenital, 19–21; *see also* Osteotomy, innominate
      diagnosis, 325
      pre-operative skeletal traction, 331
      treatment, 325–60
      results, 356
    in cerebral palsy, surgical treatment, 270
    reduction, open, operative technique, 332–53, 358
  disorders, congenital, 325–60
  flexion deformity, correction, 281
    fixed, treatment, 269
  operative procedures in cerebral palsy, 269

Hip, osteoarthritis, 367–75
  arthrodesis, 384
  arthroplasty, 386
    results, 379
  degenerative, arthroplasty in, 377–92
  knee pain in, 370
  osteotomy for, 368
  pathology, 378
  'prosthesis' arthroplasty, 385
  resection in, 384
  physiological conditions aiding reconstruction, 378
  prosthesis, in treatment of osteoarthritis, 378
  reconstruction, for osteoarthritis, 377
  rotation deformity, surgical correction, 269
  silastic prosthesis, 104
  subluxation, congenital, reduction, 325
    results of treatment, 357
    innominate osteotomy for, technique, 354
  transplantation, 251, 254
Hodgson's rongeurs, 304
Homocystinuria, 15
Howship's lacunae, 128
Humerus, articular transplant, 235
  chondrocalcinosis, 44
Hunter's syndrome, 15
Hurler's syndrome, 15

I
Iliopsoas, transplantation, 280
Immunogenetics, 5
Immunological response, effect of low temperature techniques, 218
Indomethacin in gout, 45
Inheritance, patterns, 1
Intervertebral disc, cervical, lesion, interbody fusion, 296
  lumbar, lesions, interbody fusion, 314

J
Joints, transplantation, 119, 248

K
Keratosulphate, 16
Kidney function and orthopaedic surgery, 279

INDEX

Kiel bone, 185
Klinefelter's syndrome, 13
Knee, chondrocalcinosis, 43
   deformities in spina bifida, correction, 282
   flexion, fixed, correction, 270
   osteoarthritis, arrest, 362–6
      fixed deformity in, 365
   pain, non-referred, in osteoarthritis of hip, 370
   quadriceps adhesion, prevention with silastic sheeting, 105
   silastic tibial plateau replacement, 106
   transplantation, 248, 249, 252
Kyphosis, congenital, in spina bifida, correction, 284

L

Latch bone graft, 117
Limbs, artificial, permanently attached, silicone interface, 103
   homografting, 64
   severed, reattachment, 49–78
      circulatory embarrassment, 59
      indications, 51
      postoperative management, 58
      refrigeration, 61
      restoration of nerve function, 63
      technique, 51
Locomotor disability, pathophysiology, 265
Lordo-scoliosis, lumbar, correction, 273
Lumbar disc lesions, interbody fusion, 314

M

McMurray's osteotomy, 380
Medullary intrinsic induction, 142
Meniscectomy, in osteoarthritis of knee, 366
Menisci, derangements, causing osteoarthritis of knee, 363
   microscopic appearance, 373
Merthiolate for bone sterilization, 169, 174
Metacarpal bone, articular transplant, 234
   use for grafts, 118
Metatarsal bone, use for grafts, 118
Micrognathia, genetic factors, 13
Mongolism, *see* Down's syndrome
Moore's hip prosthesis, 385
Morquio's syndrome, 15

Mosaicism, chromosomal, 6
Mucopolysaccharidoses, 15
Muscle contractility in reattachment of severed limbs, 61
   mummification in reattachment limbs, 62
   treatment in reattachment of severed limbs, 55
Muscular dystrophy, Duchenne's, pattern of inheritance, 4
Mutation, 8
Myelocele, 274
Myelomeningocele, 13, 274

N

Nerve repair with silastic sheeting, 102
   restoration of function after reattachment of severed limbs, 63
   treatment in reattachment of severed limbs, 55, 58
Neural tube defects, 25

O

Oestrogen excretion in congenital dislocation of hip, 20
Os purum, 184
Osteoarthritis, articular cartilage in, 372
   degenerative, of hip, arthroplasty in, 377–92
   of hip, 367–75
   of knee, arrest, 362–6
   pathology, 378
Osteoclastic cells, 128
Osteogenesis in bone grafts, 140
   of bone repair, 125–8
Osteogenic induction, 126
Osteoprogenitor cells, 125
Osteosynthesis by compression, 79
Osteotomy for hip dislocation and subluxation
   innominate, advantages, 360
   complications, 355
   contra-indications, 330
   errors and pitfalls, 358
   indications, 329
   in treatment of congenital hip disorders, 327–60
   object, 327
   operative technique, 332–53, 359
   post-operative management, 332

Osteotomy for osteoarthritis of hip, 88, 367, 380
   innominate, pre-operative management, 330, 358
      prerequisites, 330
      principle, 328
      results, 355
      selection of patients, 358
Osteotomy of tibia for osteoarthritis, 369
   principle, 328
Oswestry bone, grafting, 188

P

Palsy, cerebral, bracing, 266
   physiotherapy, 266
   surgical treatment, 265–74
      indications, 267
      lower limb, 269
      pre-operative assessment, 268
      upper limb, 271
Paralysis, lower limb, in spina bifida, 275
Pedicle transplants of bone and digits, 120
Pedochirodactyloplasty, 119
Periosteum, cellular biology, 121
   contribution to osteogenesis in bone graft, 140
Phenylbutazone in gout, 45
Plagiocephaly, 24
Polydactyly, 13
Polygenes, 7
Probenecid in gout, 46
β-Propiolactone for bone sterilization, 169
Prostheses, silastic, 103
Pseudogout, 37, 38
   simulating septic arthritis, 45
Pycnodysostosis, 15

R

Radiation, ionizing, for bone preservation, 169
Radius, articular transplant, 235
Refrigeration of amputated extremities, 61
Ribs, chips, effects of remodelling, 149
   use for grafts, 118
Russian lock for articular bone end fixation, 229

S

Sanfilippo syndrome, 16
Scapula, articular transplant, 237
Scoliosis, correction, operative procedure, 308
   surgical approach for, 308
   idiopathic, 21–25
   thoracic, correction, 308
Screws for bone compression, 81
Shoulder, frozen, silicone treatment, 100
   transplantation, 251
Silastics, 94
   orthopaedic applications, 101
   prostheses, 103
   tendons, 110
Silicones, 91–114
   fluid, articular cartilage protection, 100
      as floating bath for burns, 97
      as joint lubricant, 95
      for frozen shoulder, 100
      for plantar callosities, 100
      orthopaedic uses, 95
      uses, 93
   physical and chemical properties, 92
   physiological properties, 92
   toxicity, 92, 93
Skeletal traction, pre-operative, in innominate osteotomy, 331
Skin closure after reattachment of severed limbs, 55, 58
   homograft, rejection mechanism, 163
Spasticity without deformity, management, 273
Spina bifida, assessment of paralysis and deformity in, 276
   incidence, 25
   lower limb paralysis and deformity in, mechanism, 275
   orthopaedic surgery, 274–86
   treatment, principles, 277
Spine, anterior approach, 289–323
   cervico-dorsal, split sternal approach, 297
   curvature, correction, operative procedure, 308
      surgical approach, 308
   deformities in cerebral palsy, 273
   in spina bifida, correction, 284
   dorso-lumbar, anterior approach, 307
   lumbar approach, 313
   sacral, perineal approach, 321
   thoracotomy approach, 301

Spine, transoral approach, 290
 transthoracic approach, 300
 tuberculosis, anterior surgical approaches, 289–323
  surgery, complications, 321
  transthoracic approach, 300, 308
  upper lumbar approach, 312
Stump neuroma, silicone capping, 103
Sulphinpyrazone in gout, 46
Synovial fluid, microscopy with polarized light, 39
Synovitis, crystal, 38

T

Talipes calcaneo-valgus, 19
 equino-varus, 16–19
Tendons, repair with silastic sheeting, 102
 silastic, 110
 treatment in reattachment of severed limbs, 55, 58
Tenomytomy for osteoarthritis of hip, 380
Tension plates, 85
Thumb, paralytic deformities, correction, 273
Tibia, articular transplant, 242
 osteotomy, for relief of osteoarthritis, 369
Tissue incompatibility, elimination, 218
 preservation at low temperatures, 217
Trabeculae, cancellous, orientation, in grafts, 151

Transplantation immunity, 163
Trisomy, 5, 13
Tuberculosis, spinal, surgery, anterior approaches, 289–323
 complications, 321
Twins, investigations in, 11

U

Urelim in gout, 46
Uricosuric drugs, 45

V

Valgus deformity of hindfoot, correction, 271
Varus deformity of hindfoot, correction, 271
 osteotomy, intertrochanteric, 88
Vertebrae cervical, transoral approach, 289
 transthoracic approach, 300
 transthyrohyoid approach, 292
 tuberculosis, transoral surgical approach, 290
 lumbar, transthoracic approach, 300, 308
Voss's operation of tenomyotomy, 380

W

Walking education, in spina bifida patients, 285
Wound drainage with silastics, 101
Wrist chondrocalcinosis, 43
 flexion deformity, correction, 272